D0366016

Books by Corinne T. Netzer
THE CORINNE T. NETZER ANNUAL CALORIE COUNTER
THE CORINNE T. NETZER BRAND-NAME CALORIE COUNTER
THE COMPLETE BOOK OF FOOD COUNTS
THE CORINNE T. NETZER CHOLESTEROL COUNTER
THE CORINNE T. NETZER CARBOHYDRATE COUNTER
THE CARBOHYDRATE DIETER'S DIARY
THE CORINNE T. NETZER DIETER'S DIARY
THE CORINNE T. NETZER ENCYCLOPEDIA OF FOOD VALUES
THE CORINNE T. NETZER FAT COUNTER
THE CORINNE T. NETZER FIBER COUNTER
THE CORINNE T. NETZER LOW FAT DIARY
THE DIETER'S CALORIE COUNTER
THE COMPLETE BOOK OF VITAMIN & MINERAL COUNTS
CORINNE T. NETZER'S BIG BOOK OF MIRACLE CURES

THE COMPLETE BOOK OF FOOD COUNTS COOKBOOK SERIES:
100 LOW FAT SMALL MEAL AND SALAD RECIPES
100 LOW FAT VEGETABLE AND LEGUME RECIPES
100 LOW FAT SOUP AND STEW RECIPES
100 LOW FAT PASTA AND GRAIN RECIPES
100 LOW FAT FISH AND SHELLFISH RECIPES
100 LOW FAT CHICKEN AND TURKEY RECIPES

THE CORINNE T. NETZER CARBOHYDRATE COUNTER

Corinne T. Netzer

Revised Edition

A Dell Book

Published by
Dell Publishing
a division of
Random House, Inc.
1540 Broadway
New York, New York 10036

Dell books may be purchased for business or promotional use or for special sales. For information please write to: Special Markets Department,
Random House, Inc., 1540 Broadway, New York, NY 10036.

Dell® is a registered trademark of Random House, Inc., and the
colophon is a trademark of Random House, Inc.

ISBN: 0-440-23682-7

Printed in the United States of America

Published simultaneously in Canada

September 2001

10 9 8 7 6 5 4 3 2 1

OPM

Introduction

The Carbohydrate Counter is the largest compilation of carbo grams available under one cover. No matter what your aim or interest in carbohydrates might be, the information on all the foods—whether generic or brand name, fresh or frozen, even a fast-food favorite—can be found here.

Because the entries in this book are alphabetized, there is no index. I have tried to cross-reference as many items as possible, but space does not allow this in every instance. If you do not find the item you are seeking in one place, please look for it under a category—i.e., if you don't find "apple pie" under "Apple," look for it under "Pie."

If you are making comparisons, remember to compare only foods that are similar in measure. Eight ounces is not necessarily equivalent to one eight-ounce cup. Eight ounces is a measure of how much the food weighs, while an eight-ounce cup is a measure of how much space the food occupies. For example, a cup of popcorn weighs about an ounce; thus, eight ounces of popcorn would fill quite a few cups.

The data contained herein are derived from information supplied by the various food producers, processors, distributors, and food chains, and from the United States Department of Agriculture. As we go to press, this information is the most complete and accurate available.

Good luck and good eating.

C.T.N.

Abbreviations and Symbols in This Book

"	inch
<	less than
approx.	approximately
cont.	container
diam.	diameter
lb.	pound(s)
pkg.	package(s)
pkt.	packet(s)
oz	ounce(s)
tbsp.	tablespoon(s)
tsp.	teaspoon(s)
*	prepared according to basic package directions

THE
CORINNE T. NETZER
CARBOHYDRATE
COUNTER

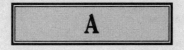

FOOD AND MEASURE   **CARBOHYDRATE GRAMS**

Abalone, meat only:

raw, 4 oz. 6.8

fried, 4 oz. 12.5

Abruzzese sausage *(Boar's Head Cinghiale),* 1 oz. ....<1.0

Acerola, fresh, raw, trimmed:

1 acerola, .2 oz. 4

1 cup 7.5

Acerola juice, fresh, 8 fl. oz. 11.6

Ackee, trimmed, 1 oz. 1.6

Acorn:

raw, shelled, 1 oz. 11.6

dried, shelled, 1 oz. 15.2

Acorn flour, full-fat, 1 oz. 15.5

Acorn squash, fresh:

raw:

    (Frieda's), ¾ cup, 3 oz. 9.0

    untrimmed, 1 lb. 35.9

    4"-diam. squash, 15.2 oz. 44.9

    cubed, 1 cup...14.6

baked, cubed, 1 cup...29.9

boiled, mashed, 1 cup..21.5

Adobo *(Goya),* ¼ tsp. 0

Aduki beans, canned *(Eden* Organic), ½ cup...........19.0

Adzuki beans:

(Arrowhead Mills), ¼ cup 29.0

mature, raw, 1 cup..117.6

mature, boiled, 1 cup...57.0

canned, sweetened, 1 cup....................................162.8

Agar, see "Seaweed"

Agnotti, gorgonzola walnut in macchiato pasta *(Cafferata),*

½ of 9-oz. pkg...36.0

Albacore, without added ingredients...............................0

Alfalfa sprouts:

(Jonathan's), 1 cup 3.0

Alfalfa sprouts *(cont.)*
1 cup 1.2
1 tbsp. 1
with dill or garlic *(Jonathan's)*, 1 cup 4.0
with onion or radish *(Jonathan's)*, 1 cup 3.0
Alfredo entree, see specific entree listings
Alfredo sauce, canned or in jar, ¼ cup, except as noted:
(Classico Di Roma) 3.0
(Five Brothers) 3.0
(Progresso Authentic), ½ cup 7.0
garlic, roasted *(Classico* Di Siena) 3.0
with mushrooms *(Five Brothers)* 3.0
sun-dried tomato *(Classico* Di Capri) 4.0
tomato *(Classico* Di Roma) 6.0
Alfredo sauce, refrigerated, ¼ cup:
(Contadina Buitoni/Contadina Buitoni Light) 5.0
(Di Giorno) 3.0
(Di Giorno Light Varieties) 9.0
mushroom *(Contadina Buitoni)* 6.0
Alfredo sauce mix, see "Pasta sauce, mix"
Allspice:
1 tbsp. 4.3
1 tsp. 1.4
Almond, shelled, except as noted:
(Beer Nuts Choice), 1 oz. 6.0
whole *(Sonoma* Organic), ¼ cup, 1.1 oz. 6.0
natural, whole or chopped *(Dole)*, ¼ cup 5.0
natural, sliced *(Dole)*, ⅓ cup 5.0
blanched:
    whole *(Dole)*, ¼ cup 5.0
    whole, 1 cup 28.9
    slivered *(Dole)*, ⅓ cup 5.0
sliced *(Planters)*, ⅓ cup 6.0
sliced or ground, 1 cup 18.8
slivered *(Planters)*, 2-oz. pkg. 11.0
dry-roasted:
    (River Queen), 1 oz., about 24 nuts 7.0
    1 oz. 5.5
    1 cup 26.6
honey-roasted:
    (Blue Diamond), 3 tbsp., 1.1 oz. 8.0

unblanched, whole kernels, 1 oz. 7.9
unblanched, whole kernels, 1 cup 40.2
oil-roasted:
   (Blue Diamond), 3 tbsp., 1.1 oz. 4.0
   salted or unsalted, 1 oz., 22 kernels.............................5.0
   salted or unsalted, whole kernels, 1 cup 27.8
roasted *(River Queen),* 3 tbsp., 1 oz. 4.0
smoked *(Planters),* 1 oz..............................6.0
Almond butter, crunchy or creamy:
(Arrowhead Mills), 2 tbsp. 7.0
salted or unsalted, 1 cup 53.1
salted or unsalted, 1 tbsp..............................3.4
Almond paste (see also "Pastry filling"):
(Solo), 2 tbsp..............................19.0
(Solo Marzipan), 2 tbsp. 25.0
1 oz..............................12.4
1 cup, firmly packed.............................108.5
Almond powder:
full-fat, 1 cup.............................14.5
partially defatted, 1 cup.............................20.7
Almond syrup *(Trader Vic's* Orgeat), 2 tbsp..............................25.0
Amaranth, whole-grain:
1 oz..............................18.8
½ cup.............................64.5
Amaranth flour *(Arrowhead Mills),* ¼ cup.............................19.0
Amaranth leaves:
raw, untrimmed, 1 lb..............................17.2
raw, 1 leaf 6
raw, 1 cup 1.1
boiled, drained, 1 cup 5.4
Amaranth seeds *(Arrowhead Mills),* ¼ cup.............................29.0
Anaheim chili, see "Pepper, chili"
Anasazi beans *(Arrowhead Mills),* ¼ cup.............................27.0
Anchovy, fresh or canned in oil 0
Anchovy paste *(Reese),* 1 tbsp. 0
Andouille sausage, see "Sausage"
Angel-hair pasta, plain:
dry, see "Pasta"
refrigerated *(Contadina Buitoni),* 1¼ cups 43.0
refrigerated *(Di Giorno),* 2 oz..............................31.0

Angel-hair pasta dish, mix:

chicken broccoli *(Lipton* Pasta & Sauce), ⅓ cup, 1 cup*...........43.0

with herbs *(Pasta Roni),* about 1 cup*..42.0

with lemon and butter *(Pasta Roni),* about 1 cup*.....................48.0

Parmesan *(Lipton* Pasta & Sauce), ⅓ cup, 1 cup*....................41.0

with Parmesan cheese *(Pasta Roni),* about 1 cup*...................40.0

Angel-hair pasta entree, frozen *(Lean Cuisine Everyday*
Favorites), 10 oz..43.0

Anise seed:

1 tbsp..3.4

1 tsp..1.0

Antelope, without added ingredients..0

Apio root, see "Celeriac"

Apple, fresh:

raw:

(Dole), 1 medium 18.0

(Dole Cameo), 1 medium, 5.4 oz..22.0

(Frieda's Lady), 5 oz...21.0

with peel, 2¾" apple...21.1

with peel, sliced, 1 cup...16.8

with peel, quartered or chopped, 1 cup.................................19.1

peeled, 1 medium, 2¾" diam., 5.3 oz.....................................19.0

peeled, sliced, 1 cup...16.3

boiled, peeled, sliced, 1 cup...23.3

microwaved, peeled, sliced, 1 cup 24.5

Apple, candied, 3-oz. apple:

(Tastee Candy) 26.0

caramel *(Tastee)*...26.0

Apple, canned:

cinnamon *(Del Monte Fruitrageous),* 4-oz. cup...........................19.0

escalloped *(White House),* ½ cup...35.0

pie spiced, in sauce *(Del Monte Fruit Pleasures),* ½ cup...........18.0

spiced rings *(Comstock),* 2 rings...7.0

sweetened, sliced, drained, unheated, 1 cup..............................34.1

sweetened, sliced, drained, heated, 1 cup..................................34.1

Apple, dehydrated:

diced *(AlpineAire),* ¾ cup 26.0

sulfured, uncooked, 1 cup...56.1

sulfured, stewed, 1 cup..38.4

Apple, dried:

flakes, unsulfured *(AlpineAire),* ½ cup...26.0

rings *(Sonoma* Organic), 11 rings, 1.4 oz.................................29.0
sulfured, uncooked, 1 cup...56.7
sulfured, uncooked, 1 ring...4.2
sulfured, stewed, 1 cup...39.1
sulfured, stewed with sugar, 1 cup 58.0
Apple, escalloped, frozen *(Stouffer's),* ½ of 12-oz. pkg..........37.0
Apple, frozen:
sliced, unheated, 1 cup..21.3
sliced, heated, 1 cup...24.7
Apple butter:
(Eden Organic), 1 tbsp. 6.0
(Lucky Leaf/Musselman's), 1 tbsp. 8.0
(Sonoma), 2 tbsp. 6.0
all varieties *(Smucker's),* 1 tbsp. 11.0
Apple chips, see "Apple snack"
Apple cider, see "Apple juice"
Apple cider, alcoholic *(Hard Core* Crisp), 12 fl. oz. 19.0
Apple chutney, see "Chutney"
Apple drink blend:
berry burst *(Dole),* 8 fl. oz. 31.0
cranberry or grape *(Mott's),* 8 fl. oz. 29.0
raspberry *(Fruit Works),* 12 fl. oz. 42.0
raspberry-blackberry *(Tropicana Twister),* 10 fl. oz..................38.0
Apple filling, see "Pastry filling" and "Pie filling"
Apple fritter, frozen *(Mrs. Paul's),* 2 pieces...........................33.0
Apple fruit square pastry, frozen *(Pepperidge Farm),* 1 piece ...27.0
Apple juice, 8 fl. oz., except as noted:
(After the Fall Special Harvest Organic) 22.0
(Eden Organic) 23.0
(Juicy Juice)...29.0
(Juicy Juice), 8.45-fl.-oz. box 31.0
(Juicy Juice), 4.23-fl.-oz. box 15.0
(Lucky Leaf Little Brown Jug Old Fashioned Cider) 31.0
(Lucky Leaf/Lincoln/Speas Farm)...31.0
(Lucky Leaf/Lucky Leaf Old Fashioned/Premium Select) 31.0
(Mott's 128 oz.)...26.0
(Mott's 16/64 oz.) 29.0
(Mott's), 11.5-fl.-oz. can 42.0
(Mott's), 10-fl.-oz. bottle 36.0
(Mott's Natural) 27.0
(Musselman's Premium Natural)..33.0

Apple juice *(cont.)*

(*Musselman's/Musselman's* Natural/Premium)............................31.0
(*R.W. Knudsen* From Concentrate) 28.0
(*R.W. Knudsen* Natural) 30.0
(*R.W. Knudsen* Organic) 30.0
(*R.W. Knudsen* Organic Aseptic) 28.0
(*Santa Cruz Organic*)..30.0
(*Season's Best*) 28.0
(*Snapple*) 44.0
(*Speas Farm* Premium Cider)...31.0
sparkling:
   (*After the Fall Harvest Moon*) 27.0
   cider (*Heinke's*)...30.0
   cider (*Lucky Leaf/Musselman's*)......................................36.0
spiced (*R.W. Knudsen* Cider and Spice)................................30.0
spiced (*Santa Cruz Organic* Cider and Spice) 30.0
Apple juice blend, 8 fl. oz., except as noted:
apricot (*R.W. Knudsen*)..30.0
banana (*R.W. Knudsen*) 30.0
boysenberry or cranberry (*R.W. Knudsen*) 30.0
cranberry (*Mott's*), 11.5-fl.-oz. can 43.0
cranberry (*R.W. Knudsen* Aseptic)..29.0
mango (*Rocket Juice Galactic Green*), 16 fl. oz. 73.0
peach, raspberry, or strawberry (*R.W. Knudsen*)....................30.0
Apple nectar (*Libby's*), 11.5-fl.-oz. can 49.0
Apple snack (see also "Fruit snack"):
(*Weight Watchers*), 1 pkg. 13.0
chips:
   (*Weight Watchers*), 1 pkg...18.0
   all varieties (*Seneca*), 1 oz...20.0
   caramel (*Tastee*), 1 oz. 22.0
rings, caramel (*Sonoma Apple-Teasers*), 10 rings, 1.4 oz. 25.0
Applesauce:
natural/unsweetened:
   (*Apple Time* Original), 4 oz...13.0
   (*Apple Time* Original), ½ cup 12.0
   (*Eden* Organic) 15.0
   (*Lucky Leaf* Old Fashioned), 4 oz. 13.0
   (*Lucky Leaf* Old Fashioned Natural/*Musselman's*
      Natural), 4-oz. cup...12.0

(Lucky Leaf Old Fashioned Natural/*Musselman's* Natural),
  6-oz. cup...18.0
(Mott's), 3.9-oz. cont..12.0
(Santa Cruz Organic Gravenstein), ½ cup..........................15.0
(Seneca 100% Natural), ½ cup......................................14.0
1 cup...27.5
cinnamon *(Apple Time* Original/*Lucky Leaf* Natural),
  ½ cup..12.0
cinnamon *(Lucky Leaf/Musselman's* Natural), 4 oz..............13.0
sweetened:
  (Lucky Leaf), 6-oz. cont. 30.0
  (Lucky Leaf/Lucky Leaf Premium), 4 oz. 22.0
  (Lucky Leaf/Musselman's 4 Pack), 4-oz. cup 21.0
  (Mott's Original), ½ cup..22.0
  (Musselman's 6 Pack), 4-oz. cup 20.0
  (Musselman's/Musselman's Premium), 4 oz..................22.0
  (Seneca Golden Delicious), ½ cup 22.0
  (Seneca/Seneca McIntosh), ½ cup 24.0
  1 cup..50.8
  chunky *(Lucky Leaf),* 4 oz. 22.0
  chunky *(Musselman's* Homestyle), 4 oz..........................25.0
  cinnamon *(Lucky Leaf),* 4-oz. cont................................21.0
  cinnamon *(Lucky Leaf/Lucky Leaf* Deluxe), 4 oz. 25.0
  cinnamon *(Lucky Leaf/Musselman's),* 6-oz. cont. 31.0
  cinnamon *(Mott's),* 4-oz. cont......................................26.0
  cinnamon *(Musselman's),* ½ cup..................................20.0
  cinnamon *(Musselman's* Deluxe), ½ cup 21.0
  cinnamon *(Musselman's/Musselman's* Deluxe), 4 oz. 25.0
  cinnamon *(Seneca),* ½ cup 24.0
Applesauce fruit blend:
all varieties:
  (Mott's Fruitsations), 4-oz. cont. 23.0
  (Mott's Rugrats), 4-oz. cont. 23.0
  (Santa Cruz Organic), ½ cup 15.0
strawberry or mixed berry *(Mott's),* 4-oz. cont. 22.0
Apricot, fresh:
(Dole), ½ cup...9.0
3 medium, 12 per lb..11.8
pitted, halves, 1 cup...17.2
pitted, sliced, 1 cup..18.3

Apricot, canned:
(Del Monte Lite), ½ cup...16.0
in water:
    whole, pitted, without skin, 1 cup 12.4
    halves, with skin, 1 cup 15.5
    halves, with skin, 1 half 2.5
in juice, halves, with skin:
    (Libby's Lite), ½ cup 13.0
    1 cup 30.1
    1 half with juice 4.4
in extra light syrup, halves, with skin, 1 cup..................30.9
in light syrup:
    (Del Monte Orchard Select), ½ cup........................21.0
    halves, with skin, 1 cup 41.7
    halves, 1 half with syrup 6.6
    almond flavor *(Del Monte),* ½ cup 22.0
in heavy syrup:
    (Del Monte), ½ cup..26.0
    whole, with skin, 1 cup..51.5
    whole, peeled *(S&W),* ½ cup 29.0
    whole, pitted, without skin, 1 cup 55.3
    halves, with skin, 1 cup 55.4
in extra heavy syrup, whole, pitted, without skin, 1 cup.............61.1
Apricot, dehydrated, sulfured:
uncooked, 1 cup 98.6
stewed, 1 cup..81.2
Apricot, dried:
(Sonoma Organic), 10 pieces, 1.4 oz............................31.0
halves, sulfured:
    uncooked, 1 half..2.2
    uncooked, 1 cup..80.3
    stewed, 1 cup 54.8
    stewed, with sugar, 1 cup..79.0
Apricot, frozen, sweetened, 1 cup.............................60.7
Apricot butter *(Simon Fischer* Golden), 2 tbsp. 25.0
Apricot drink blend *(Rocket Juice Apricot C 2001),*
    16 fl. oz. 51.0
Apricot filling, see "Pastry filling" and "Pie filling"
Apricot fruit roll, see "Fruit snack"
Apricot nectar, 8 fl. oz., except as noted:
(Goya) 31.0

(Goya 12 fl. oz.), 6 fl. oz. 29.0
(Libby's) 36.0
(Libby's), 11.5-fl.-oz. can 51.0
(Libby's), 5.5-fl.-oz. can 24.0
(R.W. Knudsen) 30.0
(Santa Cruz Organic) 30.0
canned 36.1
Apricot syrup, ¼ cup:
(Knott's Berry Farm) 52.0
(Smucker's) 52.0
Arame, see "Seaweed"
Arby's, 1 serving:
breakfast items:
    bacon, 2 strips 0
    biscuit with margarine 26.0
    croissant 28.0
    eggs, scrambled 0
    French *Toastix,* plain, 6 pieces 48.0
    ham 1.0
    maple syrup, 1.5 oz. 54.0
    sausage patty 1.0
chicken sandwiches:
    chicken bacon 'n Swiss 52.0
    chicken breast fillet 49.0
    chicken Cordon Bleu 50.0
    grilled chicken deluxe 42.0
    roast chicken club 39.0
roast beef sandwiches:
    Arby's melt with cheddar 38.0
    Arby-Q 42.0
    beef 'n cheddar 45.0
    Big Montana 44.0
    giant roast beef 43.0
    junior or regular roast beef 36.0
    super roast beef 50.0
sub sandwiches:
    French dip 43.0
    hot ham 'n Swiss 47.0
    Italian 49.0
    Philly beef 'n Swiss 52.0
    roast beef 48.0

Arby's, sub sandwiches (cont.)

turkey	49.0
light menu:	
garden salad, with crouton pkt. and 2 saltines	16.0
grilled chicken	33.0
grilled chicken salad	16.0
roast chicken deluxe	32.0
roast chicken salad	16.0
roast turkey deluxe	33.0
side salad, with crouton pkt. and 2 saltines	12.0
chicken finger snack	62.0
chicken finger meal	81.0
side items:	
curly fries, cheddar	52.0
curly fries, large	75.0
curly fries, medium	49.0
curly fries, small	40.0
homestyle fries, large	86.0
homestyle fries, medium	57.0
homestyle fries, small	46.0
Jalapeño Bites	29.0
mozzarella sticks	34.0
potato, baked, broccoli 'n cheddar	71.0
potato, baked, with butter and sour cream	65.0
potato, baked, deluxe	68.0
potato cakes, 2 pieces	21.0
onion petals	43.0
condiments:	
Arby's Sauce pkt.	3.0
BBQ dipping sauce	10.0
beef stock au jus	0
bleu cheese dressing	3.0
Bronco Berry Sauce	23.0
buttermilk ranch dressing	2.0
buttermilk ranch dressing, reduced-calorie	12.0
German mustard pkt.	0
honey French dressing	24.0
honey mustard	5.0
Horsey Sauce pkt.	3.0
Italian dressing, reduced-calorie	4.0
ketchup pkt.	3.0

mayonnaise pkt. 0

mayonnaise pkt., light 1.0

marinara sauce 4.0

Tangy Southwest Sauce 3.0

Thousand Island dressing 11.0

desserts and shakes:

    apple turnover, iced 54.0

    cherry turnover, iced 53.0

    shake, chocolate, 10.3 oz. 69.0

    shake, Jamocha, 10.3 oz. 66.0

    shake, strawberry or vanilla, 10.3 oz. 67.0

Arrowhead:

untrimmed, 1 lb. 68.8

raw, 1 large, .9-oz. corm 5.1

raw, 1 medium, .4-oz. corm 2.4

boiled, drained, 1 medium, .4-oz. corm 1.9

Arrowroot, fresh, raw:

1.2-oz. root 4.4

sliced, 1 cup 16.1

Arrowroot flour, 1 cup 112.8

Artichoke, French or globe, fresh:

raw:

    (Dole), 1 medium, 4.5 oz. 13.0

    1 large, 5.7 oz. 17.0

    1 medium, 4.5 oz. 13.5

boiled, drained, 10.6-oz. choke, 4.5 oz. edible 13.4

boiled, drained, hearts, ½ cup 9.4

Artichoke, canned, hearts, in brine:

(Progresso), 2 pieces 6.0

(Reese), 2 pieces with liquid 9.0

Artichoke, frozen:

boiled, drained, 9-oz. pkg. 22.0

boiled, drained, 1 cup 15.4

hearts *(Birds Eye),* ½ cup 8.0

Artichoke, Jerusalem, see "Jerusalem artichoke"

Artichoke, marinated:

grilled *(Antica Cucina Mediteranea),* 1 oz. 2.0

hearts *(Progresso),* 2 pieces with liquid 2.0

Artichoke, pickled, in jars *(Braswell's),* 3 pieces, 1 oz. 4.0

Artichoke dip, in jar *(Victoria),* 2 tbsp. 2.0

Artichoke salad, in jar *(Reese),* ⅓ cup 7.0
Arugula, fresh, raw:
1 oz. 1.0
½ cup...4.0
Asian pear, see "Pear, Asian"
Asparagus, fresh:
raw:
    (Dole), 5 spears, 3.3 oz. 4.0
    (Frieda's), ⅔ cup or 3 oz...4.0
    untrimmed, 1 lb...8.9
    4 spears, 3.8 oz. 2.6
    1 small spear, 5" long or less 5
boiled, drained, 4 spears, ½" diam. base 2.5
boiled, drained, ½ cup...3.8
Asparagus, canned:
(Seneca), ½ cup 3.0
(Stokely), ½ cup 3.0
all styles *(Del Monte),* ½ cup..3.0
spears:
    (Green Giant), 4.5 oz. 3.0
    14.5-oz. can...10.2
    1 spear, approx. 5" long, drained.. .4
    drained, 1 cup 6.0
    extra large *(LeSueur),* ½ cup 3.0
    extra long *(Green Giant),* 4.5 oz., about 5 spears...............3.0
spears, cut *(Green Giant),* ½ cup..3.0
spears, white *(Haddon House),* 6 spears, 4.6 oz. 3.0
Asparagus, freeze-dried *(AlpineAire),* ½ cup 4.0
Asparagus, frozen:
spears:
    (Birds Eye), 8 spears 4.0
    (Freshlike), 7 spears 3.0
    4 spears, 2 oz.. .8
cuts:
    (Birds Eye), ½ cup 4.0
    (Freshlike), ¾ cup 3.0
    (Green Giant), ⅔ cup 3.0
    (Green Giant Harvest Fresh), ⅔ cup 4.0
unprepared, 10-oz. pkg...11.6
boiled, drained, 10-oz. pkg...14.3
boiled, drained, 1 cup 8.8

Asparagus, pickled, in jar *(Hogue Farms)*, 3 spears....................1.0
Asparagus bean, see "Winged bean"
Asparagus combination, frozen *(Birds Eye* Farm Fresh
    Stir-Fry), 2 cups 16.0
Atemoya *(Frieda's)*, 3-oz. fruit 20.0
Au jus gravy:
(Franco-American), ¼ cup 2.0
(Heinz Home Style Bistro), ¼ cup......................................2.0
1 cup 6.0
Au jus gravy mix *(Knorr* Gravy Classics), 1 tsp., ¼ cup*............2.0
Aubergine, see "Eggplant"
Australian blue squash *(Frieda's)*, ¾ cup, 3 oz....................7.0
Avocado, fresh, raw:
cubed, 1 cup 11.1
puree, 1 cup 17.0
California, trimmed, 1 fruit, approx. 6 oz. 12.0
California, puréed, 1 cup 15.9
Florida, trimmed, 1 fruit, approx. 10.75 oz. 20.5
Florida, pureed, 1 cup 27.1
Avocado, cocktail *(Frieda's)*, 1.4-oz. piece.........................3.0
Avocado dip (see also "Guacamole"), 2 tbsp.:
(Kraft)..4.0
(Nalley)..3.0

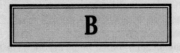

FOOD AND MEASURE **CARBOHYDRATE**

Babaganoush, see "Eggplant dip"
Bacon (see also "Breakfast strips"):
raw, 1 thick slice, 12 slices per lb. 0
raw, 3 medium slices, 20 slices per lb. 1
pan-fried, 3 medium slices, 20 slices per lb. raw 1
pan-fried, 4.5 oz. (yield from 1 lb. raw) 7
Bacon, Canadian-style:
(Boar's Head), 2 oz. 1.0
(Jones Dairy Farm), 3 slices 0
(Pillow Pack), 20 slices, 2 oz. 2.0
unheated, 2 slices, 2 oz. 1.0
unheated, 6-oz. pkg. 2.9
grilled, 2 slices, 1.6 oz. (yield from 2 oz. unheated) 6
grilled, 4.9 oz. (yield from 6-oz. pkg. unheated) 1.9
Bacon, turkey, see "Turkey bacon"
"Bacon," vegetarian:
1 oz. raw or .6 oz. cooked...1.0
frozen:
    (Lightlife Fakin Bacon), 3 slices...6.0
    (Morningstar Farms Breakfast Strips), 2 strips 2.0
    (Worthington Stripples), 2 strips...2.0
    Canadian style *(Yves* Veggie), 3 slices 2.0
Bacon bits, all varieties *(Hormel),* 1 tbsp. 0
"Bacon" bits, imitation:
(Bac'n Pieces), 1½ tbsp. 2.0
(Bac-'Os), 1½ tbsp. 2.0
Bacon-horseradish dip, 2 tbsp.:
(Kraft)...3.0
(Kraft Premium Sour Cream) 2.0
Bacon-onion dip, 2 tbsp.:
(Breakstone's) 2.0
(Kraft Premium Sour Cream) 2.0

Bagel, 1 piece, except as noted:
plain:

    (Awrey's), 4 oz..58.0
    (Awrey's), 2.6 oz...40.0
    (Awrey's), 2 oz..31.0
    (Awrey's Miniature), .9 oz................................16.0
    (Lender's) 56.0
    (Thomas' New York Style)..............................56.0
    seeded, unseeded or onion, 3" diam., 2 oz...........30.4
apple cinnamon or wildberry-blueberry *(Thomas'* New York
    Style), ½ piece 33.0
blueberry *(Awrey's),* 4 oz. 61.0
blueberry *(Thomas'* New York Style) 59.0
cinnamon or cinnamon raisin swirl *(Thomas'* New York Style) ..57.0
cinnamon raisin:

    (Awrey's), 4 oz..61.0
    (Awrey's), 2.6 oz...42.0
    (Awrey's), 2 oz..32.0
    3" diam., 2 oz..31.5
egg, 3" diam., 2 oz. 30.2
oat bran, 3" diam., 2 oz. 30.4
Bagel, frozen, 1 piece:
plain *(Sara Lee),* 2.8 oz. 43.0
blueberry *(Sara Lee),* 2.8 oz...................................41.0
cinnamon raisin *(Sara Lee),* 2.8 oz. 45.0
egg *(Sara Lee),* 2.8 oz...44.0
oat bran *(Sara Lee),* 2.8 oz. 42.0
onion *(Sara Lee),* 2.8 oz..44.0
poppyseed *(Sara Lee),* 2.8 oz. 41.0
sesame seed *(Sara Lee),* 2.8 oz. 42.0
Bagel chips:
plain *(Burns & Ricker/New York Style),* 3 chips, 1 oz................19.0
brown rice, butter sesame, or onion poppy *(Hain),* .4-oz. chip 9.0
brown rice, everything, or cinnamon raisin *(Hain),* .4-oz. chip...10.0
cinnamon raisin *(New York Style),* 3 chips, 1 oz. 20.0
garlic or sea salt *(Burns & Ricker/New York Style),* 3 chips,
    1 oz. 20.0
sesame *(Burns & Ricker/New York Style),* 3 chips, 1 oz. 19.0
snack mix *(New York Style),* ⅔ cup or 1 oz. 19.0
Bagel sandwich, with cream cheese *(Pillsbury Toaster Bagel
    Shoppe),* 1 piece 24.0

Baked beans (see also specific bean listings), ½ cup,
    except as noted:
(Allens)......29.0
(Bearitos Fat Free)......26.0
(B&M Original)......30.0
(Campbell's New England Style/Old Fashioned)......32.0
(Eden Organic)......27.0
(Greene's Farm)......32.0
(Van Camp's Original/Fat Free)......32.0
plain or vegetarian, 1 cup......52.1
bacon and onion *(B&M)*......36.0
with beef, 1 cup......45.0
brown sugar and bacon *(Campbell's)*......29.0
with franks, see "Beans and franks"
maple flavor *(B&M)*......28.0
maple sugar *(S&W)*......29.0
with onion *(Van Camp's* Southern Style)......35.0
with pork:
    (B&M)......33.0
    (Trappey's/Wagon Master)......21.0
    (Van Camp's Bold & Spicy)......23.0
    (Van Camp's Large)......22.0
    (Van Camp's Small)......23.0
    (Van Camp's Southwestern)......27.0
    peas *(East Texas Fair* Peas n' Pork)......19.0
    smoked ham *(Van Camp's)*......29.0
    sweet sauce, 1 cup......53.1
    tomato sauce *(Campbell's)*......24.0
    tomato sauce, 1 cup......49.1
sweet hickory and bacon *(Van Camp's)*......32.0
vegetarian *(B&M)*......28.0
Baking mix (see also "Biscuit mix"), all-purpose:
(Arrowhead Mills), ¼ cup......30.0
(Bisquick Original), ⅓ cup......25.0
(Bisquick Reduced Fat), ⅓ cup......27.0
(Bisquick Sweet), ⅓ cup......31.0
(Hodgson Mill Insta-Bake), ⅓ cup......25.0
("Jiffy"), ¼ cup......22.0
wheat-free *(Arrowhead Mills)*, ¼ cup......27.0
Baking powder:
(Calumet), ¼ tsp.......0

(Davis), ¼ tsp. 0
(Featherweight), ¼ tsp. 0
1 tsp. 1.1
low-sodium, 1 tsp. 2.3
Baking soda, 1 tsp. 0
Balsam pear, fresh:
(Frieda's Bitter Melon), 1 cup or 3 oz. 3.0
leafy tips:
    raw, 1 leaf 1
    raw, ½ cup 8
    boiled, drained, 1 cup 3.9
pods:
    raw, 1 balsam pear, 4.4 oz. 4.6
    raw, ½" pieces, 1 cup 3.4
    boiled, drained, ½" pieces, 1 cup 5.4
Bamboo shoots, fresh:
raw:
    untrimmed, 1 lb. 6.8
    ½" slices, 1 cup 7.8
    ½" pieces, ½ cup 4.0
boiled, drained, 5.1-oz. shoot 2.8
boiled, drained, ½" slices, 1 cup 2.3
Bamboo shoots, canned *(Chun King/La Choy)*, 2 tbsp. 1.0
Banana (see also "Plantain"):
fresh, raw:
    (Dole), 1 medium 28.0
    (Frieda's Burro/Ice Cream/Niño), 3-oz. fruit 20.0
    untrimmed, 1 lb. 69.1
    1 medium, 8¾" long 26.7
    sliced, 1 cup 35.1
    mashed, 1 cup 52.7
fresh, red, raw *(Frieda's)*, 5 oz. 33.0
Banana, baking, see "Plantain"
Banana, dehydrated or powder:
1 cup 88.3
1 tbsp. 5.5
Banana, dried *(Frieda's)*, 1 piece, 1.2 oz. 8.0
Banana chips, 1 oz. 16.6
Banana drink blend *(After the Fall Banana Casablanca),*
    8 fl. oz. 19.0
Banana milk drink *(Nesquik* Reduced Fat), 1 cup 31.0

Banana nectar *(Libby's)*, 11.5-fl.-oz. can 47.0
Banana squash *(Frieda's)*, ¾ cup, 3 oz. 7.0
Banana-strawberry juice *(R.W. Knudsen)*, 8 fl. oz. 30.0
Bananas Foster, dried *(AlpineAire)*, 2 oz. 47.0
Barbecue dip, sweet and spicy *(Kraft)*, 2 tbsp. 4.0
Barbecue glaze *(Trader Vic's Polynesian Style)*, 2 tbsp. 10.0
Barbecue pocket, frozen, 4.5-oz. piece:
(Hot Pockets) 47.0
(Ken & Robert's Veggie Pockets) 45.0
Barbecue sauce, 2 tbsp.:
(D.L. Jardine's 5-Star) 10.0
(Heinz Hearty Original) 9.0
(Heinz Old Fashioned) 10.0
(Hunt's Original) 10.0
(Hunt's Original Bold) 11.0
(KC Masterpiece Bold) 12.0
(KC Masterpiece Original) 13.0
(Kraft Char-Grill) 13.0
(Kraft Extra Rich Original) 12.0
(Kraft Original) 9.0
(Kraft Thick 'n Spicy Original) 12.0
(Sun Luck Korean Style) 7.0
(Sylvia's Original) 9.0
(Trader Vic's Polynesian Style) 3.0
all varieties *(Muir Glen Organic)* 6.0
brown sugar *(Kraft Thick 'n Spicy)* 15.0
garlic, roasted *(Kraft)* 12.0
hickory:
    (Hunt's) 12.0
    (KC Masterpiece) 13.0
    bacon *(Kraft Thick 'n Spicy)* 13.0
    and brown sugar *(Hunt's)* 18.0
    smoke *(Kraft Thick 'n Spicy)* 12.0
    smoke, regular or hot *(Kraft)* 9.0
    smoke, onion bits *(Kraft)* 11.0
honey *(Kraft/Kraft Thick 'n Spicy)* 13.0
honey, spicy or hickory *(Kraft)* 14.0
honey Dijon *(KC Masterpiece)* 10.0
honey hickory *(Hunt's)* 13.0
honey mustard:
    (Hunt's) 11.0

(Kraft)	13.0
(Kraft Thick 'n Spicy)	14.0
hot:	
(D.L. Jardine's Killer)	6.0
(Kraft)	9.0
and spicy *(Hunt's)*	11.0
Jamaican *(Helen's Tropical Exotics)*	12.0
Kansas City style *(Kraft)*	11.0
Kansas City style *(Kraft Thick 'n Spicy)*	14.0
mesquite:	
(D.L. Jardine's)	6.0
(Hunt's)	9.0
(KC Masterpiece)	13.0
smoke *(Kraft)*	9.0
smoke *(Kraft Thick 'n Spicy)*	12.0
molasses *(Kraft)*	16.0
mustard *(D.L. Jardine's* Chik'n-Lik'n)	10.0
onion bits *(Kraft)*	11.0
pecan, Texas *(D.L. Jardine's)*	7.0
pepper, see "Pepper sauce"	
teriyaki *(Kraft)*	12.0
Barley, pearled:	
dry:	
(Arrowhead Mills), ¼ cup	37.0
(Quaker Scotch), ¼ cup	37.0
(Quaker Scotch Quick), ⅓ cup	37.0
1 cup	155.5
cooked, 1 cup	44.3
Barley flakes, rolled *(Arrowhead Mills),* ⅓ cup	28.0
Barley flour or meal:	
(Arrowhead Mills Flour), ¼ cup	19.0
1 oz.	21.1
1 cup	110.3
malt flour, 1 oz.	22.2
malt flour, 1 cup	126.8
Barley malt syrup, see "Malt syrup"	
Barley sauce *(Westbrae Natural* Mellow), 1 tsp.	1.0
Basil, fresh:	
1 oz.	1.2
5 medium leaves	.1
chopped, 2 tbsp.	.2

Basil, dried, ground:
(*McCormick*), ¼ tsp. 1
1 tbsp. ... 2.7
1 tsp. 9
Baskin Robbins:
ice cream, ½ cup:
   banana-strawberry ... 17.0
   Baseball Nut ... 18.0
   berry innocent cheese, nonfat ... 24.0
   black walnut ... 13.0
   blackberry, Oregon ... 16.0
   blueberry cheesecake ... 18.0
   butter pecan, old-fashioned ... 13.0
   cherries jubilee ... 16.0
   chocolate ... 18.0
   chocolate, winter white or world-class ... 18.0
   chocolate almond ... 17.0
   chocolate cake, German ... 20.0
   chocolate chip ... 15.0
   chocolate chip cookie dough ... 20.0
   chocolate fudge ... 21.0
   chocolate mousse royale ... 20.0
   chocolate passion, triple ... 21.0
   chocolate-raspberry truffle ... 23.0
   chocolate-vanilla twist, nonfat ... 21.0
   cookies and cream ... 16.0
   egg nog ... 16.0
   English toffee ... 19.0
   espresso and cream, low fat ... 18.0
   Everybody's Favorite Candy Bar ... 20.0
   fudge brownie ... 19.0
   gold medal ribbon ... 20.0
   Heath bar, chunky ... 19.0
   Jamoca ... 14.0
   Jamoca almond fudge ... 17.0
   Jamoca swirl, nonfat ... 23.0
   lemon custard ... 16.0
   mint chocolate chip ... 15.0
   Mississippi mud ... 22.0
   peanut butter, *Reese's* ... 17.0
   peanut butter and chocolate ... 16.0

pistachio almond	13.0
pralines and cream	19.0
pumpkin pie	16.0
Quarterback Crunch	18.0
rocky road	19.0
rum raisin	18.0
strawberry, very berry	16.0
strawberry shortcake	18.0
vanilla or French vanilla	14.0

sherbet, ½ cup:

orange or rainbow	26.0
raspberry, blue	25.0
tangerine-pineapple	22.0

sorbet, ½ cup:

black tie bubbly	31.0
mixed berry lemonade	28.0
pink raspberry lemon	29.0

Bass, all varieties, without added ingredients ... 0
Batter mix, see "Pancake, mix"
Bay leaf, dried:

(McCormick), 1 leaf	.1
crumbled, 1 tbsp.	1.3
crumbled, 1 tsp.	.4

Bean casserole, dried, five-bean *(AlpineAire),* 12 oz. ... 47.0
Bean dip, 2 tbsp.:

(Fritos)	6.0
black bean *(Old El Paso)*	4.0
black bean *(Taco Bell Home Originals)*	6.0
hot *(Fritos)*	5.0
pinto bean *(Bearitos* Fat Free)	5.0

Bean dish, canned, see specific bean listings
Bean salad:

(Cedarlane Carribean), ½ cup	25.0
(Westbrae Natural Salad), ½ cup	16.0
four bean *(Hanover),* ⅓ cup	14.0
three bean *(Green Giant),* ½ cup	16.0
three bean *(Seneca),* 3 oz.	13.0

Bean sauce, spicy brown, Oriental *(House of Tsang),* 1 tsp. ... 3.0
Bean sprouts (see also "Sprouts" and specific bean listings),
fresh *(Chang Farms),* 1 cup ... 4.0

Bean sprouts, canned, 1 cup:

(Chun King)...1.0

(La Choy) 4.0

Beans, see specific listings

Beans, baked, see "Baked beans"

Beans, refried, see "Refried beans"

Beans, snap or string, see "Green beans"

Beans and franks, 1 cup, except as noted:

(Hormel Wieners), 7.5-oz. can 34.0

(Kid's Kitchen Wieners), 1 cup.............................37.0

(Van Camp's Beenee Weenee Micro) 29.0

(Van Camp's Beenee Weenee Zestee) 40.0

baked *(Van Camp's Beenee Weenee)* 49.0

barbecued *(Van Camp's Beenee Weenee)*.................36.0

chili *(Van Camp's Beenee Weenee Chilee)* 27.0

Beans and rice, see "Rice dish, mix"

Béarnaise sauce mix, dry:

(Knorr Classic Sauces), 1 tsp................................2.0

.9-oz. pkt. 14.8

8 fl. oz.* 9.9

Beechnut, dried, shelled, 1 oz. 9.5

Beef, all cuts, without added ingredients........................0

Beef, canned (see also "Beef entree, canned or packaged" and
    "Beef hash, canned"):

corned *(Libby's)*, 2 oz. 0

corned *(Hormel)*, 2 oz. 0

dried, sliced *(Hormel)*, 10 slices, 1 oz. 1.0

roast, with gravy *(Hormel)*, ½ cup..........................3.0

Beef, corned (see also "Beef, canned," "Beef hash," and "Beef
    lunch meat"), brisket, cooked:

11.3 oz. (edible yield from 1 lb. raw) 1.5

4 oz. 5

Beef, dried:

cured:

    *(Hormel Pillow Pack/*Jar), 10 slices, 1 oz. 0

    5 slices, ¾ oz. 3

    4 oz. 1.8

freeze-dried, diced *(AlpineAire)*, ⅓ cup............................0

Beef, refrigerated, cooked:

roast, au jus *(Always Tender)*, 5 oz. 3.0

sirloin filet, peppercorn flavor *(Always Tender)*, 4 oz. 2.0

sirloin filet, teriyaki flavor *(Always Tender)*, 4 oz. 4.0
steak strips, seasoned, grilled *(Louis Rich)*, 3 oz. ....<1.0
tips, with gravy *(Always Tender)*, 5 oz. 5.0
Beef, sandwich steaks, flaked, chopped, and formed:
thinly sliced, 14-oz. pkg. 1.3
thinly sliced, 2 oz. 2
"Beef," vegetarian (see also "Burger, vegetarian"):
canned:
    (Loma Linda Swiss Stake), 3.25-oz. piece 8.0
    (Worthington Vegetable Steaks), 2 pieces, 2.5 oz. 3.0
    (Worthington Prime Stakes), 3.25-oz. piece...........................4.0
frozen:
    (Worthington Stakelets), 2.5-oz. piece 6.0
    corned beef *(Worthington* Meatless), 4 slices, 2 oz. 5.0
    smoked *(Worthington* Meatless), 6 slices, 2 oz. 6.0
Beef dinner, frozen, 1 pkg.:
chicken-fried steak *(Banquet Extra Helping)*, 16 oz. 63.0
mesquite, with barbecue sauce *(Healthy Choice* Meal), 11 oz. ...38.0
oven-roasted *(Healthy Choice* Meal), 10.15 oz. 35.0
patty, char-broiled *(Healthy Choice* Meal), 11 oz. 40.0
pot roast:
    (Healthy Choice Meal), 11 oz...41.0
    Yankee *(Banquet Extra Helping)*, 14.5 oz. 33.0
    Yankee *(Swanson)*, 11.5 oz. 39.0
Salisbury steak *(Banquet Extra Helping)*, 16.5 oz. 37.0
Salisbury steak *(Healthy Choice* Meal Traditional), 11.5 oz.........48.0
Stroganoff *(Healthy Choice* Meal), 11 oz. 40.0
tips, portobello *(Healthy Choice* Meal), 11.25 oz. 34.0
Beef entree, canned or packaged:
chow mein *(Chun King* Bi-Pack), 1 cup 15.0
chow mein *(La Choy* Bi-Pack), 1 cup..11.0
pepper, 1 cup:
    (Chun King Bi-Pack)...11.0
    Oriental *(La Choy* Bi-Pack) 13.0
    steak *(Chun King/La Choy* Skillet Dinner)............................15.0
pot roast *(Dinty Moore American Classics)*, 1 bowl..................19.0
roast, with potatoes *(Dinty Moore American Classics)*, 1 bowl ..24.0
Salisbury steak *(Dinty Moore American Classics)*, 1 bowl..........28.0
stew:
    (Castleberry's Original), 1 cup...16.0
    (Chef Boyardee Microwave), 1 bowl......................................19.0

Beef entree, canned or packaged, stew *(cont.)*

    (Dinty Moore), 1 cup 18.0

    (Dinty Moore), 7.5-oz. can 15.0

    (Dinty Moore Microwave*)*, 1 cup.............................16.0

    (Dinty Moore American Classics), 1 bowl 22.0

    (Hormel Microcup Meals*)*, 1 cup............................14.0

    burger, hearty *(Dinty Moore* Microwave*)*, 1 cup...................19.0

Beef entree, dried:

barbecued, and turkey, with beans *(AlpineAire)*, 1⅛ cups..........61.0

rotini *(AlpineAire)*, 1⅛ cups..59.0

Stroganoff *(AlpineAire)*, 1 cup 37.0

Beef entree, frozen (see also "Beef, refrigerated"), 1 pkg.,
    except as noted:

brisket, sliced *(Stouffer's* Homestyle*)*, 10 oz..............................32.0

and broccoli *(Lean Cuisine Everyday Favorites)*, 8.5 oz. 40.0

broccoli and *(Stouffer's Skillet Sensations)*, ½ of 25-oz. pkg.....51.0

Burgundy, with garlic mashed potatoes *(Michelina's)*, 8.5 oz. 22.0

burrito, see "Burrito"

Cantonese, with rice *(Michelina's Yu Sing)*, 8 oz. 41.0

cheddar *(Stouffer's Skillet Sensations)*, ½ of 25-oz. pkg............58.0

chipped, creamed:

    (Banquet Hot Sandwich Toppers*)*, 4-oz. bag 8.0

    (Freezer Queen Cook-in-Pouch*)*, 4 oz....................................8.0

    (Stouffer's), ½ cup 8.0

cured, shaved, cream sauce with *(Michelina's)*, 8 oz. 40.0

enchilada, see "Enchilada entree"

ginger, with rice *(Michelina's Yu Sing)*, 8 oz. 43.0

home style *(Stouffer's Skillet Sensations)*, ½ of 25-oz. pkg. 41.0

meatballs, see "Meatball entree"

meatloaf, see "Meat loaf entree"

nacho bake *(Ortega* Family Fiesta*)*, 9 oz. ¼ pkg. 36.0

Oriental *(Lean Cuisine Cafe Classics)*, 9.25 oz. 30.0

Oriental, and peppers, with rice *(Michelina's Yu Sing)*, 8 oz.......44.0

oven-roasted *(Lean Cuisine Cafe Classics)*, 9.25 oz. 28.0

patty:

    char-broiled *(Freezer Queen* Meal*)*, 9.5 oz............................15.0

    char-broiled, gravy and *(Morton)*, 9 oz. 26.0

    char-broiled, mushroom gravy and *(Banquet* Family Size*)*,
        1 patty with gravy 6.0

    char-broiled, mushroom gravy and *(Freezer Queen* Family
        Entree*)*, 1 patty with gravy...6.0

onion gravy and *(Freezer Queen* Family Entree), ¼ pkg.,
7 oz. 12.0
with vegetables, country style *(Banquet)*, 9.5 oz. 22.0
Western style *(Banquet)*, 9.5 oz. 28.0
pepper steak:
    (Michelina's), 8.5 oz. 45.0
    green *(Stouffer's* Homestyle), 10.5 oz. 33.0
    Oriental *(Healthy Choice* Entree), 9.5 oz. 34.0
    with rice *(Michelina's)*, 8 oz. 43.0
peppercorn *(Lean Cuisine Cafe Classics)*, 8.75 oz. 32.0
and peppers, with rice:
    (Freezer Queen Deluxe Family Entree), 1 cup 38.0
    (Freezer Queen Homestyle), 8.5 oz. 35.0
pie/pot pie:
    (Banquet), 7 oz. 38.0
    (Marie Callender's), 9.5 oz. 53.0
    (Marie Callender's), ½ of 16.5-oz. pkg. 50.0
    (Stouffer's), 10 oz. 36.0
    potato-topped *(Swanson)*, 12 oz. 47.0
portobello *(Lean Cuisine Cafe Classics)*, 9 oz. 24.0
pot roast:
    (Freezer Queen Deluxe Family Entree), 1 cup 24.0
    (Freezer Queen Meal), 9.25 oz. 20.0
    (Lean Cuisine Cafe Classics), 9 oz. 25.0
    (Marie Callender's Skillet Meals), ½ of 22-oz. pkg. 33.0
    (Stouffer's Hearty Portions), 16 oz. 48.0
    and gravy, old-fashioned *(Marie Callender's* Meals), 15 oz. ...55.0
    with potato wedges *(Michelina's)*, 10 oz. 35.0
    and potatoes, browned *(Stouffer's* Homestyle), 8⅞ oz. 29.0
    Yankee *(Banquet)*, 9.4 oz. 20.0
with potatoes, roasted, and peppers *(Stouffer's Oven
Sensations)*, ½ of 24-oz. pkg. 44.0
and rice, fiesta *(Lean Cuisine Skillet Sensations)*, ½ of
24-oz. pkg. 48.0
roast *(Marie Callender's* Meals), 14.5 oz. 30.0
Salisbury steak:
    (Banquet), 9.5 oz. 28.0
    (Lean Cuisine Cafe Classics), 9.5 oz. 29.0
    (Lean Cuisine Hearty Portions Meal), 15.5 oz. 40.0
    (Stouffer's Homestyle), 9⅝ oz. 27.0
    brown gravy and *(Banquet* Family Size), 1 patty with gravy....7.0

Beef entree, frozen, Salisbury steak *(cont.)*

gravy and *(Banquet* Hot Sandwich Toppers), 5-oz. bag 8.0

gravy and *(Freezer Queen* Cook-in-Pouch), 5 oz. 8.0

gravy and *(Freezer Queen* Family Entree),

1 patty with gravy 6.0

gravy and *(Morton),* 9 oz..24.0

and gravy *(Michelina's),* 8 oz..21.0

and gravy, with shells and cheese *(Michelina's),* 10.5 oz. ...34.0

with pasta shells *(Stouffer's Hearty Portions),* 16 oz. 43.0

sirloin, and gravy *(Marie Callender's* Meals), 14 oz..............51.0

with whipped potato *(Freezer Queen* Homestyle), 8.5 oz. 26.0

sandwich, see "Beef sandwich/pocket"

sirloin:

peppercorn, with noodles *(Michelina's),* 8.5 oz. 33.0

roasted, supreme *(Michelina's),* 8 oz. 34.0

roasted, supreme, with noodles *(Michelina's),* 8.5 oz. 33.0

sliced, in gravy with noodles *(Boston Market),* 14 oz. 50.0

sliced *(Banquet),* 9 oz. 19.0

sliced, gravy and:

(Banquet Hot Sandwich Toppers), 4-oz. bag 5.0

(Freezer Queen Cook-in-Pouch), 4 oz. 5.0

(Freezer Queen Deluxe Family Entree), ⅔ cup 6.0

(Freezer Queen Meal), 9 oz...17.0

brown gravy *(Banquet* Family Size), 2 slices with gravy 5.0

steak:

chicken-fried *(Banquet),* 10 oz. 39.0

chicken-fried, and gravy *(Marie Callender's* Meals), 15 oz. ...50.0

chicken-fried, and gravy, mashed potatoes *(Marie Callender's*

Family), 1 patty with gravy, ½ cup potatoes.....................47.0

country-fried *(Stouffer's Hearty Portions),* 16 oz. 61.0

stew, hearty *(Banquet* Family Size), 1 cup 18.0

Stroganoff:

(Lean Cuisine Hearty Portions Meal Homestyle), 14.25 oz. ..44.0

(Marie Callender's Skillet Meals), ½ of 22-oz. pkg................31.0

(Marie Callender's Skillet Meals), ¼ of 35-oz. pkg. 25.0

(Stouffer's Homestyle), 9¾ oz...37.0

(Stouffer's Skillet Sensations), ¼ of 40-oz. pkg. 38.0

and noodles *(Marie Callender's* Meals), 13 oz. 59.0

teriyaki, with rice *(Lean Cuisine Skillet Sensations),* ½ of

24-oz. pkg...48.0

teriyaki, with rice *(Yu Sing),* 8 oz. 51.0

tips:

    français *(Healthy Choice* Entree), 9.5 oz.............................40.0

    in mushroom sauce *(Marie Callender's* Meals), 13.6 oz........39.0

    Southern *(Lean Cuisine Cafe Classics)*, 8.75 oz. 37.0

and tomatoes, chunky *(Stouffer's* Homestyle), 10 oz. 35.0

tortilla bake *(Ortega* Family Fiesta), 10 oz., ¼ pkg.....................52.0

and vegetables, savory *(Lean Cuisine Skillet Sensations)*,

    ½ of 24-oz. pkg..38.0

Beef entree mix*, frozen:

beefy noodle *(Green Giant Create a Meal!)*, 1¼ cups 31.0

and broccoli stir-fry *(Green Giant Create a Meal!)*, 1⅓ cups 15.0

cheesy pasta and vegetable *(Green Giant Create a Meal!)*,

    1¼ cups 29.0

with garlic potatoes *(Birds Eye Steak Voila!)*, 1 cup 26.0

stew, homestyle *(Green Giant Create a Meal!)*, 1 cup.................24.0

Szechuan stir-fry *(Green Giant Create a Meal!)*, 1¼ cups...........20.0

Beef fat..0

Beef gravy, ¼ cup, except as noted:

(Boston Market Classic) 3.0

(Franco-American) 4.0

(Franco-American Fat Free) 5.0

(Franco-American Slow Roasted Regular/Fat Free).....................4.0

savory *(Heinz* Fat Free) 3.0

Beef hash, corned *(Jones Dairy Farm)*, 2 oz. 5.0

Beef hash, canned, 1 cup, except as noted:

corned:

    (Libby's) 33.0

    (Mary Kitchen)..22.0

    (Mary Kitchen), 7.5-oz. can 19.0

    (Mary Kitchen 50% Less Fat) 25.0

    (Stagg) 29.0

roast *(Mary Kitchen)* 22.0

Beef hash, dried, roast *(AlpineAire* All American), 1 cup 28.0

Beef jerky, see "Sausage sticks"

Beef kidney, see "Kidney"

Beef lunch meat, 2 oz., except as noted:

(Carl Buddig Lean), 2.5-oz. pkg...1.0

(Carl Buddig Lean), 9 slices, 2 oz. 1.0

cooked *(Boar's Head* No Salt) 0

corned beef:

    (Black Bear)...2.0

Beef lunch meat *(cont.)*

    (Carl Buddig Lean), 2.5-oz. pkg. 1.0
    (Carl Buddig Lean), 9 slices, 2 oz. 1.0
    (Hansel 'n Gretel Healthy Deli) 2.0
    (Healthy Choice) 0
    brisket *(Russer)* 0
    brisket or round *(Boar's Head)* 0
    loaf, jellied 0
    zesty *(Healthy Choice* Hearty Deli Flavor), 4 slices, 1.8 oz. 1.0
cured:
    jellied 0
    chopped, smoked, 1-oz. slice 5
    thin-sliced, 5 slices, ¾ oz. 1.2
loaf, 1-oz. slice 8
London broil, flame-seared *(Hansel 'n Gretel Healthy Deli)* 2.0
pepper-seasoned, eye round *(Boar's Head)* 0
peppered *(Sara Lee* Deli Choice), 3 slices, 2.2 oz. 0
peppered, roast *(Sara Lee)* 1.0
roast/oven-roasted:
    (Black Bear) 0
    (Boar's Head No Salt) 0
    (Russer), 2 oz. 0
    (Sara Lee Deli Choice), 2 slices, 1.6 oz. 0
    Cajun *(Boar's Head)* 0
    Cajun *(Healthy Choice)* 1.0
    chopped, formed *(Healthy Choice)*, 1-oz. slice 1.0
    chopped, formed *(Healthy Choice Deli Traditions)*, 6 slices,
        1.9 oz. 1.0
    flame-roasted *(Sara Lee)* 1.0
    Italian style *(Boar's Head)* 2.0
    Italian style *(Healthy Choice)* 1.0
    Italian style, top round *(Hansel 'n Gretel Healthy Deli)* 1.0
    medium *(Healthy Choice)* 2.0
    medium rare *(Healthy Choice)* 1.0
    top round *(Boar's Head* Deluxe) 0
    top round *(Boar's Head* Deluxe Cap-Off) .... <1.0
    top round *(Sara Lee)* 1.0
    top round or well done *(Hansel 'n Gretel Healthy Deli)* 0
    structured *(Healthy Choice)* 0
Beef pie, see "Beef entree, frozen"

Beef sandwich/pocket, 1 piece, except as noted:

barbecued *(Hormel Quick Meal),* 4.3 oz. 38.0

and cheddar *(Hot Pockets),* 4.5 oz. 44.0

cheeseburger:

    (Hormel Quick Meal), 4.8 oz. 36.0

    (Hot Pockets), 4.5 oz. 41.0

    bacon *(Hormel Quick Meal),* 5 oz. 34.0

    mini *(Kid's Kitchen),* 2 pieces, 4.8 oz. 44.0

fajita *(Hot Pockets),* 4.5 oz. 37.0

hamburger *(Hormel Quick Meal),* 4.3 oz. 34.0

potato top *(Mrs. Patterson's Aussie Pie),* 5.5 oz. 33.0

steak, cheese:

    (Deli Stuffs), 4.5 oz. 40.0

    jalapeño *(Hot Pockets),* 4.5 oz. 37.0

    Philly steak *(Croissant Pockets),* 4.5 oz. 40.0

    Philly steak *(Healthy Choice Hearty Handfuls),* 6.1 oz. 47.0

    Philly steak *(Healthy Choice Hearty Handfuls),* 6.1 oz. 50.0

    Philly steak *(Lean Pockets),* 4.5 oz. 43.0

    Philly steak *(Toaster Breaks Melts),* 2.2 oz. 20.0

Beef sauce, see "Steak sauce" and specific listings

Beef seasoning mix:

pot roast/sauerbraten *(Knorr Recipe Classics),* 1 tbsp. 6.0

stew *(Adolph's Meal Makers),* 1 tbsp. 3.0

stew *(Knorr Recipe Classics),* 1⅓ tbsp. 6.0

Beef stew, see "Beef entree"

Beer, 12 fl. oz.:

regular 13.2

light 4.6

Beer beans, see "Edamame"

Beet, fresh:

(Frieda's), ½ cup, 3 oz. 8.0

raw:

    untrimmed, 1 lb. 30.4

    1 beet, 2" diam., 2.9 oz. 7.8

    sliced, 1 cup 13.0

boiled, drained, 2 beets, 2" diam., 3.5 oz. 10.0

boiled, drained, sliced, ½ cup 8.5

Beet, canned:

all styles *(Seneca),* ½ cup 7.0

whole, julienne, or sliced *(S&W),* ½ cup 7.0

whole or sliced *(Green Giant),* ½ cup 8.0

Beet, canned *(cont.)*
sliced *(Del Monte)*, ½ cup 8.0
diced, drained, 1 cup...11.3
shredded, drained, 1 cup 14.0
Harvard:
    (Green Giant), ⅓ cup...15.0
    (Seneca), ½ cup..21.0
    sliced, 1 cup 44.7
pickled:
    (Greenwood Sweet & Tangy)*, ½ cup 24.0
    (Seneca), 1 oz. 4.0
    crinkle style *(Del Monte)*, ½ cup 19.0
    sliced, 1 cup 37.0
Beet greens, fresh:
raw:
    untrimmed, 1 lb..10.1
    1 leaf 1.3
    1" pieces, 1 cup 1.5
boiled, drained, 1" pieces, 1 cup 7.9
boiled, drained, 1" pieces, ½ cup 3.9
Berliner, beef and pork, 1 oz......................................7
Berry, see specific listings
Berry juice blend, 8 fl. oz.:
(After the Fall Oregon Berry).....................................25.0
(Mott's)...29.0
nectar *(Santa Cruz Organic)*.......................................30.0
Berry juice drink blend:
(WhipperSnapple Power Berry Smoothie)*, 10 fl. oz. 40.0
black and blue *(WhipperSnapple)*, 10 fl. oz. 40.0
punch *(Tropicana)*, 8 fl. oz. 32.0
Biryani paste, see "Curry paste"
Biscuit (see also "Roll"):
(Arnold Old Fashioned)*, 2 pieces 18.0
buttermilk *(Awrey's* Round/Country)*, 2 oz........................31.0
Biscuit, refrigerated, 1 piece, except as noted:
(Grands! Crescent)*, 2.6 oz......................................29.0
(Grands! Homestyle)*, 2 oz. 24.0
(Pillsbury Country)*, 3 pieces, 2.25 oz..........................29.0
buttermilk:
    (Grands!), 2 oz. 24.0
    (Grands! Reduced Fat)*, 2 oz. 26.0

(Hungry Jack Flaky Layers), 1.2 oz.	14.0
(Pillsbury), 3 pieces, 2.25 oz.	29.0
corn *(Grands!)*, 2.2 oz.	28.0

flaky:

(Grands!), 2.2 oz.	25.0
(Hungry Jack Flaky Layers/*Butter Tastin'* Flaky Layers), 1.2 oz.	14.0
honey butter *(Hungry Jack* Flaky Layers), 1.2 oz.	17.0

plain or buttermilk:

lower-fat, 2" diam.	10.9
lower-fat, baked, 2¼" diam.	11.6
higher-fat, 2½" diam.	13.1
higher-fat, baked 2½" diam.	12.8
mixed-grain, 2½" diam.	20.9
Southern style *(Grands!)*, 2 oz.	23.0

Biscuit mix (see also "Baking mix"):

(Arrowhead Mills), ¼ cup	23.0
("Jiffy"), ¼ cup	22.0
(Kentucky Kernel), ¼ cup	28.0
plain or buttermilk, 3"-diam. biscuit*	27.6
buttermilk *("Jiffy")*, ⅓ cup	29.0

Bitter melon, see "Balsam pear"

Black beans, mature:

dry:

(Frieda's), ⅓ cup, 3 oz.	20.0
(Goya), ¼ cup	23.0
1 cup	121.0
boiled, 1 cup	40.8

turtle:

dry *(Arrowhead Mills)*, ¼ cup	28.0
dry, 1 cup	116.4
boiled, 1 cup	45.0

Black beans, canned, ½ cup:

(Allens)	19.0
(Eden Organic)	18.0
(Joan of Arc)	18.0
(Progresso)	17.0
(Walnut Acres Organic Farms)	20.0
(Westbrae Natural)	16.0
baked *(Bearitos* Fat Free)	22.0
with ginger and lemon *(Eden* Organic)	21.0

Black beans, canned *(cont.)*

seasoned *(Trappey's),* ½ cup 20.0
turtle *(Hain),* ½ cup 17.0

Black bean dip, see "Bean dip"

Black bean salsa, see "Salsa"

Black bean sauce, in jar, 1 tbsp.:

(Ka•Me) 3.0
garlic *(Lee Kum Kee)* 3.0
spicy garlic or with shiitake mushrooms *(Annie Chun's)* 4.0

Blackberries, fresh, raw, 1 cup 18.4

Blackberries, canned:

(Allens), ½ cup 13.0
in light syrup *(Oregon),* ½ cup 29.0
in heavy syrup, 1 cup 59.1

Blackberries, frozen:

unsweetened, 18-oz. pkg. 79.9
unsweetened, 1 cup 23.7

Blackberry filling, see "Pie filling"

Blackberry syrup, ¼ cup:

(Knott's Berry Farm) 52.0
(Smucker's) 52.0

Black-eyed peas:

fresh or frozen, see "Cowpeas"
mature, 1 cup 32.7

Black-eyed peas, canned, ½ cup, except as noted:

fresh shell *(Allens/East Texas Fair/Dorman)* 21.0
fresh shell, with jalapeño *(Trappey's)* 20.0

mature:

   (Allens) 18.0
   (Eden Organic) 16.0
   (Joan of Arc) 16.0
   (Shari Ann's Organic) 17.0
   with bacon *(Allens/Sunshine)* 20.0
   with bacon *(Trappey's)* 19.0
   with bacon and jalapeños *(Trappey's)* 19.0
   with pork, 1 cup 39.7

Black-eyed peas, frozen:

(Birds Eye Southern),* ½ cup 21.0
(Seabrook Farms), ½ cup 21.0

Blintz, frozen:

apple, blueberry, or cherry *(Empire* Kosher), 2 pieces, 4.4 oz. 36.0

cheese *(Empire* Kosher), 2 pieces, 4.4 oz. 29.0
"cheese," nondairy:
   (Tofutti Mintz's), 2-oz. piece 15.0
    apple danish, blueberry, or cherry *(Tofutti* Pillows),
     2.25-oz. piece 2.0
potato *(Empire* Kosher), 2 pieces, 4.4 oz. 32.0
potato *(Ratner's),* 2.2-oz. piece 17.0
Blood sausage, .9-oz. slice 3
Bloody Mary mixer:
(D.L. Jardine's Red Snapper), 3 fl. oz. 5.0
(Mr & Mrs T), 8 fl. oz. 9.0
(Mr & Mrs T Rich & Spicy) 11.0
(Tabasco), 8 fl. oz. 11.0
(Trader Vic's Spicy), 4 fl. oz. 6.0
Blue squash, see "Australian blue squash"
Blueberries, fresh:
1 pint 56.8
1 cup 20.5
Blueberries, canned:
in light syrup *(Oregon),* ½ cup 26.0
in heavy syrup *(S&W),* ⅓ cup 16.0
in heavy syrup, 1 cup 56.5
Blueberries, dried:
(Frieda's), ¼ cup, 1.4 oz. 33.0
(Sonoma), ¼ cup, 1.4 oz. 33.0
freeze-dried, ½ oz. 17.0
Blueberries, frozen:
unsweetened, 20-oz. pkg. 69.0
unsweetened, unthawed, 1 cup 18.9
sweetened, 10-oz. pkg. 62.2
sweetened, thawed, 1 cup 50.5
Blueberry filling, see "Pastry filling" and "Pie filling"
Blueberry juice *(After the Fall* Maine Coast), 8 fl. oz. 25.0
Blueberry syrup:
(Estee), ¼ cup 20.0
(Knott's Berry Farm), 1 fl. oz. 30.0
(Maple Grove Farms), ¼ cup 62.0
(Smucker's), ¼ cup 52.0
Bluefish, without added ingredients 0
Boar, wild, without added ingredients 0

Bocconcini dish, mix, four-cheese Parmesano *(Land O Lakes International Pasta Collection),* 2.5 oz. 43.0
Bockwurst, raw, 2.3-oz. link 3
Bok choy, see "Cabbage, bok choy"
Bologna (see also "Turkey bologna"), 2 oz., except as noted:
  (Boar's Head) ....<1.0
  (Boar's Head Lower Sodium) 0
  (Hansel 'n Gretel Healthy Deli) 3.0
  (Hebrew National Presliced), 4 slices, 2 oz. 1.0
  (Johnsonville Ring/Beef) 1.0
  (Oscar Mayer Fat Free), 1-oz. slice 2.0
  (Oscar Mayer Thick Cut), 2-oz. slice 2.0
  (Russer/Russer Light) 3.0
  beef:
    (Boar's Head) 0
    (Oscar Mayer), 1.4-oz. slice 1.0
    (Russer/Russer Light) 3.0
    .8-oz. slice 2
    Lebanon, .8-oz. slice 6
  beef and pork, .8-oz. slice 6
  garlic *(Boar's Head)* 1.0
  garlic *(Oscar Mayer),* 1.4-oz. slice 1.0
  garlic or jalapeño *(Russer)* 3.0
  German:
    (Black Bear) 1.0
    (Hansel 'n Gretel Healthy Deli) 3.0
    (Russer Wunderbar) 5.0
  Lebanon *(Russer)* 1.0
  pork, .8-oz. slice 2
  turkey, pork, and beef *(Healthy Choice),* 1-oz. slice 3.0
  turkey, pork, and beef *(Healthy Choice Deli Traditions),*
    4 slices, 2 oz. 5.0
"Bologna," vegetarian, frozen *(Worthington Bolono),*
  3 slices, 2 oz. 2.0
Boniato *(Frieda's),* 3 oz. 24.0
Bonito, meat only, raw, 4 oz. 5
Borage, fresh, raw, 1" pieces, 1 cup 2.7
Boston Market, 1 serving:
entrees:
  chicken, ½ chicken, with skin 4.0
  chicken, dark meat, ¼ chicken, with skin 2.0

chicken, dark meat, ¼ chicken without skin............................1.0
chicken, white meat, ¼ chicken, with or without skin.............2.0
chicken, Southwest savory, 1 portion 26.0
chicken, teriyaki, dark or white meat, ¼ chicken
    with skin 17.0
chicken, triple-topped, 1 portion 20.0
chicken drumstick or wing, *Tabasco* barbecued, 1 piece 4.0
chicken pot pie, 1 pie 61.0
chicken salad, chunky, ¾ cup 3.0
ham, lean, *Boston Hearth,* 5 oz. 9.0
meat loaf and brown gravy, 7 oz. 19.0
meat loaf and chunky tomato sauce, 8 oz. 22.0
turkey breast, rotisserie, 5 oz. 1.0
sandwiches, 1 piece:
    chicken, barbecued...84.0
    chicken, with cheese and sauce 72.0
    chicken, without cheese or sauce.......................................62.0
    chicken salad 63.0
    ham, with cheese and sauce 72.0
    ham, without cheese or sauce..66.0
    meat loaf, with cheese..95.0
    meat loaf, without cheese...86.0
    pastry sandwich, barbecued chicken....................................56.0
    pastry sandwich, broccoli, chicken cheddar.........................45.0
    pastry sandwich, ham and cheddar......................................47.0
    pastry sandwich, Italian chicken..43.0
    turkey, with cheese and sauce..68.0
    turkey, without cheese or sauce 61.0
    turkey, open-faced 61.0
    turkey club..64.0
sides, hot:
    apples, hot cinnamon, ¾ cup 56.0
    baked beans, barbecued, ¾ cup...48.0
    black beans and rice, 1 cup..45.0
    broccoli cauliflower au gratin, ¾ cup 14.0
    broccoli with red peppers, ¾ cup..5.0
    broccoli rice casserole, ¾ cup 26.0
    butternut squash, ¾ cup 25.0
    carrots, honey-glazed, ¾ cup...35.0
    chicken gravy, 1 oz. 2.0
    corn, whole-kernel, ¾ cup...30.0

Boston Market, sides, hot (cont.)

green bean casserole, ¾ cup	10.0
green beans, ¾ cup	5.0
macaroni and cheese, ¾ cup	32.0
potatoes, mashed, homestyle, ¾ cup	24.0
potatoes, mashed, homestyle, and gravy, ¾ cup	26.0
potatoes, new, ¾ cup	25.0
potato planks, oven roasted, 5 planks	32.0
red beans and rice, 1 cup	45.0
rice pilaf, ⅔ cup	32.0
spinach, creamed, ¾ cup	11.0
squash casserole, ¾ cup	20.0
stuffing, savory, ¾ cup	44.0
sweet potato, baked, 1 piece	94.0
sweet potato casserole, ¾ cup	39.0
vegetables, steamed, ⅔ cup	7.0
zucchini marinara, ¾ cup	7.0

sides, cold:

applesauce, chunky cinnamon, ¾ cup	62.0
bean salad, coyote, ¾ cup	24.0
Caesar side salad, 4 oz.	7.0
coleslaw, ¾ cup	30.0
cranberry-walnut relish, ¾ cup	84.0
fruit salad, ¾ cup	15.0
potato salad, old-fashioned, ¾ cup	30.0

baked goods:

apple pie, cinnamon, ⅕ pie	46.0
brownie, 1 piece	47.0
chocolate chip cookie, 1 piece	48.0
corn bread, 1 loaf	33.0

Bouillon (see also "Bouillon concentrate"):

barbecue, hickory *(Wyler's Shakers* Bouillon & Seasoning),

1 tsp.	2.0

beef/beef flavor:

(Herb-ox), 1 cube or 1 tsp.	<1.0
(Herb-ox Instant Broth & Seasoning), 1 pkt.	<1.0
(Herb-ox Instant Broth & Seasoning Low Sodium), 1 pkt.	2.0
(Knorr), ½ cube.	<1.0
(Maggi Instant), 1 tsp.	0
(Wyler's), 1 cube	1.0
(Wyler's Granules), 1 tsp.	0

(Wyler's Reduced Sodium), 1 cube 1.0
(Wyler's Sodium Free), 1 tsp. 2.0
(Wyler's Shakers Bouillon & Seasoning), 1 tsp. 1.0
(Wyler's Shakers Bouillon & Seasoning Reduced Sodium),
   1 tsp. 2.0
(Wyler's/MBT Instant Broth), 1 pkt. 2.0
(Wyler's/MBT Instant Broth Very Low Sodium), 1 pkt. 3.0
beef and French onion *(Wyler's Shakers* Bouillon & Seasoning),
   1 tsp. 0
chicken/chicken flavor:
   (Herb-ox), 1 cube or 1 tsp. ....<1.0
   (Herb-ox Instant Broth & Seasoning), 1 pkt. ....<1.0
   (Herb-ox Instant Broth & Seasoning Low Sodium), 1 pkt. 2.0
   (Knorr), ½ cube ....<1.0
   (Maggi Instant), 1 tsp. 1.0
   (Wyler's), 1 cube 1.0
   (Wyler's Granules), 1 tsp. 0
   (Wyler's Reduced Sodium), 1 cube 1.0
   (Wyler's Sodium Free), 1 tsp. 2.0
   (Wyler's Shakers Bouillon & Seasoning Reduced Sodium),
      1 tsp. 2.0
   (Wyler's/MBT Instant Broth), 1 pkt. 2.0
   (Wyler's/MBT Instant Broth Very Low Sodium), 1 pkt. 3.0
chicken garlic and herb, with parsley, or Southwestern
   (Wyler's Shakers Bouillon & Seasoning), 1 tsp. 1.0
fish *(Knorr)*, ½ cube 0
Italian, zesty *(Wyler's Shakers* Bouillon & Seasoning), 1 tsp. 2.0
vegetable:
   (Herb-ox), 1 cube ....<1.0
   vegetarian *(Knorr)*, ½ cube 1.0
   vegetarian *(Maggi)*, 1 cube 0
Bouillon concentrate, 2 tsp.:
beef *(Knorr)* 1.0
chicken *(Knorr)* ....<1.0
Bow tie pasta dish, mix:
and beans, with savory herb sauce *(Knorr)*, ⅔ cup 47.0
cheese, Italian *(Lipton* Pasta & Sauce), ¾ cup 38.0
with chicken-flavored vegetable sauce *(Knorr)*, ⅓ cup 20.0
chicken primavera *(Lipton* Pasta & Sauce), ¾ cup 40.0
and red lentils *(Marrakesh Express* Pasta & Sauce),
   ⅓ cup, 1 cup* 39.0

Bow tie pasta entree, frozen, and chicken *(Lean Cuisine Cafe Classics)*, 9½ oz...32.0
Boysenberries, fresh, see "Blackberries"
Boysenberries, canned:
in light syrup *(Oregon)*, ½ cup 27.0
in heavy syrup, 1 cup...57.1
Boysenberries, frozen:
unsweetened, 10-oz. pkg. 34.6
unsweetened, 1 cup 16.1
Boysenberry nectar *(R.W. Knudsen)*, 8 fl. oz. 33.0
Boysenberry syrup, ¼ cup:
(Knott's Berry Farm)..25.0
(Maple Grove Farms) 61.0
(Smucker's)..52.0
Bran, see "Cereal" and specific grains
Bratwurst:
(Boar's Head), 4-oz. link...0
grilled:
   (Johnsonville Original/Beer/Irish Garlic/German
     Brand/Low Fat), 3-oz. link..1.0
   cheddar *(Johnsonville)*, 3-oz. link 2.0
   cocktail *(Johnsonville* Brat Bites), 6 links, 2 oz. 1.0
   honey and garlic *(Johnsonville)*, 3-oz. link.......................5.0
   onion or roasted garlic *(Johnsonville)*, 3-oz. link 1.0
   patty *(Johnsonville)*, 3.3-oz. patty...................................1.0
   precooked *(Johnsonville)*, 2.71-oz. link............................2.0
   smoked, pork or beef *(Johnsonville)*, 2.7-oz. link 2.0
pork, 3-oz. link 1.8
pork and beef, 2.5-oz. link 2.1
turkey *(Butterball)*, 3.8-oz. link...2.0
Braunschweiger (see also "Liverwurst"):
(Boar's Head Lite), 2 oz. 1.0
(Russer/Russer Light), 2 oz..3.0
all varieties, except with onion *(Jones Dairy Farm)*, 2 oz............1.0
with onion *(Jones Dairy Farm)*, 2 oz..2.0
Brazil nuts, shelled:
1 oz., 6–8 kernels...3.6
1 cup 17.9
Bread (see also "Wraps"):
black *(Wild's)*, 1.4-oz. slice 20.0
bran *(Arnold Bran'nola* Original), 1.34-oz. slice 19.0

bran *(Shiloh Farms)*, 1.25-oz. slice...16.0
buttermilk *(Arnold* Country), 1.34-oz. slice.......................20.0
buttermilk, sweet *(Pepperidge Farm Farmhouse)*,
    1.5-oz. slice...22.0
cinnamon *(Arnold)*, 1-oz. slice.....................................16.0
cinnamon raisin, see "raisin," below
cinnamon swirl *(Pepperidge Farm)*, 1-oz. slice...........................15.0
egg, 1.4-oz. slice...19.5
French or Vienna, including sourdough, 1.2-oz. slice.................18.2
Italian:
    (Bakery Light), 2 slices, 1.5 oz..21.0
    (Pepperidge Farm), 1.1-oz. slice 15.0
    (Pepperidge Farm Light Style), ⅔-oz. slice............................9.0
    1.1 oz.-slice...15.0
kamut, sprouted Egyptian *(Shiloh Farms)*, 1.4-oz. slice 18.0
mountain, see "Wrap"
multigrain:
    (Pepperidge Farm Crunchy Grains), 1.2-oz. slice 15.0
    seven-grain *(Arnold)*, 1.34-oz. slice 20.0
    seven-grain *(Pepperidge Farm)*, 1.4-oz. slice.........................18.0
    seven-grain *(Pepperidge Farm* Light Style), ⅔-oz. slice 9.0
    nine-grain *(Great Harvest)*, 1.8-oz. slice................................23.0
    nine-grain *(Pepperidge Farm)*, 1.2-oz. slice 15.0
    twelve-grain *(Arnold)*, 1.34-oz. slice 20.0
    twelve-grain *(Arnold Bran'nola)*, 1.34-oz. slice 19.0
    mixed, whole-grain, or seven-grain, 1.1-oz. slice..................14.8
    sprouted *(Shiloh Farms* Firehouse Unsliced), 2-oz. slice 29.0
    sprouted *(Shiloh Farms* Sandwich Loaf), 1.2-oz. slice..........17.0
    sprouted five-grain *(Shiloh Farms)*, 1.4-oz. slice 19.0
    sprouted five-grain *(Shiloh Farms* Hearth), 2-oz. slice..........28.0
    sprouted seven-grain *(Shiloh Farms)*, 1.4-oz. slice...............19.0
    sprouted ten-grain *(Shiloh Farms)*, 2 slices, 2 oz. 26.0
Navajo fry:
    5"-diam. piece, 3.2 oz. 48.0
    10½"-diam. piece, 5.6 oz...85.3
nut *(Arnold* Health Nut), 1.34-oz. slice......................................20.0
nut *(Arnold Bran'nola* Nutty Grain), 1.34-oz. slice 19.0
oat:
    (Arnold Bran'nola Country), 1.34-oz. slice 19.0
    crunchy *(Pepperidge Farm)*, 1.4-oz. slice...............................17.0

Bread, oat *(cont.)*

honey *(Pepperidge Farm)*, 1.2-oz. slice	15.0
nut *(Arnold* Oatnut), 1.34-oz. slice	19.0

oat bran:

(Arnold), 2 slices, 2.3 oz.	30.0
(Shiloh Farms), 1.4-oz. slice	18.0
1.1-oz. slice	11.9
reduced-calorie, .8-oz. slice	9.5

oatmeal:

(Bakery Light), 2 slices, 1.5 oz.	21.0
(Pepperidge Farm Light Style), ⅔-oz. slice	9.0
(Pepperidge Farm Old Fashioned), 1.2-oz. slice	15.0
(Wild's European Style), 1-oz. slice	13.0
1-oz. slice	13.1
reduced-calorie, .8-oz. slice	10.0
soft *(Pepperidge Farm Farmhouse)*, 1.5-oz. slice	21.0

pita:

onion *(Sahara)*, 2-oz. piece	32.0
wheat, unbleached *(Cedarlane)*, 2-oz. piece	31.0
wheat, whole *(Cedarlane)*, 2-oz. piece	31.0
wheat, whole *(Sahara)*, 2-oz. piece	26.0
wheat, whole *(Sahara* Mini), 1-oz. piece	13.0
wheat, whole, 6½"-diam. piece, 2.1 oz.	35.2
wheat, whole, 4"-diam. piece, 1 oz.	15.4
white *(Sahara)*, 2-oz. piece	29.0
white *(Sahara* Mini), 1-oz. piece	14.0
white, 6½"-diam. piece, 2.1 oz.	33.4
white, 4"-diam. piece, 1 oz.	15.6

potato:

(Arnold Country), 1.34-oz. slice	20.0
golden *(Pepperidge Farm)*, 1.4-oz. slice	18.0
golden *(Pepperidge Farm Farmhouse)*, 1.5-oz. slice	21.0

protein, .7-oz.-slice	8.3

pumpernickel:

(Arnold), 1.1-oz. slice	15.0
(Pepperidge Farm Dark Pump), 1.1-oz. slice	15.0
(Wild's Hearty), 1.4-oz. slice	20.0
(Wild's Westphalian), 1-oz. slice	14.0
.9-oz. slice	12.4

raisin:

cinnamon *(Great Harvest)*, 1.8-oz. slice	24.0

cinnamon swirl *(Pepperidge Farm)*, 1-oz. slice 14.0
cinnamon swirl *(Sun•Maid)*, 1-oz. slice...........................14.0
enriched, 1.1-oz. slice 16.7
whole-wheat *(Shiloh Farms)*, 2 slices, 2 oz..........................30.0
rice bran, 1-oz. slice...11.7
rye:
(Arnold Real Jewish Melba Thin), 2 slices, 1.4 oz.............20.0
(Wild's Bauernbrot), 1.3-oz. slice 17.0
(Wild's Party), 3 slices, 1.1 oz..14.0
1.1-oz. slice 15.5
reduced-calorie, .8-oz. slice...9.3
seeded *(Arnold* Real Jewish), 1.1-oz. slice........................15.0
seeded or unseeded *(Levy* Real Jewish), 1.1-oz. slice 16.0
unseeded *(Pepperidge Farm* Deli), 1-oz. slice 15.0
sourdough, sprouted five-grain *(Shiloh Farms* Unsliced), 2 oz...28.0
spelt *(Shiloh Farms)*, 1.4-oz. slice 21.0
sunflower:
(Great Harvest), 1.8-oz. slice..21.0
(Wild's), 1.4-oz. slice...20.0
seed, whole-wheat *(Shiloh Farms)*, 2 slices, 2 oz. 23.0
wheat:
(Pepperidge Farm Light Style), ⅔-oz. slice...............................9.0
(Pepperidge Farm Old Fashioned), 1.2-oz. slice 16.0
(Pepperidge Farm Very Thin), 3 slices, 1.6 oz.......................21.0
(Shiloh Farms Butter Hearth Unsliced), 2 oz. 28.0
(Shiloh Farms Homestyle), 2 slices, 2 oz. 29.0
.9-oz. slice..11.8
bran, 1.3-oz. slice..17.2
germ, 1-oz. slice..13.5
golden *(Bakery Light)*, 2 slices, 1.5 oz. 20.0
reduced-calorie, .8-oz. slice..10.0
sesame *(Pepperidge Farm)*, 1.4-oz. slice 17.0
winter *(Arnold Best)*, 1.1-oz. slice.....................................13.0
wheat, whole:
(Arnold Brick Oven 100%), 2 slices, 1.7 oz...........................22.0
(Pepperidge Farm 100% Stoneground), 1.2-oz. slice 16.0
(Pepperidge Farm Thin), .9-oz. slice 11.0
(Shiloh Farms), 2 slices, 2 oz..26.0
1-oz. slice 12.9
honey *(Great Harvest)*, 1.8-oz. slice 23.0

Bread *(cont.)*

wheat and rye, sprouted, with onion *(Shiloh Farms)*, 2 slices,
   2 oz. 26.0
wheatberry, .9-oz. slice 11.8
white:
   (Arnold Brick Oven), 2 slices, 1.7 oz. 25.0
   (Arnold Brick Oven Big Slice), 1.2-oz. slice 17.0
   (Bakery Light Premium), 2 slices, 1.5 oz. 21.0
   (Great Harvest), 1.8-oz. slice..22.0
   (Pepperidge Farm Original), .9-oz. slice 13.0
   (Pepperidge Farm Sandwich), 2 slices, 1.6 oz. 23.0
   (Pepperidge Farm Toasting), 1.1-oz. slice 16.0
   (Pepperidge Farm Very Thin), 3 slices, 1.6 oz......................24.0
   (Pepperidge Farm Farmhouse Hearty), 1.5-oz. slice 20.0
   (Sunbeam Small Family), 2 slices, 1.4 oz. 21.0
   1-oz. slice 14.0
   reduced-calorie, .8-oz. slice..10.2
white cheddar garlic *(Great Harvest)*, 1.8-oz. slice 18.0
whole-grain *(Wild's)*, 1-oz. slice..14.0
Bread, brown, canned:
1.6-oz. slice..19.5
plain or raisin *(B&M)*, ½" slice, 2 oz. 29.0
Bread, frozen or refrigerated:
(Pillsbury Homestyle Loaf), ⅑ pkg. 25.0
cornbread and honey butter *(Marie Callender's)*, 1 piece, 1 tbsp.
   honey butter 28.0
French loaf *(Pillsbury)*, ⅕ pkg. 27.0
garlic original or Parmesan and Romano *(Marie Callender's)*,
   1 piece..23.0
Bread, mix:
cheese and herb *(Hodgson Mill* European), ¼ cup....................21.0
corn bread:
   (Arrowhead Mills), ¼ cup..24.0
   (Aunt Jemima Easy Mix), ⅛ pkg.* 24.0
   (Ballard), ⅛ pkg.* 23.0
   (Hodgson Mill), ¼ cup 28.0
   (Kentucky Kernel), ¼ cup...24.0
   2.1-oz. piece*..28.9
   jalapeño *(Hodgson Mill)*, ¼ cup 21.0
herb, Italian *(Fleischmann's* Bread Machine Mix), ⅓ cup,
   ⅛ loaf*..29.0

mixed-grain, nine-grain *(Hodgson Mill)*, ¼ cup 22.0
oatmeal, honey *(Fleischmann's* Bread Machine Mix), ⅓ cup,
  ⅛ loaf* 33.0
potato bread *(Hodgson Mill)*, ¼ cup 23.0
rye *(Arrowhead Mills)*, ⅓ cup 33.0
rye, caraway *(Hodgson Mill)*, ¼ cup 22.0
sourdough *(Fleischmann's* Bread Machine Mix), ⅓ cup,
  ⅛ loaf* 29.0
spelt or multigrain *(Arrowhead Mills)*, ⅓ cup 31.0
wheat, stoneground *(Fleischmann's* Bread Machine Mix),
  ⅓ cup, ⅛ loaf* 32.0
wheat, whole *(Arrowhead Mills)*, ⅓ cup 31.0
wheat, whole, honey *(Hodgson Mill)*, ¼ cup 22.0
white:
  (Arrowhead Mills), ⅓ cup 31.0
  (Hodgson Mill Wholesome), ¼ cup 22.0
  country *(Fleischmann's* Bread Machine Mix), ⅓ cup,
    ⅛ loaf* 31.0
Bread, mix, sweet (see also "Muffin, mix"), 1/12 loaf*, except as
  noted:
apple cinnamon *(Fleischmann's* Bread Machine Mix), ⅓ cup,
  ⅛ loaf* 32.0
banana *(Betty Crocker* Quick) 25.0
cinnamon raisin *(Fleischmann's* Bread Machine Mix), ⅓ cup,
  ⅛ loaf* 33.0
cinnamon streusel *(Betty Crocker* Quick), 1/14 loaf* 28.0
corn, see "Bread, mix"
cranberry *(Pillsbury* Quick) 30.0
cranberry-orange *(Betty Crocker* Quick) 29.0
cranberry-orange *(Fleischmann's* Bread Machine Mix), ⅓ cup,
  ⅛ loaf* 33.0
lemon poppyseed *(Betty Crocker* Quick) 25.0
Bread, stuffed, see "Focaccia, stuffed," and specific sandwich
  listings
Bread crumbs:
all-purpose or Italian *(Arnold)*, ¼ cup 19.0
plain:
  (Progresso), ¼ cup 19.0
  dry, 1 oz. 20.6
  dry, 1 cup 78.3
Italian style *(Contadina)*, ¼ cup 19.0

Bread crumbs *(cont.)*
Italian style *(Progresso)*, ¼ cup 20.0
seasoned, dry, 1 oz. 20.0
seasoned, dry, 1 cup 84.5
white:
    fresh, cubes, 1 cup 17.3
    fresh, crumbs, 1 cup 22.3
    toasted, cubes, 1 cup 17.3
    toasted, crumbs, 1 cup 22.3
Bread stick:
(Stella D'oro Original/Sodium Free), 1 piece 7.0
4½"-long piece, .2 oz. 3.4
all varieties *(Real Torino* Grissini), 5 pieces, .5 oz. 12.0
all varieties *(Stella D'oro* Snack Stix), 4 pieces 11.0
onion *(Stella D'oro)*, 1 piece 6.0
sesame *(Stella D'oro)*, 1 piece 7.0
Bread stick, refrigerated:
(Pillsbury), 2 pieces 25.0
garlic, with herb-garlic topping *(Pillsbury)*, 2 pieces, 2.1 oz.......25.0
Breadfruit, fresh, raw:
¼ small, approx. 3.5 oz. 26.0
trimmed, 1 cup 59.7
Breadfruit seeds, roasted, 1 oz. 11.4
Breadnut tree seeds:
fresh, raw, 1 oz. 13.1
dried, 1 oz. 22.5
dried, 1 cup 127.0
Breakfast dish, see specific listings
Breakfast sandwich, frozen, 1 piece:
cheese, egg, and ham or sausage *(Pillsbury Toaster*
    Scrambles), 1.7 oz. 14.0
egg, with sausage and cheese *(Croissant Pockets)*, 4.5 oz. 38.0
English muffin, with patty *(Morningstar Farms Scrambles)*,
    5.1 oz. 32.0
English muffin, with patty and cheese *(Morningstar Farms)*,
    6 oz. 35.0
Western *(Pillsbury Toaster Scrambles)*, 1.7 oz. 17.0
Breakfast strips (see also "Bacon"):
beef, cured, 12-oz. pkg. 2.4
beef, cured, 3 slices 5

pork, cured:
    raw or unheated, 12-oz. pkg..2.4
    raw or unheated, 3 slices 5
    cooked, 12-oz. pkg. 1.8
    cooked, 3 slices.. .4
Breakfast syrup, see "Pancake syrup" and specific listings
Breyers Ice Cream Parlor, ½ cup:
apple pie with cinnamon 21.0
banana split..22.0
Black Forest..22.0
candy bar sundae...21.0
Chips Ahoy! chocolate chip cookie 19.0
chocolate malt, double...21.0
coffee and cream...18.0
English toffee...23.0
Hershey's milk chocolate with almonds 21.0
ice cream sandwich..21.0
marble mint chip..23.0
Mississippi mud...23.0
Oreo cookies and cream 19.0
raspberry cobbler 21.0
Reese's peanut butter cups 22.0
strawberry shortcake 25.0
Broad beans, fresh:
immature, 1 bean... .9
immature, 1 cup...12.8
in pod, 1 pod, .2 oz...1.1
in pod, 1 cup...22.2
Broad beans, mature:
raw *(Frieda's* Fava Beans), ¾ cup, 3 oz. 50.0
raw, 1 cup...87.5
boiled, 1 cup...33.4
Broad beans, mature, canned:
(Progresso Fava Beans), ½ cup...20.0
1 cup...31.8
Broccoli, fresh:
raw:
    (Andy Boy), 1 medium stalk..8.0
    (Dole), 1 medium stalk, 5.3 oz. 8.0
    untrimmed, 1 lb...14.5
    1 floret.. .6

Broccoli, raw *(cont.)*

　florets *(Mann's Broccoli Wokly)*, 4 oz........................7.0
　florets, 1 cup 3.7
　4-oz. stalk..6.0
　chopped, 1 cup 4.6
raw, baby *(Mann's Broccolini)*, 8 stalks, 2.9 oz. 6.0
boiled, drained, 1 large stalk, 11"–12" long 14.2
boiled, drained, 1 medium stalk, 7½"–8" long 9.1

Broccoli, Chinese:

raw *(Frieda's Gai Lan)*, 1 cup, 3 oz. 3.0
cooked, 1 cup 3.3

Broccoli, freeze-dried *(AlpineAire)*, ½ cup 4.0

Broccoli, frozen:

spears:

　(Birds Eye), 3 spears.....................................4.0
　(Freshlike), 2 spears.....................................4.0
　(Green Giant), 3.5 oz., approx. 3 spears 4.0
　(Seneca), 1 cup 4.0
　unprepared, 10-oz. pkg. 15.2
　boiled, drained, 10-oz. pkg. 13.4
　boiled, drained, ½ cup 4.9

florets:

　(Birds Eye), 5 pieces 4.0
　(Seabrook Farms Petite), 4 pieces........................4.0
　baby *(Birds Eye)*, 1 cup 4.0

chopped:

　(Birds Eye), ⅓ cup 5.0
　(Freshlike), ½ cup 4.0
　(Green Giant), ¾ cup 4.0
　unprepared, 10-oz. pkg. 13.6
　unprepared, 1 cup 7.5
　boiled, drained, 1 cup......................................9.8

cuts:

　(Birds Eye), ½ cup 5.0
　(Freshlike), 1 cup..4.0
　(Freshlike Stir-Fry), 1 cup..............................5.0

in butter sauce, spears *(Green Giant)*, 4 oz................7.0

in cheese sauce:

　(Birds Eye), ½ cup 7.0
　(Freezer Queen Family Side Dish), ⅔ cup.................12.0

(Green Giant), ⅔ cup 9.0
Broccoli combination, fresh (see also "Broccoli salad"), 4 oz.:
and carrots *(Mann's)*..7.0
and carrots, snap peas, celery *(Mann's Broccoli Wokly* Stir-fry) ..7.0
and cauliflower, baby carrots *(Mann's* Vegetable Medley) 8.0
Broccoli combination, frozen (see also "Vegetables, mixed"):
(Birds Eye/Freshlike Baby Broccoli Blend), 1 cup 8.0
(Seneca Normandy), 1 cup 5.0
beans, onions, red peppers *(Birds Eye* Farm Fresh), ½ cup.........6.0
carrots, water chestnuts *(Birds Eye* Farm Fresh), ½ cup..............7.0
cauliflower:
    (Birds Eye Farm Fresh), ½ cup 4.0
    carrots *(Birds Eye* Farm Fresh), ½ cup 5.0
    carrots, cheese sauce *(Birds Eye),* ½ cup 7.0
    carrots, cheese sauce *(Green Giant),* ⅔ cup.........................11.0
    red peppers *(Birds Eye* Farm Fresh), ½ cup 5.0
corn, red peppers *(Birds Eye* Farm Fresh), ½ cup.....................12.0
pasta, cauliflower, carrots, in cheese sauce *(Freezer Queen*
    Family Side Dish), ⅔ cup..14.0
potatoes, carrots *(Birds Eye* French Country Style), ⅔ cup........10.0
red peppers, onion, mushrooms *(Birds Eye* Farm Fresh), ½ cup ...5.0
stir-fry *(Birds Eye* Farm Fresh), 1 cup......................................5.0
stir-fry *(Seneca),* 1 cup 6.0
Broccoli dish, frozen:
au gratin *(Stouffer's),* ½ cup...8.0
pancake *(Dr. Praeger's),* 1.3-oz. cake.......................................8.5
pot pie *(Amy's),* 7.5 oz...46.0
Broccoli rabe, fresh *(Frieda's* Rapini), 3 oz. 4.0
Broccoli rabe, frozen *(Seabrook Farms),* 1 cup 4.0
Broccoli salad, fresh:
with carrots, red cabbage *(Mann's Broccoli Cole Slaw Broccoli*
    Hearts), 4 oz...6.0
and cauliflower hearts, carrots, red cabbage *(Mann's Rainbow*
    Salad Broccoli Hearts), 4 oz. 6.0
with dressing, corn chips *(Mann's Broco Taco),* 1 cup.................7.0
oriental crunch, with dressing *(Mann's)*....................................10.0
Broccoli sprouts, fresh:
(Brocco Sprouts), 1 oz., about ½ cup 1.0
(Jonathan's), 1 cup 5.0
clover with *(Jonathan's),* 1 cup...4.0
Broccoli-cheese croissant *(Sara Lee),* 3.7-oz. piece.................30.0

Broccoli-cheese pocket, frozen, 1 piece:
(Amy's), 4.5 oz. 37.0
(Pepperidge Farm), 3.7 oz. 18.0
cheddar *(Ken & Robert's* Veggie Pockets), 4.5 oz. 38.0
Broiling sauce, see "Grilling sauce"
Broth, see "Bouillon" and "Soup"
Brown gravy, with onions *(Franco-American),* ¼ cup 4.0
Brown gravy mix:
(Hain), 2 tsp. 3.0
(Knorr Gravy Classics), 2 tsp. or ¼ cup* 3.0
(Loma Linda Gravy Quik), 1 tbsp. 4.0
dry, 1 tsp. 3.6
onion, see "Lyonnaise gravy mix"
Brownie, 1 piece, except as noted:
(Hostess Brownie Bites), 3 pieces, 1.3 oz. 21.0
(Little Debbie Christmas Tree), 1.4 oz. 26.0
(Little Debbie Cosmic), 2.2 oz. 40.0
(Little Debbie Lights), 1.9 oz. 29.0
(Little Debbie Loaves), 2.1 oz. 31.0
2-oz. piece 35.8
chocolate *(Awrey's* Decadent), 1.9 oz. 31.0
chocolate-peanut *(Awrey's* Sensation), 1.9 oz. 27.0
fudge:
    (Little Debbie), 2.2 oz. 39.0
    (Little Debbie Singles), 2.5 oz. 46.0
    nut *(Awrey's),* 1.8 oz. 28.0
Brownie, frozen or refrigerated, 1 piece:
bar, chocolate *(Nestlé Toll House)* 26.0
bar, walnut *(Nestlé Toll House)* 23.0
Brownie mix, 1 piece*, except as noted:
(Arrowhead Mills) 27.0
(Arrowhead Mills Fat Free) 28.0
(Arrowhead Mills Wheat Free) 26.0
(Estee), 2 pieces* 23.0
2" square, .8-oz. 12.0
caramel swirl *(Pillsbury),* 1/14 pkg. 23.0
cheesecake swirl *(Pillsbury),* 1/18 pkg. 19.0
chocolate:
    chunk *(Betty Crocker* Supreme) 25.0
    dark *(Betty Crocker* Pouch) 27.0
    dark, fudge *(Betty Crocker* Supreme) 24.0

    dark, with syrup *(Betty Crocker Hershey Supreme* 25.0
    double *(Pillsbury)*, 1/16 pkg. 23.0
    German *(Betty Crocker Supreme)* 29.0
frosted *(Betty Crocker Supreme)* 30.0
fudge:
    (Betty Crocker Original Supreme 20 Pack) 27.0
    (Betty Crocker Pouch) 27.0
    (Betty Crocker Supreme 12 Pack) 30.0
    (Betty Crocker Supreme Family Size 20 Pack) 24.0
    (Betty Crocker Supreme Megapack/4 Pouches/20 Pack) 25.0
    ("Jiffy"), 1/5 cup 28.0
    (Pillsbury), 1/18 pkg. 26.0
    (Sweet Rewards Low Fat), 1/18 pkg. 27.0
    (Sweet Rewards Reduced Fat) 27.0
    hot *(Betty Crocker Supreme)* 23.0
    rich *(Pillsbury One Step)*, 1/12 pkg. 13.0
    swirl, hot *(Pillsbury)*, 1/14 pkg. 23.0
    peanut butter chunk *(Betty Crocker Reese's Pieces)* 23.0
    turtle *(Betty Crocker)* 23.0
    walnut *(Betty Crocker Supreme)* 22.0
Bruschetta, frozen, pesto, mozzarella, and tomato
    (Cedarlane), 1.3-oz. piece 10.0
Brussels sprouts:
raw:
    (Dole), 1 cup or 3.1 oz. 8.0
    1 sprout, .7 oz. 1.7
    1 cup 7.9
boiled, drained, 1 sprout, 3/4 oz. 1.8
boiled, drained, 1/2 cup 6.8
Brussels sprouts, frozen:
(Birds Eye), 11 sprouts 7.0
(Birds Eye Southern), 6 sprouts 7.0
(Freshlike), 6 sprouts 5.0
unprepared, 10-oz. pkg. 22.4
boiled, drained, 1 cup 12.9
baby, in butter sauce *(Green Giant)*, 2/3 cup 9.0
Brussels sprouts, frozen, combination, cauliflower, carrots
    (Birds Eye Farm Fresh), 1/2 cup 7.0
Buckwheat:
1 oz. 20.3
1 cup 121.6

Buckwheat flour:
(Arrowhead Mills), ¼ cup 21.0
(Hodgson Mill), ⅓ cup..33.0
whole-groat, 1 oz. 20.0
whole-groat, 1 cup..84.7
Buckwheat groats:
brown *(Arrowhead Mills),* ¼ cup 30.0
roasted, dry, 1 cup..122.9
roasted, cooked, 1 cup..33.5
Bulgur, dry:
uncooked:
    (Arrowhead Mills), ¼ cup...............................33.0
    1 oz. 21.5
    1 cup 106.2
    with soy grits *(Hodgson Mill),* ¼ cup.............24.0
cooked, 1 cup...33.8
Bulgur dish mix, pilaf *(Casbah),* ¾ cup 36.0
Bulgur salad, see "Tabouli salad"
Bun, see "Roll"
Bun, sweet, 1 piece:
cheese...28.8
cinnamon, with raisins...42.2
honey *(Hostess),* 4 oz. 34.0
honey *(Little Debbie* Singles), 4 oz. 55.0
Bun, sweet, frozen or refrigerated, 1 piece, except as noted:
cinnamon:
    (Sara Lee), 2.7 oz. 41.0
    cream cheese icing *(Pillsbury)* 23.0
    iced *(Grands!/Grands!* Extra Rich), 3.5-oz. piece.....52.0
    iced *(Pillsbury),* 1.7-oz. piece........................26.0
    iced *(Pillsbury* Reduced Fat), 1.6-oz. piece.....24.0
honey *(Morton)*..35.0
honey, mini *(Morton)*...19.0
Burbot, without added ingredients................................0
Burdock root:
raw:
    (Frieda's Gobo Root), ¾ cup, 3 oz. 15.0
    1 root, 5.5 oz. 27.1
    1" pieces, 1 cup...20.5
boiled, drained:
    5.9-oz. root...35.1

2⅓-oz. root 14.0
1" pieces, 1 cup 26.4
Burger, see "Beef sandwich/pocket" and specific restaurant listings
Burger, vegetarian, canned:
(Loma Linda Redi-Burger), ⅝" slice................................7.0
(Loma Linda Vege-Burger), ¼ cup.................................2.0
(Worthington), ¼ cup 2.0
Burger, vegetarian, frozen, 1 patty, except as noted:
(Amy's All American), 2.5 oz...19
(Dr. Praeger's California/Bombay), 2.8 oz. 9.5
(Harvest Burgers), 3.2 oz..8.0
(Hempeh Burger), 1 oz...12.0
(Ken & Robert's), 2.5 oz. 26.0
(Morningstar Farms Garden Grille), 2.5 oz. 18.0
(Morningstar Farms Garden Veggie Pattie), 2.4 oz. 9.0
(Morningstar Farms Ground Meatless), ½ cup................4.0
(Morningstar Farms Better'n Burgers), 2.75 oz. 8.0
(Morningstar Farms Grillers), 2.25 oz.............................5.0
(Morningstar Farms Harvest Burgers Original), 3.2 oz. 8.0
(Morningstar Farms Quarter Prime), 3.4 oz. 6.0
(Morningstar Farms/Natural Touch Hard Rock Café), 3 oz. 18.0
(Natural Touch Garden Veggie Pattie), 2.4 oz. 8.0
(Natural Touch Vegan), 2.75 oz......................................6.0
(Tofutti Quit Beef'n), 2.5 oz...8.0
(Worthington FriPats), 2.25 oz..4.0
(Yves Burger), 3 oz. 9.0
black bean, spicy *(Morningstar Farms),* 2.75 oz. 16.0
black bean, spicy *(Natural Touch),* 2.75 oz. 15.0
black bean and mushroom *(Yves),* 3 oz...........................13.0
California *(Amy's Veggie),* 2.5 oz....................................19.0
with cheese *(Dr. Praeger's Royale),* 3 oz.......................11.5
with cheese, soy *(Tofutti Quit Beef'n),* 2.5 oz.................8.0
Chicago *(Amy's Veggie),* 2.5 oz.....................................20.0
crumbles *(Morningstar Farms),* ⅔ cup.............................4.0
crumbles *(Morningstar Farms Burger Recipe),* ½ cup......5.0
grilled *(Fantastic Foods Nature's Burger Original),* 2.5 oz. 23.0
Italian style *(Harvest Burgers),* 3.2 oz..............................8.0
Italian style *(Morningstar Farms Harvest Burgers),* 3.2 oz. 8.0
oven-roasted *(Morningstar Farms),* 2.4 oz. 9.0
red pepper, roasted, and garlic *(Fantastic Foods
    Nature's Burger),* 2.5 oz. 20.0

Burger, vegetarian, frozen *(cont.)*
Southwestern:
    (Harvest Burgers), 3.2 oz. 9.0
    (Morningstar Farms), 3.2 oz. 9.0
    black bean *(Fantastic Foods Nature's Burger),* 2.5 oz. 20.0
Texas *(Amy's* Veggie), 2.5 oz. 15.0
tofu *(Natural Touch* Okara), 2.25 oz. 4.0

Burger, vegetarian, mix:
(Loma Linda Patty Mix), ⅓ cup 7.0
(Loma Linda Vita Burger), ¼ cup chunks or 3 tbsp. granules 6.0
(Worthington GranBurger), 3 tbsp. 3.0

Burger King, 1 serving:
breakfast dishes:
    biscuit..35.0
    biscuit with egg...37.0
    biscuit with sausage...36.0
    biscuit with sausage, egg, and cheese 37.0
    cini-minis, without vanilla icing, 4 rolls..............................51.0
    Croissan'wich, with sausage and cheese............................21.0
    Croissan'wich, with sausage, egg, and cheese.....................23.0
    French toast sticks, 5 pieces 51.0
    hash browns, large...42.0
    hash browns, small...25.0
breakfast components:
    bacon or ham 0
    A.M. Express dip 21.0
    A.M. Express jam, grape 7.0
    A.M. Express jam, strawberry 8.0
    vanilla icing, 1 oz..20.0
    Land O Lakes whipped classic blend....................................0
sandwiches, with or without mayo:
    bacon cheeseburger..27.0
    bacon double cheeseburger 28.0
    Big King...28.0
    BK Big Fish 59.0
    BK Broiler chicken 45.0
    cheeseburger/double cheeseburger....................................27.0
    chicken 54.0
    Chick'N Crisp..37.0
    Double Whopper/Double Whopper with cheese....................47.0
    hamburger..27.0

Whopper/Whopper with cheese 47.0
Whopper Jr./Whopper Jr. with cheese.....................28.0
sandwich condiments:
Bull's Eye barbecue sauce, ½ oz. 5.0
ketchup, ½ oz...4.0
King sauce, ½ oz...2.0
tartar sauce, 1.5 oz...0
Chicken Tenders:
  4 pieces 9.0
  5 pieces 11.0
  8 pieces 17.0
dipping sauces, 1 oz.:
  barbecue...9.0
  honey-flavored...23.0
  honey mustard 10.0
  ranch 2.0
  sweet and sour..11.0
side orders:
  french fries, king size 74.0
  french fries, medium 50.0
  french fries, small...32.0
  onion rings, king size 74.0
  onion rings, medium 46.0
dessert and shakes:
  Dutch apple pie...39.0
  shake, chocolate, medium...................................75.0
  shake, chocolate, small 58.0
  shake, vanilla, medium 73.0
  shake, vanilla, small 56.0
  shake, syrup added, chocolate, medium 105.0
  shake, syrup added, chocolate, small...................72.0
  shake, syrup added, strawberry, medium..............104.0
  shake, syrup added, strawberry, small 72.0
Burger sandwich, vegetarian, and cheese *(Morningstar Farms Stuffed Sandwich)*, 4.5-oz. piece.................................40.0
Burrito, frozen or refrigerated, 1 piece:
bean, black *(Amy's)*, 6 oz..54.0
bean and cheese:
  (Amy's), 6 oz. 43.0
  (Las Campanas), 4 oz.......................................41.0
  (Patio), 5 oz..46.0

Burrito *(cont.)*
bean and rice *(Amy's)*, 6 oz. 48.0
bean, rice, and cheese *(Cedarlane)*, 5.9 oz. 48.0
beef, red hot *(Las Campanas)*, 4 oz. 39.0
beef and bean:
    (Las Campanas), 4 oz. 39.0
    hot *(Patio)*, 5 oz. 43.0
    mild or medium *(Patio)*, 5 oz. 45.0
    red hot chili *(Patio)*, 5 oz. 42.0
breakfast *(Amy's)*, 6 oz. 38.0
chicken *(Las Campanas)*, 4 oz. 36.0
chicken *(Patio)*, 5 oz. 44.0
vegetable, roasted, cheese *(Cedarlane)*, 6 oz. 48.0
Burrito dinner kit:
(Chi-Chi's), 2 shells and seasonings 52.0
(Ortega), 1 shell, ⅛ seasoning 29.0
bean *(Taco Bell Home Originals* Ultimate), 1 burrito* ...34.0
Burrito entree, frozen, chicken breast con queso *(Healthy*
    Choice Entree), 10.55-oz. pkg. 60.0
Burrito seasoning mix:
(Chi-Chi's), ¼ pkg. 6.0
(Lawry's Spices & Seasonings), 1 tbsp. 6.0
Butter (see also "Margarine"):
(Land O Lakes), 1 tbsp. 0
1 cup or 8 oz. ....<.1
1 tbsp. 0
whipped, 1 cup ....<.1
whipped, 1 tbsp. 0
Butter, honey *(Land O Lakes)*, 1 tbsp. 4.0
"Butter," soy, roasted *(Natural Touch)*, 2 tbsp. 10.0
Butter beans, see "Lima beans"
Butterbur, fresh:
raw, 1 stalk, .2 oz. 2
raw, 1 cup 3.4
Butterbur, canned:
3 stalks, 1.6 oz. 2
chopped, 1 cup 5
Butterfish, without added ingredients 0
Buttermilk, see "Milk"

Butternut, dried, shelled:
1 oz. 3.4
1 cup 14.5
Butternut squash, fresh:
(Frieda's), ¾ cup, 3 oz. 7.0
raw, cubed, 1 cup..16.4
baked, cubed, 1 cup...21.5
Butternut squash, frozen:
unprepared, 12-oz. pkg. 49.0
boiled, drained, mashed, 1 cup 24.1
Butterscotch, see "Candy"
Butterscotch baking chips:
(Hershey's), 1 tbsp. 10.0
(Nestlé Morsels), 1 tbsp..9.0
1 oz. 19.0
1 cup 114.1
Butterscotch syrup (Smucker's Sundae), 2 tbsp. 25.0
Butterscotch topping, 2 tbsp.:
(Kraft)..28.0
(Mrs. Richardson's) 30.0
(Smucker's Spoonable) 31.0
Butterscotch-caramel topping (Smucker's Special Recipe),
    2 tbsp. 30.0

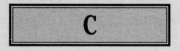

C

FOOD AND MEASURE	CARBOHYDRATE GRAMS

Cabbage:
raw:
    untrimmed, 1 lb...19.5
    1 head, 5¾" diam., approx. 2.5 lbs. 49.3
    chopped, 1 cup...4.8
    shredded, 1 cup..3.8
    shredded, ½ cup 1.9
boiled, drained:
    1 head, 2.8 lbs...56.3
    1 head, 9.2 oz..11.7
    shredded, ½ cup 3.3
Cabbage, bok choy:
raw:
    (Frieda's), 1 cup or 3 oz. 2.0
    untrimmed, 1 lb...8.7
    1.9-lb. head...18.3
    shredded, 1 cup..1.5
boiled, drained, shredded, 1 cup..............................3.0
baby *(Frieda's),* ⅔ cup, 3 oz. 2.0
Cabbage, dehydrated, diced *(AlpineAire),* ½ cup 13.0
Cabbage, Napa:
raw *(Frieda's),* 1 cup, 3 oz....................................3.0
cooked, 1 cup 2.4
Cabbage, pe-tsai:
raw, untrimmed, 1 lb..13.6
raw, shredded, 1 cup..2.5
boiled, drained, 1 leaf...3
boiled, drained, shredded, 1 cup...............................2.9
Cabbage, pickled, spicy, see "Kimchee"
Cabbage, red:
raw:
    untrimmed, 1 lb..22.2
    chopped, 1 cup..5.4
    shredded *(Dole Classic),* 3 oz..............................5.0

shredded, 1 cup..4.3
boiled, drained, 1 leaf...1.0
boiled, drained, shredded, ½ cup 3.5
Cabbage, red, sweet and sour, in jar *(Greenwood),* ½ cup 24.0
Cabbage, savoy:
raw:
   (Frieda's Salad Savoy), ⅔ cup, 3 oz.......................5.0
   untrimmed, 1 lb...22.1
   shredded, 1 cup..4.3
boiled, drained, shredded, 1 cup......................7.8
Cabbage, stuffed, entree, frozen *(Lean Cuisine Everyday Favorites),* 9½ oz..25.0
Cabbage, Tuscan *(Frieda's),* ⅔ cup or 3 oz. 5.0
Cabbage salad, see "Coleslaw"
Cactus pad, see "Nopale"
Cactus pear, see "Prickly pear"
Caesar salad, see "Salad"
Cake:
angel food, ¹⁄₁₂ of 9"-diam. cake, 1 oz. 6.2
banana, iced *(Entenmann's),* ⅛ cake 40.0
banana, sheet *(Awrey's),* ¹⁄₂₄ cake 40.0
banana chocolate chip *(Awrey's* Marquise 9"), ¹⁄₁₆ cake 39.0
Black Forest, torte *(Awrey's* 8"), ¹⁄₁₂ cake 42.0
Boston cream, ⅙ cake, 3.2 oz...........................39.5
butter *(Entenmann's* Sunshine), ⅙ cake 43.0
butter loaf *(Entenmann's* All Butter), ⅙ cake 30.0
carrot, cream-cheese-iced, 2 layer *(Awrey's* 9"), ¹⁄₁₆ cake 48.0
carrot, sheet *(Awrey's* Supreme), ¹⁄₂₄ cake..........50.0
cheesecake, see "Cheesecake"
cherries cordial *(Awrey's* Marquise 9"), ¹⁄₁₆ cake 29.0
chocolate:
   (Awrey's Marquise Killer 9"), ¹⁄₁₆ cake...................41.0
   chocolate-frosted, ⅛ of 18 oz. cake, 2¼ oz. 34.9
   creme-filled, chocolate-iced *(Entenmann's),* ⅛ cake.............42.0
   double, buttercream, 3-layer *(Awrey's* 9"), ¹⁄₁₆ cake...............47.0
   double, buttercream, 2-layer *(Awrey's* 8"), ¹⁄₁₆ cake...............38.0
   double, sheet *(Awrey's),* ¹⁄₂₄ cake 45.0
   double, torte *(Awrey's* 8"), ¹⁄₁₂ cake 53.0
   fudge, chocolate-iced *(Entenmann's),* ⅛ cake.........39.0
   German, buttercream, 3-layer *(Awrey's* 9"), ¹⁄₁₆ cake 45.0
   German, sheet *(Awrey's),* ¹⁄₂₄ cake 40.0

Cake, chocolate *(cont.)*

    loaf *(Entenmann's* Light Fat Free), ⅛ cake 29.0
    tropical *(Awrey's* Marquise 9"), 1/16 cake 34.0
    white-iced, 2-layer *(Awrey's* 8"), 1/16 cake 35.0
chocolate chip crumb loaf *(Entenmann's)*, ⅛ cake 32.0
chocolate peanut *(Awrey's* Marquise Fantasy 9"), 1/16 cake 38.0
coconut buttercream, sheet *(Awrey's)*, 1/24 cake....................41.0
coconut buttercream, yellow, 3-layer *(Awrey's* 9"), 1/16 cake 46.0
coffee cake:
    (Entenmann's Light Fat Free), ⅑ cake 36.0
    cheese, ⅙ of 16-oz. cake 33.7
    creme-filled, with chocolate frosting, ⅙ of 19-oz. cake,
        3.2 oz...48.4
    fruit, ⅛ cake, 1¾ oz. 25.8
crumb *(Entenmann's* Ultimate), 1/10 cake................................32.0
devil's food, marshmallow-iced *(Entenmann's)*, ⅛ cake 38.0
devil's food, marshmallow-iced *(Entenmann's* Light Fat Free),
    ⅙ cake...45.0
(Entenmann's Louisiana Crunch Light Fat Free), ⅙ cake............48.0
espresso, French *(Awrey's* Marquise 9"), 1/16 cake 30.0
fruit, 1.5-oz. piece 26.5
fudge, cherry, with chocolate frosting, ⅛ cake, 2.5 oz. 27.0
gingerbread, see "Bread mix, sweet"
golden:
    fudge-iced *(Entenmann's)*, ⅛ cake....................................40.0
    fudge-iced *(Entenmann's* Light Fat Free), ⅛ cake 45.0
    loaf *(Entenmann's* Light Fat Free), ⅛ cake 30.0
lemon *(Awrey's* Marquise Whisper 9"), 1/16 cake.........................33.0
lemon, buttercream, 3-layer *(Awrey's* 9"), 1/16 cake 38.0
lemon-coconut *(Entenmann's)*, ⅛ cake 37.0
marble loaf *(Entenmann's* All Butter), ⅛ cake............................26.0
Neapolitan, torte *(Awrey's* 8"), 1/12 cake....................................41.0
orange, buttercream, 3-layer *(Awrey's* 9"), 1/16 cake 43.0
orange, sheet *(Awrey's* Frosty), 1/24 cake....................................42.0
peach, Georgia *(Awrey's* Marquise 9"), 1/16 cake.........................34.0
pound:
    1/12 of 12-oz. cake 14.9
    1/10 of 10.6-oz. cake 15.6
    butter, 1/12 of 12-oz. cake 13.8
    butter, 1/10 of 10.6-oz. cake 14.6
    fat-free, 1/12 of 12-oz. cake..17.3

raisin loaf *(Entenmann's)*, ⅛ cake..33.0
raspberries and cream *(Awrey's* Marquise 9"), ¹⁄₁₆ cake..............34.0
raspberry *(Awrey's* Marquise Extraordinaire 9"), ¹⁄₁₆ cake...........48.0
raspberry-nut *(Awrey's* Marquise 9"), ¹⁄₁₆ cake............................35.0
red velvet *(Awrey's* Marquise 9"), ¹⁄₁₆ cake 34.0
sour cream loaf *(Entenmann's)*, ⅛ cake 24.0
sponge, uniced, ¹⁄₁₂ of 16-oz. cake..23.2
sponge, uniced, sheet *(Awrey's)*, ¹⁄₂₄ cake 28.0
strawberry, torte *(Awrey's* Supreme 8"), ¹⁄₁₂ cake.......................39.0
yellow:
    chocolate-frosted, ⅛ of 18-oz. cake....................................35.5
    vanilla-frosted, ⅛ of 18-oz. cake..37.6
    white-iced, sheet *(Awrey's)*, ¹⁄₂₄ cake 40.0
    yellow-iced, 2 layer *(Awrey's* 8"), ¹⁄₁₆ cake 35.0
Cake, frozen:
carrot *(Oregon Farms)*, ⅙ cake..37.0
cheesecake, see "Cheesecake, frozen or refrigerated"
chocolate:
    fudge, 3-layer *(Pepperidge Farm)*, ⅛ cake 31.0
    German, layer *(Sara Lee)*, ⅛ cake 35.0
    layer, double *(Sara Lee)*, ⅛ cake 33.0
    mousse cake *(Sara Lee)*, ⅕ cake 37.0
coconut, 3-layer *(Pepperidge Farm)*, ⅛ cake 35.0
coffee cake:
    (Sara Lee Reduced Fat), ⅙ cake..28.0
    butter streusel *(Sara Lee)*, ⅙ cake 25.0
    crumb *(Sara Lee)*, ⅛ cake...32.0
    pecan *(Sara Lee)*, ⅙ cake...24.0
    raspberry *(Sara Lee)*, ⅙ cake..27.0
coconut layer *(Sara Lee)*, ⅛ cake 33.0
corn, sweet *(El Torito)*, ⅓ cup..33.0
devil's food, 3-layer *(Pepperidge Farm)*, ⅛ cake.........................34.0
fudge golden layer *(Sara Lee)*, ⅛ cake.......................................34.0
fudge stripe, 3-layer *(Pepperidge Farm)*, ⅛ cake.......................31.0
golden, chocolate-frosted, 3-layer *(Pepperidge Farm)*,
    ⅛ cake...33.0
pound:
    (Sara Lee Reduced Fat), ¼ cake..42.0
    all-butter *(Sara Lee)*, ¼ cake 38.0
    all-butter *(Sara Lee* Family Size), ⅙ cake...........................36.0
    chocolate swirl *(Sara Lee)*, ¼ cake 42.0

Cake, frozen, pound *(cont.)*
    strawberry swirl *(Sara Lee)*, ¼ cake............................44.0
strawberry shortcake layer *(Sara Lee)*, ⅛ cake.............27.0
vanilla layer *(Sara Lee)*, ⅛ cake 32.0
Cake, mix, 1/12 cake*, except as noted:
angel food:
    (Pillsbury)...31.0
    (SuperMoist Easy Pouch)*, ¼ pkg. 37.0
    chocolate swirl or confetti *(SuperMoist)*.................34.0
    white *(SuperMoist* One Step)..................................32.0
    white *(SuperMoist* Traditional) 30.0
banana *(Pillsbury Moist Supreme)*.................................35.0
brownie with mini kisses *(Betty Crocker Stir 'n Bake)*, ⅙ pkg....36.0
butter pecan *(SuperMoist)*...35.0
butter recipe *(Pillsbury Moist Supreme)*........................35.0
carrot *(SuperMoist)*, 1/10 cake* 42.0
carrot, with cream cheese *(Betty Crocker Stir 'n Bake)*,
    ⅙ pkg...46.0
cheesecake, see "Cheesecake, mix"
cherry chip *(SuperMoist)*, 1/10 cake* 41.0
chocolate:
    (Estee), ⅕ pkg. 36.0
    (Pillsbury Moist Supreme) 34.0
    butter recipe *(SuperMoist)*....................................35.0
    with creamy fudge swirls *(SuperMoist)*, ⅑ cake*....32.0
    fudge *(SuperMoist)*...35.0
    German *(Duncan Hines Moist Deluxe)* 32.0
    German *(SuperMoist)*...36.0
    milk *(SuperMoist)*...34.0
    swirl, double *(SuperMoist)*....................................35.0
chocolate chip *(SuperMoist)*..35.0
coffee cake:
    (Aunt Jemima Easy Mix), ⅛ pkg. 26.0
    chocolate chip swirl *(Pillsbury* Quick Bread & Coffee
      Cake Mix), 1/16 cake* 24.0
    cinnamon streusel *(Betty Crocker Stir 'n Bake)*, ⅙ pkg. 36.0
    cinnamon streusel *(Pillsbury)*, 1/16 cake* 36.0
    cinnamon swirl *(Pillsbury* Quick Bread & Coffee Cake
      Mix) 32.0
corn, sweet *(Chi-Chi's)*, ½ cup 22.0
corn, sweet *(El Torito)*, ⅛ pkg. 22.0

devil's food:
    ("Jiffy"), ⅕ pkg. 40.0
    (Pillsbury Moist Supreme) 33.0
    (SuperMoist) 35.0
    (Sweet Rewards Reduced Fat) 36.0
    with chocolate frosting *(Betty Crocker Stir 'n Bake),*
    ⅙ pkg. 42.0
fudge marble *(SuperMoist),* ¹⁄₁₀ cake* 43.0
Funfetti (Pillsbury Moist Supreme) 36.0
gingerbread *(Betty Crocker* Classic Cake & Cookie Mix),
    ⅛ cake* 39.0
golden yellow *("Jiffy"),* ⅕ pkg. 41.0
lemon *(Pillsbury Moist Supreme)* 35.0
lemon *(SuperMoist)* 36.0
party swirl *(SuperMoist)* 35.0
pineapple *(SuperMoist)* 35.0
pineapple upside-down *(Betty Crocker* Classic), ⅙ cake* 64.0
pound *(Betty Crocker* Classic), ⅛ cake* 45.0
rainbow chip *(SuperMoist),* ¹⁄₁₀ cake* 41.0
red velvet *(Duncan Hines Moist Deluxe)* 33.0
sour cream, white *(SuperMoist),* ¹⁄₁₀ cake* 41.0
spice *(SuperMoist)* 35.0
strawberry *(SuperMoist),* 35.0
strawberry swirl *(SuperMoist),* ¹⁄₁₀ cake* 41.0
vanilla, French *(Pillsbury Moist Supreme)* 24.0
vanilla, French or golden *(SuperMoist)* 35.0
white:
    (Estee), ⅕ pkg. 38.0
    ("Jiffy"), ⅕ pkg. 41.0
    (SuperMoist) 34.0
    (Sweet Rewards Reduced Fat) 36.0
    chocolate swirl *(SuperMoist)* 34.0
yellow:
    (Pillsbury Moist Supreme) 35.0
    (SuperMoist) 35.0
    (Sweet Rewards Reduced Fat) 37.0
    butter recipe *(SuperMoist)* 36.0
    with chocolate frosting *(Betty Crocker Stir 'n Bake),*
    ⅙ pkg. 43.0
    with creamy fudge swirls *(SuperMoist),* ⅑ cake* 32.0

Cake, snack (see also "Cookie" and specific listings):

apple *(Little Debbie* Flips), 1.2 oz...24.0
banana *(Little Debbie* Twins), 2.2 oz. 39.0
banana-nut *(Little Debbie* Loaves), 2.2 oz......................31.0
banana-nut *(Little Debbie* Loaves Singles), 3.9 oz. 62.0
blueberry *(Little Debbie* Loaves), 2 oz. 29.0
blueberry *(Little Debbie* Loaves Singles), 4 oz......................58.0
Boston creme *(Drake's),* 1.5-oz. cake 25.0
cherry cordial *(Little Debbie),* 1.3 oz..................................23.0
cherry creme *(Little Debbie* Holiday Cake Roll), 2.2 oz...............38.0
chocolate:
    (Little Debbie Easter Basket Cakes), 2.4 oz. 40.0
    (Little Debbie Fall Party Cake/Holiday Snack Cake), 2.4 oz. ..41.0
    (Little Debbie Snack Cakes), 2.5 oz......................44.0
    German, cookie ring *(Little Debbie),* 1 oz....................18.0
    creme-filled *(Drake's Devil Dogs),* 1.2-oz. cake...................26.0
    creme-filled *(Drake's Ring Dings),* 2 cakes, 2.7 oz............43.0
    creme-filled *(Drake's Ring Dings* Mini), 5 cakes, 2.6 oz........45.0
    creme-filled *(Drake's Yodels),* 2 cakes, 2.2 oz. 34.0
    creme-filled *(Hostess Ho-Hos),* 3 cakes, 3 oz. 50.0
    creme-filled *(Hostess Suzy-Q),* 2 oz.........................35.0
    creme-filled *(Little Debbie* Swiss Cake Rolls), 2.2 oz. 38.0
    creme-filled *(Little Debbie* Swiss Rolls Singles), 2.7 oz. 47.0
    peanut butter–filled *(Drake's Funny Bones),* 2 pieces,
      2.5 oz...41.0
    vanilla *(Little Debbie* Be My Valentine), 2.2 oz. 38.0
chocolate chip cake *(Little Debbie),* 2.4 oz. 41.0
chocolate chip cake *(Little Debbie* Singles), 2 oz.......................34.0
cinnamon, with crumb topping, 2 oz. 26.6
cinnamon roll *(Little Debbie* Singles), 4 oz. 56.0
coconut *(Little Debbie* Rounds), 1.2 oz................................23.0
coffee cake:
    (Drake's), 1.2-oz. cake..20.0
    (Drake's Mini), 4 pieces, 1.76 oz..............................32.0
    (Little Debbie Big Snacks), 3.4 oz.............................64.0
    apple *(Little Debbie),* 2.1 oz. 39.0
    crumb *(Hostess),* 1.1 oz..19.0
creme-filled, with chocolate frosting, 1.75 oz. 30.2
cupcake:
    chocolate, creme-filled *(Drake's Yankee Doodles),*
      2 cakes, 2 oz...33.0

chocolate, creme-filled *(Entenmann's* Light Fat Free),
2 oz. 39.0
chocolate, creme-filled *(Hostess),* 1.8 oz. 39.0
chocolate, creme-filled *(Little Debbie),* 1.6 oz. 26.0
fudge *(Entenmann's),* 2.2 oz...................................33.0
golden, creme-filled *(Drake's Sunny Doodles),* 2 cakes,
2 oz. 33.0
golden, creme-filled, chocolate-iced *(Hostess),* 1.9 oz..........33.0
lemon, orange or strawberry *(Little Debbie),* 1.7 oz.............29.0
orange, creme-filled, orange-iced *(Hostess),* 1.5 oz.............27.0
date-nut bar *(Awrey's),* 1.23-oz. cake 20.0
devil's food:
   (Little Debbie Devil Cremes), 1.7 oz. 29.0
   (Little Debbie Devil Creme Singles), 3.2 oz. 56.0
   (Little Debbie Devil Squares), 2.2 oz. 39.0
fruit and cereal bars *(Little Debbie* Blastin'/Rappin'), 1.4 oz. 28.0
fudge cake, frosted *(Little Debbie),* 1.5 oz. 25.0
fudge cake, frosted *(Little Debbie* Singles), 2 oz........................34.0
fudge rounds:
   (Little Debbie), 1.2 oz. 23.0
   (Little Debbie Big Snacks), 2 oz. 38.0
   (Little Debbie Singles), 2.5 oz. 48.0
   (Little Debbie Singles), 3 oz. 58.0
golden, creme-filled:
   (Hostess Twinkies), 1.5 oz. 25.0
   (Hostess Twinkies Low Fat), 1.5 oz. 27.0
   (Little Debbie Golden Cremes), 1.5 oz......................26.0
   (Little Debbie Golden Cremes Singles), 3 oz. 52.0
jelly creme pie *(Little Debbie),* 1.2 oz.........................23.0
lemon or raspberry *(Little Debbie* Angel Cakes), 1.6 oz..............29.0
(Little Debbie Christmas Tree Cakes Singles), 2 oz.....................36.0
(Little Debbie Easter Puffs), 1.2 oz. 24.0
(Little Debbie Fancy Cakes), 2.4 oz............................42.0
(Little Debbie Star Crunch), 1.1 oz.............................22.0
(Little Debbie Star Crunch Singles), 2.2 oz. 44.0
(Little Debbie Zebra Cakes), 2.6 oz. 45.0
(Little Debbie Zebra Cakes Singles), 3 oz....................53.0
marshmallow:
   (Little Debbie Supremes), 1.1 oz. 22.0
   crispy bars *(Little Debbie),* 1.3 oz. 26.0
   pie, banana *(Little Debbie),* 1.5 oz............................30.0

Cake, snack, marshmallow *(cont.)*

    pie, banana *(Little Debbie Singles)*, 2.75 oz. 40.0

    pie, chocolate *(Little Debbie)*, 1.4 oz. 27.0

    pie, chocolate *(Little Debbie Singles)*, 2.75 oz. 39.0

  nutty bars:

    (Little Debbie), 2.1 oz. 32.0

    (Little Debbie Big Snacks), 1.5 oz. 25.0

    (Little Debbie Singles), 1.9 oz. 31.0

    (Little Debbie Singles), 2.5 oz. 44.0

    wafer crisps *(Little Debbie)*, 2 oz. 32.0

  oatmeal:

    (Little Debbie Lights), 1.3 oz. 29.0

    and creme *(Little Debbie)*, 1.3 oz. 26.0

    creme pie *(Little Debbie Big Snacks)*, 1.9 oz. 37.0

    creme pie *(Little Debbie Singles)*, 2.5 oz. 48.0

    pie, peanut butter and jelly *(Little Debbie)*, 1.1 oz. 22.0

  peanut butter bars *(Little Debbie)*, 1.9 oz. 32.0

  peanut clusters *(Little Debbie)*, 1.4 oz. 23.0

  pecan spinwheels:

    (Drake's), 1 oz. 16.0

    (Little Debbie), 1 oz. 16.0

    (Little Debbie Singles), 2 oz. 33.0

    or cinnamon *(Aunt Fanny's)*, 1 oz. 16.0

  pumpkin *(Little Debbie Delights)*, 1.2 oz. 24.0

  raisin creme pie *(Little Debbie)*, 1.2 oz. 23.0

  raisin creme pie *(Little Debbie Singles)*, 2.3 oz. 43.0

  sponge, creme-filled, 1.5-oz. cake 27.2

  strawberry shortcake rolls *(Little Debbie)*, 2.2 oz. 41.0

  vanilla *(Little Debbie Be My Valentine Singles)*, 2.8 oz. 46.0

  vanilla *(Little Debbie Easter Basket/Fall Party/Holiday Snack*

    Cake), 2.5 oz. 43.0

Cake, snack, mix (see also specific listings):

  chocolate–peanut butter bat *(Betty Crocker Supreme)*, 1 bar* ...26.0

  cookie bar *(Betty Crocker Hershey Supreme)*, 1 bar* 21.0

  date bar *(Betty Crocker Classic)*, ⅟₁₂ pkg. 23.0

  layer dessert bar, easy *(Betty Crocker Supreme)*, 1 bar* 21.0

  lemon bar *(Betty Crocker Sunkist Supreme)*, 1 bar* 24.0

Calabaza *(Frieda's)*, ½ cup, 3 oz. 2.0

Calamari, see "Squid"

Calamari dish, frozen:

crisps, breaded *(Acadian Gourmet)*, 12 pieces, 3.1 oz. 19.0

in tomato sauce *(Plumpy)*, 1 cup...............................12.0
Calves' liver, see "Liver"
Camouflage melon *(Frieda's)*, 1 cup, 5 oz. 13.0
Candy:
almond, chocolate-covered *(Chocolate World)*, 11 pieces,
   1.3 oz. 18.0
assorted:
   (Lindt Champs Elysees Tin), 4 pieces, 1.5 oz.................23.0
   (Lindt Napolitains), .2-oz. piece..................................3.0
   (Lindt Swiss Tradition Deluxe 4.93 oz.), 4 pieces, 1.5 oz.....20.0
   (Lindt Swiss Tradition Deluxe 17.6 oz.), 4 pieces, 1.5 oz.....21.0
(Baby Ruth), 2.1-oz. bar..36.0
(Baby Ruth Fun Size), 1-oz. bar 17.0
(Bittyfinger), 2 bars, 1.3 oz. 27.0
butter rum:
   (LifeSavers Bag/Large Pieces), 4 pieces 15.0
   (LifeSavers Roll), 2 pieces.....................................5.0
   (Nestlé Nips), 2 pieces, .5 oz....................................11.0
(Butterfinger), 2.1-oz. bar.......................................44.0
(Butterfinger Fun Size), .75-oz. bar..........................15.0
(Butterfinger BB's), 1.7-oz. bag...............................34.0
(Butterfinger Treasures), 3 pieces, 1.2 oz. 23.0
butterscotch:
   (Estee No Sugar), 2 pieces.....................................12.0
   hard *(Land O Lakes)*, 3 pieces, .6 oz. 17.0
   hard *(TasteTations)*, 3 pieces, .6 oz. 12.0
(Candy Bar Factory), 3-oz. pkg.................................47.0
candy cane, fruit punch *(Jolly Rancher)*, .7-oz. piece 18.0
candy corn *(Blueberry Hill)*, 22 pieces, 1.4 oz. 37.0
caramel:
   (Caramello), 1.2-oz. bar..22.0
   (Hershey's Classic), 6 pieces, 1.3 oz.......................27.0
   (Nestlé Nips), 2 pieces, .5 oz...................................11.0
   (Rolo), 1.9-oz. pkg. 36.0
   (Treasures), 3 pieces, 1.2 oz. 22.0
   chocolate-coated *(Milk Duds)*, 1.8-oz. box.............37.0
   chocolate-filled *(Hershey's* Classic), 6 pieces, 1.3 oz. 26.0
   fudge *(Hershey's Sweet Escapes)*, .7-oz. bar 13.0
   hard *(TasteTations)*, 3 pieces, .6 oz. 12.0
   and peanut butter, crispy *(Hershey's Sweet Escapes)*,
      .7-oz. bar 13.0

Candy *(cont.)*

vanilla and chocolate *(Estee* No Sugar), 5 pieces..................26.0

cherry, see "fruit/fruit-flavored," below

chocolate:

    (Nestlé Nips), 2 pieces, .5 oz..................11.0

    (Twizzlers Twists), 3 pieces, 1.5 oz. 32.0

    parfait *(Nestlé Nips),* 2 pieces, .5 oz. 10.0

    regular or mint *(TasteTations),* 3 pieces, .6 oz. 12.0

chocolate, assorted *(Godiva),* about 3 pieces, 1.5 oz. 27.0

chocolate, assorted *(Hershey's* Miniatures), 2.25-oz. pkg. 37.0

chocolate, bittersweet:

    (Lindt Surfin Bar), 14 blocks, 1.4 oz. 21.0

    with hazelnuts *(Lindt* Bar), 14 blocks, 1.4 oz. 18.0

    with hazelnuts *(Perugina Baci),* 4 pieces, 1.4 oz. 19.0

chocolate, candy-coated:

    (M&M's Singles), 1.7-oz. bag..................34.0

    almond *(M&M's* Singles), 1.3-oz. bag..................21.0

    crispy *(M&M's* Singles), 1.5-oz. bag..................30.0

    peanut *(M&M's* Singles), 1.75-oz. bag..................30.0

    peanut butter *(M&M's* Singles), 1.6-oz. bag 27.0

chocolate, dark:

    (Dove), 1.3-oz. bar 22.0

    (Estee No Sugar), 7 squares, 1.4 oz..................23.0

    (Hershey's Special Dark), 1.4-oz. bar 24.0

    (Hershey's Special Dark Miniatures), 5 pieces, 1.5 oz...........25.0

    almond *(Hershey's Nuggets),* 4 pieces, 1.3 oz. 19.0

chocolate, milk:

    (Cadbury's Dairy), 9 blocks, 1.4 oz. 24.0

    (Dove), 1.3-oz. bar 22.0

    (Estee No Sugar), 7 squares, 1.4 oz..................17.0

    (Hershey's), 1.5-oz. bar 25.0

    (Hershey's Giant Kiss), 1/8 pkg., 1.4 oz. 23.0

    (Hershey's Hugs), 9 pieces, 1.4 oz. 23.0

    (Hershey's Hugs and Kisses), 9 pieces, 1.4 oz..................24.0

    (Hershey's Kisses), 1.5-oz. pkg. 24.0

    (Hershey's Nuggets), 4 pieces, 1.4 oz. 23.0

    (Hershey's Symphony), 1.5-oz. bar 24.0

    (Lindt Excellence Bar 3 oz.), 14 blocks, 1.4 oz....................21.0

    (Lindt Excellence Bar 3.5 oz.), 4 squares, 1.4 oz. 13.0

    (Lindt Mocca Bar), 14 blocks, 1.4 oz. 21.0

    (Lindt Swiss Milk Bar), 14 blocks, 1.4 oz..................22.0

(Nestlé), 1.45-oz. bar..26.0
almond *(Cadbury's* Roast), 9 blocks, 1.4 oz...........21.0
almond *(Estee* No Sugar), 7 squares, 1.4 oz.........16.0
almond *(Hershey's)*, 1.4-oz. bar.............................20.0
almond *(Hershey's Bites)*, 17 pieces, 1.4 oz. 20.0
almond *(Hershey's Kisses)*, 9 pieces, 1.4 oz. 21.0
almond *(Hershey's Nuggets)*, 4 pieces, 1.3 oz. 20.0
almond *(Lindt* Bar), 5 pieces, 1.5 oz. 20.0
almond *(Lindt* Swiss Milk Bar), 12 blocks, 1.4 oz....18.0
caramel *(Lindt* Bar), 5 pieces, 1.4 oz....................23.0
cherry *(Lindt* Bar), 5 pieces, 1.4 oz. 25.0
cookies and mint *(Hershey's)*, 1.5-oz. bar..............27.0
crisps *(Buncha Crunch)*, 1.4-oz. bag......................26.0
crisps *(Cadbury's* Krisp), 9 blocks, 1.4 oz.............25.0
crisps *(Estee* No Sugar), 7 squares, 1.25 oz. 29.0
crisps *(Krackel)*, 1.4-oz. bar.................................26.0
crisps *(Nestlé Crunch)*, 1.55-oz. bar 29.0
crisps *(Nestlé Crunch* Fun Size), 4 bars, 1.4 oz. 26.0
eggs, candy-coated *(Hershey's)*, 1.55-oz. pkg. 30.0
fruit and nut *(Cadbury's)*, 9 blocks, 1.4 oz. 24.0
fruit and nut *(Chunky)*, 1.4-oz. bar........................24.0
fruit and nut *(Estee* No Sugar), 7 squares, 1.4 oz. ..18.0
fruit and nut mix *(Estee* No Sugar), ¼ cup..............19.0
hazelnut *(Lindt* Swiss Milk Bar), 14 blocks, 1.4 oz. ..18.0
orange *(Lindt* Bar), 5 pieces, 1.4 oz. 24.0
peanut *(Mr. Goodbar)*, 1.7-oz. bar..........................25.0
pistachio *(Lindt)*, 5 pieces, 1.4 oz. 19.0
raisins and almonds *(Hershey's Nuggets)*, 4 pieces,
    1.4 oz..23.0
raisins, hazelnuts, and almonds *(Lindt* Bar), 12 blocks,
    1.4 oz..22.0
raspberry *(Lindt* Bar), 5 pieces, 1.4 oz....................24.0
strawberry *(Lindt* Bar), 5 pieces, 1.4 oz. 23.0
toffee, almond *(Hershey's Symphony)*, 1.5-oz. bar 22.0
toffee and almonds *(Hershey's Nuggets)*, 4 pieces, 1.3 oz....20.0
truffles, see "truffles," below
chocolate, white:
    (Lindt Swiss Bar), 14 blocks, 1.4 oz. 22.0
    cookies *(Hershey's Cookie 'n' Cream)*, 1.5-oz. bar ...25.0
    cookies *(Hershey's Cookies 'n' Cream* Bites), 18 pieces,
        1.4 oz..23.0

Candy, chocolate, white *(cont.)*

cookies *(Hershey's Cookies 'n' Cream Nuggets)*, 4 pieces,
1.3 oz...21.0

crisps *(Nestlé Crunch)*, 1.4-oz. bar 23.0

cinnamon *(Breath Savers)*, 1 piece 2.0

coconut, chocolate-coated:

(Hershey's Pot of Gold), 2.75-oz. bar 36.0

(Mounds), 1.9-oz. pkg...31.0

almond *(Almond Joy)*, 1.7-oz. pkg.....................................29.0

almond *(Almond Joy Bites)*, 18 pieces, 1.4 oz. 22.0

almond *(Almond Joy Bits)*, 1 tbsp., .5 oz...........................7.0

coffee *(Nestlé Nips)*, 2 pieces, .5 oz.....................................10.0

cookie bar:

caramel *(Twix)*, 2 bars, 2 oz. 37.0

caramel *(Twix)*, 1-oz. bar...18.0

peanut butter *(Twix)*, 2 bars, 1.8 oz. 28.0

peanut butter *(Twix)*, .52-oz. bar 8.0

(5th Avenue), 2-oz. bar 38.0

fruit/fruit-flavored:

all flavors:

(Amazin' Fruit Bears & Scares), 1.5-oz. bag....................32.0

(Chuckles), 4 pieces, 1.6 oz..37.0

(Creme Savers), 3 pieces 11.0

(Delites Orchard Fruits/Delites Summer Blend),
5 pieces...15.0

(Drops), 13 pieces, 1.4 oz..35.0

(Drops Soft), 13 pieces, 1.4 oz..35.0

(Estee No Sugar), 5 pieces 16.0

(Estee Gummy Bears), 17 pieces.....................................30.0

(Fruit Chews Intense!), 2.06-oz. pkg. 51.0

(Fruit Chews Intense! 7 oz.), 11 pieces 36.0

(Gummi Bears), 1.4-oz. pkg...24.0

(Gummi Jujubes), 45 pieces, 1.4 oz.................................24.0

(GummiSavers Five Flavor), 1.5-oz. pkg..........................32.0

(GummiSavers Tangy Fruits), 10 pieces 30.0

(GummiSavers Crystal Craze), 1.5-oz. pkg......................34.0

(Jolly Rancher Chews), 2-oz. pkg....................................48.0

(Jolly Rancher Gummis), 1.7-oz. pkg...............................36.0

(Jolly Rancher Hard), 3 pieces, .6 oz..............................17.0

(Jolly Rancher Jolly Beans), 25 pieces, 1.4 oz. 33.0

(Jolly Rancher Jolly Jellies), 1.3-oz. pkg.........................28.0

(Jujubes), 1.5-oz. box..32.0
(Jujyfruits), 2.1-oz. box 51.0
(Jujyfruits Soft), 15 pieces, 1.4 oz.......................32.0
(Jujyfruits & Friends), 3 boxes, 1.3 oz.................28.0
(LifeSavers Bag/Large Pieces), 4 pieces.............16.0
(LifeSavers Fruit Chews), 11 pieces 36.0
(LifeSavers Roll), 2 pieces..................................5.0
(Mexican Hats), 10 pieces, 1.4 oz. 30.0
(Sour Dudes), 2-oz. bag 48.0
(Twizzlers Twist-n-Fill), 1-oz. piece....................21.0
apple, cherry or watermelon *(Chewmongous),* .6-oz.
  piece 15.0
apple rings, gummy *(Estee* No Sugar), 5 pieces 28.0
berries, wild *(GummiSavers),* 1.5-oz. pkg.............33.0
cherry *(Nibs),* 27 pieces, 1.4 oz. 31.0
cherry *(Switzer* Bites), 18 pieces, 1.4 oz...............31.0
cherry *(Twizzlers Pull-n-Peel),* 3 pieces, 1.3 oz.....27.0
gumdrops *(Estee* No Sugar), 23 pieces 36.0
gumdrops, 10 pieces, 1.3 oz. 35.6
jelly beans:
  (Estee Gourmet No Sugar), 26 pieces 24.0
  10 large, 1 oz...26.4
  10 small, .4...10.2
paradise punch, pink lemonade or red razz
  (Twizzlers Pull-n-Peel), 1 piece, 1.2 oz...............26.0
strawberry *(Twizzlers* Twists), 1.7-oz. pkg............38.0
tropical fruit *(Estee* No Sugar), 5 pieces...............16.0
watermelon *(Jolly Rancher),* .4-oz. bar 9.0
graham, milk chocolate *(Flipz),* 9 pieces, 1 oz. 19.0
gum, chewing, all flavors:
  (Carefree), 1 piece 2.0
  (Doublemint/Juicy Fruit/Big Red/Wrigley's Spearmint) 2.0
  (Fruit Stripe), 1 piece 2.0
  (LifeSavers Ice Breakers), 1 piece 2.0
  (Stick Free), 1 piece..2.0
  bubble:
    (Bubble Yum), 1 piece 6.0
    (Bubble Yum Sugarless), 1 piece 3.0
    (Eggums), 2 pieces...3.0
    (Rain•Blo), .2-oz. piece.................................4.0
    (Rain•Blo Jumblo), .5-oz. piece....................11.0

Gum, chewing, bubble *(cont.)*
    (Rain•Blo Mega Eggs), 2.2-oz. piece 51.0
    (Screaming Sour), 1 piece.....................................4.0
    (Super Bubble), 1 piece......................................4.0
gumdrops or gummy, see "fruit/fruit-flavored," above
halvah, plain, 1 oz. 17.1
hard, see "fruit/fruit-flavored" and specific candy listings
(Hershey-ets Pastel),* 2.2-oz. pkg........................44.0
(Hershey's Pot of Gold Cameo Angel/Egg/Heart), 2 pieces,
    1.4 oz. 22.0
honey *(Bit-O-Honey),* 1.7-oz. bar 40.0
(Hot Dollars Soft), 15 pieces, 1.4 oz...................32.0
jellybeans, see "fruit/fruit-flavored," above
licorice:
    (Diamond), 10 pieces, 1.4 oz. 31.0
    (Switzer Bites), 18 pieces, 1.4 oz. 31.0
    (Twizzlers Bites), 16 pieces, 1.4 oz...............30.0
    (Twizzlers Twists), 2.5-oz. pkg. 55.0
    candy-coated *(Good & Fruity),* 1.75-oz. box 45.0
    candy-coated *(Good & Plenty),* 1.75-oz. box 43.0
    fruit-flavored, see "fruit/fruit-flavored," above
    gumdrops *(Estee* No Sugar), 11 pieces...............36.0
lollipop, all flavors *(Jolly Rancher),* .6-oz. piece 16.0
malted milk balls:
    (Whoppers), .75-oz. pouch 16.0
    (Whoppers Eggs), 6 pieces, 1.3 oz. 27.0
    (Whoppers Mini Eggs), 1.7-oz. pkg..................36.0
(Mars Almond Bar), 1.75-oz. bar 31.0
marshmallows:
    10 pieces, ¼ oz. 5.7
    miniature, 1 cup 40.7
    chocolate-covered, eggs *(Hershey's),* .9-oz. piece 17.0
(Milky Way), 2-oz. bar...41.0
(Milky Way Lite), 1.57-oz. bar 34.0
(Milky Way Midnight), 1.75-oz. bar 36.0
mint:
    (LifeSavers Crist O Mint/Chill O Mint Roll), 2 pieces....5.0
    (LifeSavers Pep O Mint Bag/Large Pieces), 4 pieces....16.0
    (LifeSavers Pep O Mint Roll), 3 pieces.................5.0
    (York Bites), 15 pieces, 1.4 oz........................31.0
    (York Peppermint Patti), 1.4-oz. pkg. 32.0

all varieties *(Breath Savers)*, 1 piece 2.0
assorted *(Estee No Sugar)*, 5 pieces 16.0
chocolate flavor *(Estee No Sugar)*, 7 squares, 1.4 oz..........23.0
peppermint, hard *(TasteTations)*, 3 pieces, .6 oz.............15.0
peppermint swirl *(Estee No Sugar)*, 3 pieces 14.0
mocha *(Nestlé Crunch)*, 1.3-oz. bar 21.0
(Nestlé Turtles), 2 pieces, 1.2 oz. 20.0
nonpareils *(Sno Caps)*, 2.3-oz. box.....................................48.0
nuts *(Hershey's Pot of Gold* All Nuts), 1.5 oz. 22.0
(Oh Henry!), .9-oz. bar..16.0
(100 Grand), 1.5-oz. pkg..30.0
peanut, caramel *(PayDay)*, 1.8-oz. bar 29.0
peanut brittle *(Estee No Sugar)*, ⅓ box 28.0
peanut butter, chocolate:
    (Estee Cups No Sugar), 5 pieces.....................................19.0
    (Flipz), 8 pieces, 1 oz. 17.0
    (Hershey's Sweet Escapes), .7-oz. bar 13.0
    (Reese's Bites), 16 pieces, 1.4 oz...............................22.0
    (Reese's Cup), 2 pieces, 1.2-oz. pkg. 19.0
    (Reese's Cup Miniatures), 1.6-oz. pkg..........................26.0
    (Reese's Egg), 1.2-oz. pkg. 19.0
    (Reese's Pieces), 1.6-oz. pkg..26.0
    (Reese's NutRageous), 1.9-oz. bar 29.0
    (ReeseSticks), .6-oz. piece...9.0
    (Treasures), 4 pieces, 1.5 oz. 22.0
    crispy rice *(Hershey's* Snack Size), 3 bars, 1.5 oz............27.0
    crunchy *(Reese's* Cookie Cup), .6-oz-pkg....................10.0
    crunchy *(Reese's* Cookie Cup Miniatures), 5 pieces, 1.4 oz. ...23.0
peanut butter parfait *(Nestlé Nips)*, 2 pieces, .5 oz......................10.0
peanuts, chocolate-covered:
    (Estee No Sugar), ¼ cup 23.0
    (Goobers), 1.38-oz. bag 20.0
    10 pieces, 1.4 oz. 19.8
    1 cup 73.6
pecan caramel cluster *(Hershey's Pot of Gold)*, 2-oz. pkg. 31.0
peppermint, see "mint," above
popcorn, see "Popcorn, popped"
pretzels, chocolate-coated:
    (Estee No Sugar), 7 pieces..19.0
    milk *(Flipz)*, 8 pieces, 1 oz..19.0
    white fudge *(Flipz)*, 7 pieces, 1 oz. 19.0

Candy *(cont.)*

raisins, chocolate-covered:

    (Estee No Sugar), ¼ cup 27.0

    (Raisinets), 1.58-oz. bag 31.0

    10 pieces, .4 oz. 6.8

    1 cup 122.9

    semisweet *(Nestlé)*, 1⅓ tbsp. 11.0

raisins, cinnamon-yogurt-coated *(AlpineAire)*, 2.5 oz. 50.0

(Red Hot Dollars), 15 pieces, 1.4 oz. 34.0

(Red Hot Dollars Bulk), 6 pieces, 1.5 oz. 36.0

(Robin Eggs), 8 pieces, 1.4 oz. 31.0

(Robin Eggs Mini), 1.8-oz. box 40.0

(Sixlets), 1.7-oz. pkg. 36.0

(Snickers), 2-oz. bar 35.0

(Snickers Munch), 1.4-oz. bar 17.0

(Snoballs), 11 pieces, 1.4 oz. 31.0

soy nuts, chocolate-dipped *(Tofutti* Totally Nuts), 1 oz. 30.0

(SweeTarts Mini Chewy), 23 pieces, .5 oz. 13.0

(SweeTarts/Spree), 8 pieces, .5 oz. 14.0

(Spree Mini Chewy), 19 pieces, .5 oz. 13.0

(3 Musketeers), 2.13-oz. bar 46.0

taffy, all flavors *(Mighty Bite)*, 5 pieces 39.0

toffee:

    (Estee No Sugar), 5 pieces 16.0

    (Heath Bites), 15 pieces, 1.4 oz. 25.0

    (Heath Bits/Bits 'O Brickle), 1 tbsp., .5 oz. 9.0

    (Heath English), 1.4-oz. bar 24.0

    (Skor), 1.4-oz. bar 23.0

    butter, nuts *(Frito-Lay* Nothing But Nuts), 1.1 oz. 9.0

(Top Secret), 2.2-oz. bar 35.0

truffles:

    assorted *(Godiva)*, about 2 pieces, 1.5 oz. 24.0

    assorted *(Hershey's Pot of Gold)*, 1.5 oz. 26.0

    assorted *(Lindt* Gourmet), 2 balls, 1.2 oz. 14.0

    dark *(Lindt* Lindor Bar), 7 pieces, 1.4 oz. 16.0

    dark or white *(Lindt* Lindor), .4-oz. ball 5.0

    milk, amaretto, orange, peanut butter, or hazelnut *(Lindt*

        Lindor), .4-oz. ball 5.0

    mint *(Lindt* Lindor), .4-oz. ball 4.0

    white *(Lindt* Lindor Bar), 7 pieces, 1.4 oz. 17.0

vanilla *(Breath Savers)*, 1 piece 1.0

vanilla almond café *(Nestlé Nips)*, 2 pieces, .5 oz......10.0
wafer, chocolate (see also "cookie bar," above):
   (Hershey's Sweet Escapes Triple), .7-oz. bar......13.0
   (Kit Kat), 4 pieces, 1.5-oz. bar......27.0
   (Kit Kat Bites), 15 pieces, 1.4 oz. 25.0
   chunky *(Kit Kat)*, 1.9-oz. bar......35.0
(Whatchamacallit), 1.7-oz. bar......30.0
(Wonderball), 1-oz. ball......21.0
(Wunderbeans), 1.5-oz. box......37.0
(Zagnut), 1.7-oz. bar......31.0
(Zero), 1.8-oz. bar......36.0
Cane syrup, 1 tbsp. 13.4
Cannellini beans, see "Kidney beans"
Cannelloni dinner, frozen *(Amy's)*, 9-oz. pkg......34.0
Cannelloni entree, frozen, cheese *(Lean Cuisine Everyday Favorites)*, 9⅛-oz. pkg. 28.0
Cantaloupe, fresh, raw:
(Dole), ¼ melon......11.0
½ of 5" melon 22.3
balls, 1 cup 14.8
cubed, 1 cup 13.4
Capers, in jar:
(Crosse & Blackwell), 1 tbsp......1.0
drained, 1 tbsp. 4
Capicola, see "Ham lunch meat"
Capon:
roasted, whole, 1 capon, 3.1 lbs......6
roasted, without added ingredients, 4 oz. 0
Capon giblets:
raw, 1 oz. 4
simmered, 4 oz. 9
simmered, chopped or diced, 1 cup 1.1
Caponata, see "Eggplant, in jar"
Cappuccino, see "Coffee, flavored, mix" and "Coffee, iced"
Carambola, fresh, raw:
(Frieda's Starfruit), 5 oz. 11.0
untrimmed, 1 lb. 33.7
1 medium, 4.7 oz. 9.9
sliced, 1 cup 8.5
cubed, 1 cup 10.7
Carambola, dried *(Frieda's* Starfruit), ⅓ cup, 1.4 oz. 29.0

Caramel apple, see "Apple, candied"
Caramel custard, see "Pudding and pie filling mix"
Caramel syrup *(Smucker's Sundae),* 2 tbsp. 25.0
Caramel topping, 2 tbsp.:
(Hershey's Chocolate Shoppe Fat Free)............................25.0
(Kraft)..28.0
(Mrs. Richardson's Fat Free)..32.0
(Smucker's Microwave Squeeze Fat Free)........................28.0
(Smucker's Spoonable)..31.0
(Smucker's Magic Shell) 13.0
butterscotch, see "Butterscotch-caramel topping"
hot *(Smucker's* Spoonable)...29.0
Caraway seeds:
1 tbsp...3.1
1 tsp. 9
Carbonara sauce mix, see "Pasta sauce, mix"
Cardamom, ground:
1 tbsp...4.0
1 tsp...1.4
Cardoon, fresh:
raw:
   (Frieda's), 1 cup or 3 oz. 4.0
   untrimmed, 1 lb..10.9
   shredded, 1 cup...8.7
boiled, drained, 4 oz..6.0
Carissa, fresh, raw:
untrimmed, 1 lb. 53.2
trimmed, 1 fruit, .7 oz. 2.7
sliced, 1 cup...20.4
Carl's Jr., 1 serving:
breakfast items:
   bacon, 2 strips...0
   burrito 26.0
   eggs, scrambled 1.0
   English muffin with margarine 27.0
   French Toast Dips, without syrup..................................42.0
   quesadilla 27.0
   sausage, 1 patty...2.0
   sourdough 32.0
   Sunrise Croissant/Sandwich, without bacon or sausage.......28.0

sandwiches:

Carl's bacon Swiss crispy chicken	66.0
Carl's Catch Fish Sandwich	50.0
Carl's ranch crispy chicken	66.0
Carl's Western Crispy Chicken Sandwich	91.0
Charbroiled BBQ Chicken Sandwich	37.0
Charbroiled Chicken Club Sandwich	33.0
Charbroiled Santa Fe Chicken Sandwich	32.0
Charbroiled Sirloin Steak Sandwich	52.0
charbroiled sirloin steak	50.0
Double Western Bacon Cheeseburger	64.0
famous bacon cheeseburger	51.0
hamburger, *Carl's Famous Star*	49.0
hamburger, *Super Star*	50.0
hamburger Jr.	34.0
Western Bacon Cheeseburger	63.0
sourdough bacon cheeseburger, regular or double	37.0
spicy chicken sandwich	47.0

sandwich cheese, American or Swiss style	0

side dishes:

chicken stars, 6 pieces	15.0
CrissCut Fries	43.0
French fries	37.0
hash brown nuggets	32.0
onion rings	53.0
zucchini	37.0

Great Stuff potatoes:

plain, without margarine	68.0
bacon and cheese	76.0
broccoli and cheese	74.0
sour cream and chives	70.0

salad, *Charbroiled Chicken Salad-to-Go*	12.0
salad, *Garden Salad-to-Go*	4.0

salad dressings, 2 oz.:

blue cheese	1.0
French, fat-free	16.0
house	3.0
Italian, fat-free	4.0
Thousand Island	5.0

breads/sauces:

breadsticks	7.0

Carl's Jr., breads/sauces (cont.)
BBQ sauce or mustard sauce 11.0
croutons 5.0
grape jelly or strawberry jam...9.0
honey sauce 22.0
salsa 2.0
sweet n' sour sauce..12.0
table syrup 21.0
bakery/desserts:
blueberry muffin 49.0
bran raisin muffin 61.0
cheese Danish 49.0
chocolate cake 49.0
chocolate chip cookie 49.0
strawberry swirl cheesecake 30.0
shake, small:
chocolate 74.0
strawberry 77.0
vanilla 54.0
Carnival squash *(Frieda's)*, ¾ cup, 3 oz. 7.0
Carob drink mix, powder:
1 tbsp. 11.2
prepared with milk, 8 fl. oz. 22.5
Carob flour, 1 cup 91.6
Carp, without added ingredients...0
Carrot, fresh:
raw:
(Dole), 7" long, 1-¼" diam. 8.0
(Green Giant), 1 medium...8.0
untrimmed, 1 lb. 41.0
1 medium, 7½" long, 2.8 oz. 7.3
chopped, 1 cup..13.0
grated, 1 cup 11.2
shredded *(Dole Classic)*, 3 oz. 9.0
shredded, ½ cup 5.6
raw, baby:
(Grimmway), 3 oz. 9.0
1 large, .5 oz...1.2
1 medium, .4 oz. 8
peeled *(Dole Classic Mini)*, 3 oz. 9.0
peeled *(Mann's)*, 3 oz. 9.0

peeled, cut *(Green Giant)*, 3 oz..8.0
peeled, crinkle-cut *(Mann's)*, 3 oz. 9.0
raw, gold *(Frieda's)*, ⅔ cup, 3 oz. 9.0
boiled, drained:
    1 medium, 1.6 oz. 4.8
    1 tbsp. 1.0
    sliced, ½ cup...8.2
Carrot, canned or in jar:
all styles *(Seneca)*, ½ cup...6.0
baby, whole:
    (Greenleaf), ½ cup 4.0
    (Reese), ½ cup 3.0
    (Twin Tree Gardens Belgian), 20 pieces, 4.5 oz.........5.0
sliced:
    (Allens/Crest Top), ½ cup 8.0
    (Del Monte), ½ cup 8.0
    16-oz. can..24.4
    ½ cup..6.6
    drained, 1 cup..8.1
julienne slice *(S&W* French Style), ½ cup 5.0
mashed, drained, 1 cup..12.6
Carrot, dehydrated, diced *(AlpineAire)*, ½ cup 17.0
Carrot, frozen:
(Seneca), ¾ cup..6.0
baby, whole:
    (Birds Eye), ½ cup 9.0
    (Birds Eye Baby Singles), ⅔ cup 6.0
    (Freshlike), ⅔ cup 6.0
    cut *(Green Giant)*, ¾ cup...7.0
sliced:
    (Birds Eye), ½ cup 9.0
    (Freshlike), ⅔ cup 6.0
    boiled, drained, 1 cup...12.0
honey-glazed *(Green Giant)*, 1 cup...................................13.0
Carrot, peas, corn, dried *(Sonoma* Vital Veggies), ½ cup.........23.0
Carrot chips *(Hain)*, 1 oz. 18.0
Carrot juice, 8 fl. oz.:
(Hollywood) 27.0
(Santa Cruz Organic)..30.0
canned 21.9

Carrot juice, with fruit juices *(cont.)*
   (After the Fall 24 Karrot)..29.0
   (AriZona Crazy Berry)...26.0
   (AriZona Crazy Cocktail)..27.0
Casaba, fresh, raw:
untrimmed, 1 lb. 16.9
whole, 3.6-lb. melon 101.7
1/10 of 7¾" melon 10.2
cubed, 1 cup 10.5
Casava, fresh, raw:
14.4-oz. root 155.2
1 cup 78.4
Cashews:
(Beer Nuts Select), 1 oz. 8.0
(Frito-Lay), 3 tbsp., 1 oz. 7.0
(Nabisco Fancy), 1 oz. 8.0
(Planters Fancy), 1 oz. 8.0
(Planters Salted), 2-oz. pkg. 16.0
(Planters Salted), 1 oz. 8.0
(River Queen Fancy), ¼ cup or 1.2 oz. 10.0
(River Queen Halves), ¼ cup or 1.2 oz. 9.0
halves *(Nabisco),* 1 oz. 7.0
halves *(Planters),* 1 oz. 7.0
dry-roasted:
   (River Queen), 1 oz., about 20 nuts 9.0
   1 oz. 9.3
   whole or halves, 1 cup 44.8
honey-roasted:
   (Planters), 2-oz. pkg. 23.0
   (Planters), 1 oz. 11.0
   (River Queen), ¼ cup or 1.2 oz. 12.0
oil-roasted, 1 oz. 8.1
oil-roasted, whole or halves, 1 cup 37.1
and peanuts, see "Peanut and cashew mix"
Cashew butter, salted or unsalted:
1 tbsp. 4.4
creamy or crunchy *(Arrowhead Mills),* 2 tbsp. 8.0
Catfish, channel:
without added ingredients..0
breaded, fried, 1 fillet, 3.1-oz. 7.0

Catfish entree, frozen, uncooked:

fillet, Cajun style or lemon pepper *(Farm Fresh Catfish),*
  4 oz. 2.0

nuggets, breaded *(Farm Fresh Catfish),* 4 oz. 24.0

Catjang:

raw, 1 oz. 16.9

boiled, ½ cup 17.5

Catsup, see "Ketchup"

Cauliflower, fresh:

raw:

  (Andy Boy), ⅙ medium head 5.0

  (Dole), ⅙ medium head, 3.5 oz. 5.0

  untrimmed, 1 lb. 8.7

  florets *(Mann's Cauliettes),* 4 oz. 6.0

  3 florets, approx. 5 oz. 2.9

  1" pieces, 1 cup 5.2

boiled, drained, 3 florets, 1.9 oz. 2.2

boiled, drained, 1" pieces, ½ cup 2.6

green:

  raw, ⅕ head 5.7

  raw, 1 floret 1.5

  raw, 1" pieces, ½ cup 3.0

  cooked, 1" pieces, ½ cup 3.9

Cauliflower, frozen:

(Birds Eye), ½ cup 4.0

(Seneca), 1 cup 3.0

unprepared, 10-oz. pkg. 13.9

unprepared, 1" pieces, ½ cup 3.1

boiled, drained, 1" pieces, 1 cup 6.8

florets *(Freshlike),* 4 pieces 3.0

florets *(Green Giant),* 1 cup 4.0

in cheese sauce *(Green Giant),* ½ cup 7.0

Cauliflower combination, frozen:

broccoli, see "Broccoli combination"

carrots, snow peas *(Birds Eye Farm Fresh),* ½ cup 6.0

Cavatappi pasta dish, mix, sun-dried tomato–basil pesto
  (Land O Lakes International Pasta Collection), 2.5 oz. 47.0

Caviar (see also "Roe"), 1 tbsp.:

black or red.. .6

lumpfish or salmon *(Romanoff)*.......................................0

whitefish, black *(Romanoff)*..1.0

Caviar spread, see "Taramosalata"
Cayenne, see "Pepper"
Ceci, see "Chickpeas"
Celeriac:
raw:
    (Frieda's Celery Root), ¾ cup, 3 oz. 8.0
    untrimmed, 1 lb..35.9
    trimmed, ½ cup...10.4
boiled, drained, pieces, 1 cup 9.1
Celery, fresh:
raw:
    (Dole), 2 medium stalks, 3.9 oz. 5.0
    untrimmed, 1 lb..14.7
    7½" stalk, 1.6 oz. 1.5
    strips, 1 cup 4.5
    diced, 1 cup...4.4
boiled, drained, 2 stalks, 2.7 oz. 3.0
boiled, drained, diced, 1 cup 6.0
Celery, Chinese, fresh *(Frieda's* Kun Choy), 1 cup, 3 oz..............3.0
Celery, dehydrated, diced *(AlpineAire),* ½ cup...........................5.0
Celery, dried:
seed, 1 tbsp. 2.7
seed, 1 tsp. 8
Celery, frozen *(Seneca),* ¾ cup...3.0
Celery root or knob, see "Celeriac"
Celery seed, see "Celery, dried"
Cellophane noodles, see "Noodles, Chinese"
Celtus, fresh, raw, 1 leaf, .3 oz. 3
Cereal, ready-to-eat (see also specific grains):
amaranth flakes *(Arrowhead Mills),* 1 cup 23.0
amaranth flakes *(Health Valley),* ¾ cup 24.0
bran:
    (Kellogg's All-Bran Original), ½ cup..................................23.0
    (Kellogg's All-Bran Bran Buds), ⅓ cup..............................24.0
    (Kellogg's All-Bran Extra Fiber), ½ cup 20.0
    (Multi-Bran Chex), 1 cup 49.0
    (Nabisco 100% Bran), ⅓ cup...23.0
    apple cinnamon *(Health Valley),* ⅓ cup..............................41.0
    flakes *(Arrowhead Mills),* 1 cup 18.0
    flakes *(Kellogg's Complete* Wheat Bran), ¾ cup 23.0
    flakes *(Post),* ¾ cup..24.0

flakes, with flax *(New Morning)*, 1 cup.................................21.0
raisin *(Arrowhead Mills)*, 1 cup 41.0
raisin *(Erewhon)*, 1 cup 40.0
raisin *(Health Valley)*, ⅓ cup 40.0
raisin *(Health Valley* Flakes), 1¼ cups............................47.0
raisin *(Kellogg's)*, 1 cup...45.0
raisin *(Kellogg's Raisin Bran Crunch)*, 1 cup.....................44.0
raisin *(Post)*, 1 cup...47.0
raisin *(Skinners)*, 1 cup..41.0
raisin *(Total)*, 1 cup..41.0
raisin *(Wheaties)*, 1 cup..44.0
raisin, with flax *(New Morning)*, 1 cup 22.0
raisin nut *(General Mills* Raisin Nut Bran), ¾ cup.............41.0
buckwheat flakes, maple *(Arrowhead Mills)*, 1 cup...................35.0
corn:
   (Barbara's Puffins), ¾ cup 23.0
   (Cap'n Crunch), ¾ cup...23.0
   (Cocoa Puffs), 1 cup..26.0
   (Corn Chex), 1 cup 26.0
   (Confetti), ¾ cup..24.0
   (Health Valley Crunch-Ems!), 1¼ cups 27.0
   (Kellogg's Corn Pops), 1 cup....................................28.0
   (Post Toasties), 1 cup..24.0
   with almonds and raisins *(New Morning Ginseng Crunch)*,
     ¾ cup 22.0
   chocolate and vanilla *(Cocomotion)*, ¾ cup 22.0
   cinnamon *(Barbara's Puffins)*, ¾ cup..........................26.0
   flakes *(Arrowhead Mills)*, 1 cup..................................30.0
   flakes *(Country* Corn Flakes), 1 cup 26.0
   flakes *(Erewhon)*, 1¼ cups...45.0
   flakes *(Kellogg's Corn Flakes)*, 1 cup.........................24.0
   flakes *(Total)*, 1⅓ cups...24.0
   flakes, blue *(Health Valley)*, ¾ cup.............................24.0
   flakes, with flax *(New Morning)*, 1 cup.......................26.0
   flakes, frosted *(Barbara's)*, 1 cup 27.0
   flakes, frosted *(Kellogg's Cocoa Frosted Flakes)*, ¾ cup 28.0
   flakes, frosted *(Kellogg's Frosted Flakes)*, ¾ cup 28.0
   flakes, fruit juice–sweetened *(Barbara's)*, 1 cup 26.0
   flakes, honey-frosted *(New Morning)*, 1 cup 25.0
   nuts and honey *(Kellogg's Honey Crunch Corn Flakes)*,
     ¾ cup 26.0

Cereal, ready-to-eat, corn *(cont.)*

    peanut butter *(Cap'n Crunch)*, ¾ cup 22.0
    puffed *(Arrowhead Mills)*, 1 cup...11.0
    puffed *(Health Valley)*, 1 cup 26.0
corn and amaranth *(Erewhon Aztec)*, 1 cup 26.0
corn and rice *(Kellogg's Crispix)*, 1 cup 25.0
corn and rice flakes *(Breadshop's)*, ¾ cup 26.0
flax *(Health Valley* Golden), ½ cup..38.0
granola:
    (AlpineAire Fat Free), ½ cup...38.0
    (Kellogg's Low Fat with Raisins), ⅔ cup...........................48.0
    (Kellogg's Low Fat without Raisins), ½ cup 39.0
    (New Morning Oatiola Granola Clusters), ¾ cup................42.0
    all varieties *(Health Valley)*, ⅔ cup..................................42.0
    almond *(AlpineAire)*, ½ cup 41.0
    almond and raisins *(Breadshop's* Granola Crunchy Oat
        Bran), ½ cup 31.0
    apple almond crisp *(AlpineAire)*, 1½ cups 55.0
    blueberry-honey, with milk *(AlpineAire)*, ¾ cup 65.0
    fruit *(Nature Valley* Low Fat), ⅔ cup 44.0
    oats and honey *(Quaker* 100% Natural), ½ cup 31.0
    oats, honey, and raisins *(Quaker* 100% Natural), ½ cup...34.0
    raisins *(Quaker* Low Fat 100% Natural), ⅔ cup.................44.0
    raspberry and cream *(Breadshop's* Granola), ½ cup.............32.0
    strawberry-honey *(AlpineAire)*, 1 cup................................65.0
kamut:
    (Breadshop's Kamut'n Honey), 1 cup 22.0
    (New Morning Kamutios), 1 cup 23.0
    flakes *(Arrowhead Mills)*, 1 cup..25.0
    flakes *(Erewhon Kamut)*, ⅔ cup..25.0
    puffed *(Arrowhead Mills)*, 1 cup..11.0
millet, puffed *(Arrowhead Mills)*, 1 cup....................................12.0
multigrain (see also "granola," above):
    (Banana Nut Crunch), 1 cup 43.0
    (Basic 4), 1 cup 42.0
    (Berry Berry Kix), ¾ cup 26.0
    (Blueberry Nut Crunch), 1¼ cups 43.0
    (Breadshop's Cinnamon Grins), ¾ cup 25.0
    (Cinnamon Grahams), ¾ cup 26.0
    (Cinnamon Toast Crunch), ¾ cup 24.0
    (Cranberry Almond Crunch), 1 cup 44.0

(Fiber One), ½ cup	24.0
(French Toast Crunch), ¾ cup	26.0
(Golden Grahams), ¾ cup	25.0
(Grape-Nuts), ½ cup	47.0
(Harmony), 1¼ cups	44.0
(Health Valley Honey Crunches and Flakes), ¾ cup	31.0
(Honey Nut Chex), ¾ cup	26.0
(Honey Nut Clusters), 1 cup	46.0
(Honeycomb), 1⅓ cups	26.0
(Kaboom), 1¼ cups	24.0
(Kellogg's Apple Jacks), 1 cup	30.0
(Kellogg's Froot Loops), 1 cup	28.0
(Kellogg's Marshmallow Blasted Froot Loops), 1 cup	27.0
(Kellogg's Müeslix), ⅔ cup	40.0
(Kellogg's Product 19), 1 cup	25.0
(Kix), 1⅓ cups	26.0
(Multigrain Cheerios), 1 cup	24.0
(New Morning Fruit-e-o's), 1 cup	25.0
(New Morning GinkgOs), 1 cup	21.0
(Quaker Life), ¾ cup	25.0
(Team Cheerios), 1 cup	25.0
(Total Whole Grain), ¾ cup	23.0
(Trix), 1 cup	27.0
(Waffle Crisp), 1 cup	24.0
(Wafflers Original), ⅔ cup	26.0
almond crunch with raisins *(Healthy Choice)*, 1 cup	45.0
brown sugar and oat *(Total)*, ¾ cup	23.0
brown sugar squares, toasted *(Healthy Choice)*, 1 cup	44.0
cinnamon *(Wafflers)*, ⅔ cup	26.0
cocoa *(Barbara's* Crunch Stars), 1 cup	26.0
cocoa *(Pebbles)*, ¾ cup	26.0
dates, raisins, walnuts *(Fruit & Fibre)*, 1 cup	42.0
flakes *(Arrowhead Mills)*, 1 cup	29.0
flakes *(Grape-Nuts)*, ¾ cup	24.0
flakes *(Healthy Choice)*, ¾ cup	26.0
flakes *(Kellogg's Smart Start)*, 1 cup	43.0
flakes *(Kellogg's Special K Plus)*, 1 cup	47.0
flakes, fiber *(Health Valley)*, ¾ cup	23.0
flakes, fiber 7 *(Health Valley)*, ¾ cup	24.0
flakes, honey fiber 7 *(Health Valley)*, ¾ cup	27.0
fruit and nut *(Kellogg's Just Right)*, 1 cup	49.0

Cereal, ready-to-eat, multigrain *(cont.)*

fruity *(Barbara's* Organic Fruity Punch), 1 cup	26.0
fruity *(Pebbles)*, ¾ cup	24.0
honey *(Barbara's* Crunch Stars), 1 cup	26.0
honey-roasted *(Breadshop's* Puffs'n Honey), ¾ cup	21.0
honey-roasted *(Breadshop's* Health Nuggets), ½ cup	38.0
maple *(Wafflers)*, ⅔ cup	26.0
pecan *(Great Grains)*, ⅔ cup	38.0
raisins and almonds *(Fruit & Fibre)*, 1 cup	42.0
raisins, dates, pecans *(Great Grains)*, ⅔ cup	39.0
vanilla-nut *(Wafflers)*, ⅔ cup	26.0

oat:

(Alpha-Bits), 1 cup	27.0
(Arrowhead Mills Nature O's), 1 cup	24.0
(Cheerios), 1 cup	22.0
(Frosted Cheerios), 1 cup	26.0
(Honey Bunches of Oats), ¾ cup	25.0
(Honey Nut Cheerios), 1 cup	24.0
(Lucky Charms), 1 cup	25.0
(New Morning Oatios Original), 1 cup	21.0
(Quaker Oatmeal Squares), 1 cup	43.0
(Quaker Toasted Oatmeal Original), 1 cup	40.0
all varieties *(Health Valley SoyO's)*, ⅓ cup	31.0
almond *(Honey Bunches of Oats)*, ¾ cup	24.0
almond *(Oatmeal Crisp)*, 1 cup	42.0
apple *(Health Valley* Crunch O's), ¾ cup	25.0
apple cinnamon *(Barbara's* Toasted O's), ¾ cup	24.0
apple cinnamon *(Cheerios)*, ¾ cup	25.0
apple cinnamon *(New Morning Oatios)*, 1 cup	21.0
apple cinnamon *(Oatmeal Crisp)*, 1 cup	45.0
blueberry *(New Morning Oatiola)*, 1 cup	41.0
chocolate-frosted *(New Morning Oatios)*, 1 cup	37.0
cinnamon *(Quaker Life)*, ¾ cup	26.0
cinnamon *(Quaker* Oatmeal Squares), 1 cup	47.0
fruit juice-sweetened *(Barbara's* Breakfast O's), 1 cup	22.0
honey *(Health Valley* Crunch O's), ¾ cup	26.0
honey and almond *(New Morning Oatios)*, 1 cup	22.0
honey-nut *(Barbara's* Toasted O's), ¾ cup	23.0
honey-nut *(Quaker* Toasted Oatmeal), 1 cup	40.0
marshmallow *(Alpha-Bits)*, 1 cup	25.0
raisin *(Oatmeal Crisp)*, 1 cup	44.0

shredded *(Barbara's Shredded Spoonfuls),* ¾ cup...............23.0
shredded, bite-size *(Barbara's),* 1¼ cup......................46.0
sweetened *(Arrowhead Mills Nature O's),* 1 cup 31.0
oat bran (see also "bran," above):
    (Health Valley Flakes), ¾ cup 24.0
    (Health Valley Oat Bran O's), ¾ cup 23.0
    (Kellogg's Cracklin' Oat Bran), ¾ cup........................35.0
    (Quaker), 1¼ cups...43.0
    almond crunch *(Health Valley),* ½ cup 34.0
    flakes *(Arrowhead Mills),* 1 cup............................24.0
    flakes *(Kellogg's Complete),* ¾ cup 23.0
    flakes *(New Morning Ultimate Oat Bran),* 1 cup 21.0
    flakes, raisin *(Health Valley),* ¾ cup 26.0
oat and corn, with apple *(Erewhon Apple Stroodles),* ¾ cup......25.0
oat and corn, with banana *(Erewhon Banana O's),* ¾ cup 26.0
oats and wheat bran *(Country Inn Specialties Green Gables
Inn* Blend), ½ cup 37.0
rice:
    (Health Valley Crunch-Ems), 1¼ cups.......................26.0
    (Kellogg's Cocoa Krispies), ¾ cup 27.0
    (Kellogg's Razzle Dazzle Rice Krispies), ¾ cup 25.0
    (Kellogg's Rice Krispies), 1¼ cups..........................29.0
    (Kellogg's Rice Krispies Treats), ¾ cup 26.0
    (Kellogg's Special K), 1 cup...............................23.0
    (Rice Chex), 1¼ cups 27.0
    brown *(Erewhon* Original Crispy Brown Rice), 1 cup.............25.0
    brown *(Erewhon Rice Twice),* ¾ cup..........................26.0
    brown *(New Morning* Crispy Rice), 1 cup 23.0
    brown, cocoa *(New Morning* Crispy Rice), 1 cup................45.0
    brown, fruit juice-sweetened *(Barbara's* Crisps), 1 cup........25.0
    flakes *(Arrowhead Mills),* 1 cup.............................19.0
    puffed *(Arrowhead Mills),* 1 cup............................14.0
    puffed, fortified, 1 cup....................................12.6
spelt flakes *(Arrowhead Mills),* 1 cup..........................23.0
wheat:
    (Frosted Wheaties), ¾ cup 27.0
    (Golden Crisp), ¾ cup 25.0
    (Wheat Chex), 1 cup 40.0
    (Wheaties), 1 cup 24.0
    flakes *(Arrowhead Mills),* 1 cup............................37.0
    flakes *(Erewhon),* 1 cup....................................42.0

Cereal, ready-to-eat, wheat *(cont.)*

    flakes, with dates, raisins and walnuts *(Erewhon Fruit'n
        Wheat)*, ¾ cup 39.0
    puffed *(Arrowhead Mills)*, 1 cup..13.0
    puffed *(Kellogg's Smacks)*, ¾ cup 24.0
    puffed, fortified, 1 cup..9.6

wheat, shredded:

    (Arrowhead Mills), 1 cup...41.0
    (Barbara's), 2 pieces, 1.4 oz. 31.0
    (Post The Original Shredded Wheat), 2 biscuits 38.0
    (Post The Original Shredded Wheat 'n Bran), 1¼ cups.........47.0
    (Post The Original Shredded Wheat Spoon Size), 1 cup 41.0
    (Quaker), 3 biscuits...50.0
    bite-size *(Honey Nut Shredded Wheat)*, 1 cup 43.0
    frosted, bite-size *(Nabisco)*, 1 cup 44.0
    sweetened *(Arrowhead Mills)*, 1 cup 44.0

wheat, whole:

    biscuits *(Kellogg's Honey Frosted Mini-Wheats* Bite Size)*,
        24 biscuits 48.0
    biscuits *(Kellogg's Mini-Wheats* Frosted Original)*,
        5 biscuits 41.0
    biscuits, apple cinnamon *(Kellogg's Mini-Wheats)*, ¾ cup....44.0
    biscuits, blueberry *(Kellogg's Mini-Wheats)*, ¾ cup..............43.0
    biscuits, frosted *(Kellogg's Mini-Wheats* Bite Size)*,
        24 biscuits 48.0
    biscuits, raisin *(Kellogg's Mini-Wheats)*, ¾ cup 42.0
    biscuits, strawberry *(Kellogg's Mini-Wheats)*, ¾ cup............40.0
    with flaxseed *(Uncle Sam)*, 1 cup...38.0
    and rice flakes *(Country Inn Specialties Greyfield Inn
        Blend)*, ¾ cup 38.0
    and rice flakes *(Country Inn Specialties Inn at Ormsby Hill
        Blend)*, 1 cup 49.0

wheat bran, see "bran," above

Cereal, cooking/hot, dry, except as noted:

barley:

    (Arrowhead Mills Bits O Barley), ⅓ cup 33.0
    (Erewhon Barley Plus), ¼ cup 37.0
    banana nut *(Fantastic Foods* Cup)*, 1.6 oz. 39.0

couscous, 1 cont.:

    apple cinnamon *(Marrakesh Express Cocorico!)*...................55.0
    banana or blueberry *(Marrakesh Express Cocorico!)*............54.0

peach *(Marrakesh Express Cocorico!)* 59.0
strawberry *(Marrakesh Express Cocorico!)* 50.0
farina, see "wheat," below
multigrain:
    (Fantastic Foods Heart Grains Cup), 2.4 oz. 52.0
    (Quaker), ½ cup 29.0
    three-grain, maple raisin *(Fantastic Foods* Cup), 1.8 oz. 42.0
    four-grain plus flax *(Arrowhead Mills),* ¼ cup......................28.0
    five-grain *(AlpineAire* Instant), 1 cup...................................48.0
    five-grain, fruit and nut *(AlpineAire* Instant), 1 cup..............47.0
    seven-grain, regular or wheat-free *(Arrowhead Mills),*
      ⅓ cup...25.0
    ten-grain *(Health Valley* Terrific Ten Grain!), 1 pkg. 41.0
    with apricots *(Fantastic Foods* Hearty Grains Cup), 2.3 oz....50.0
    banana-nut bread or raspberry Danish *(Harvest Mornings),*
      1 pkt. 32.0
    blueberry muffin *(Harvest Mornings),* 1 pkt. 31.0
oat, instant, fortified:
    1-oz. pkt. 17.9
    prepared with water, 1 cup 23.9
    bran and raisins, 1.5-oz. pkt..30.4
    cinnamon and spice, 1.6-oz. pkt. 35.9
    cinnamon and spice, prepared with water, 1 cup 52.3
    cinnamon and spice, prepared with water, 1 tbsp...................3.3
    raisins and spice, 1.5-oz. pkt...31.7
    raisins and spice, prepared with water, 1 cup 48.5
    raisins and spice, prepared with water, 1 tbsp. 3.0
oat, regular, quick, or instant, nonfortified:
    ⅓ cup..18.1
    prepared with water, 1 cup...25.3
    prepared with water, ¾ cup...18.9
    prepared with water, 1 tbsp..1.6
oat bran:
    (Hodgson Mill), ¼ cup 23.0
    (Quaker), ½ cup 25.0
    with toasted wheat germ *(Erewhon),* ⅓ cup 31.0
oatmeal/oats:
    (Arrowhead Mills Instant), 1-oz. pkt...................................20.0
    (H-O Instant Regular), 1-oz. pkt...19.0
    (Quaker Instant Oatmeal), 1-oz. pkt. 19.0
    (Quaker Old Fashioned/Quick Oats), ½ cup 27.0

Cereal, cooking/hot, oatmeal/oats *(cont.)*

apple raisin *(Erewhon* Instant), 1 pkt. 26.0
apple cinnamon *(Erewhon* Instant), 1 pkt. 24.0
apple cinnamon *(Fantastic Foods* Cup), 1.7 oz. 37.0
apple cinnamon *(H-O* Instant Variety Pack), 1.2-oz. pkt. 26.0
apple cinnamon *(Quaker* Instant Oatmeal), 1 pkt. 27.0
banana or blueberry flavor *(Quaker* Fruit & Cream Instant
    Oatmeal), 1 pkt. 26.0
cinnamon and brown sugar *(H-O* Instant Variety Pack),
    1.5-oz. pkt. 32.0
cinnamon spice *(Quaker* Instant Oatmeal), 1 pkt. 36.0
cookies and cream *(Quaker* Instant Oatmeal), 1 pkt. 31.0
cranberry *(Arrowhead Mills* Instant), 1 pkt. 24.0
cranberry-orange *(Fantastic Foods* Cup), 1.7 oz. 38.0
maple *(Maypo),* ½ cup 37.0
maple, apple-spiced *(Arrowhead Mills* Instant), 1 pkt. 25.0
maple brown sugar *(H-O* Instant), 1.5-oz. pkt. 32.0
maple brown sugar *(Quaker* Instant Oatmeal), 1 pkt. 33.0
maple spice *(Erewhon* Instant), 1 pkt. 25.0
with oat bran *(Erewhon* Instant), 1 pkt. 25.0
peaches and cream *(Quaker* Instant Oatmeal), 1 pkt. 27.0
raisin spice *(Quaker* Instant Oatmeal), 1 pkt. 33.0
raisins, dates, and walnuts *(Erewhon* Instant), 1 pkt. 24.0
raisins, dates, and walnuts *(Quaker* Instant Oatmeal), 1 pkt. 27.0
raisins and spice *(H-O* Instant), 1.5-oz. pkt. 31.0
strawberries and cream *(Quaker* Instant Oatmeal), 1 pkt. 27.0
sweet and mellow *(H-O* Instant Variety Pack), 1.2-oz. pkt. ...30.0
rice:
    (Arrowhead Mills Rice and Shine), ¼ cup 32.0
    (Cream of Rice/Creme de Arroz), ¼ cup 38.0
    (Lundberg Purely Organic Hot 'n Creamy), ⅓ cup 43.0
    brown *(Erewhon* Brown Rice Cream), ¼ cup 36.0
    cinnamon raisin *(Lundberg* Hot 'n Creamy), ⅓ cup 42.0
    sweet almond *(Lundberg* Hot 'n Creamy), ⅓ cup 40.0
wheat:
    (Arrowhead Mills Bear Mush), ¼ cup 33.0
    (Cream of Wheat), 3 tbsp. 25.0
    (Cream of Wheat Instant), 1 pkt. 21.0
    (Wheat Hearts), ¼ cup 26.0
    (Wheatena), ⅓ cup 33.0
    baked apple cinnamon *(Cream of Wheat* Instant), 1 pkt. 30.0

berries *(Fantastic Foods* Wheat N' Berries Cup), 1.7 oz. 40.0
brown sugar cinnamon *(Cream of Wheat* Instant), 1 pkt. 29.0
cracked *(Arrowhead Mills)*, ¼ cup 29.0
cracked *(Hodgson Mill)*, ¼ cup 26.0
farina *(H-O Cream Farina* Quick), 3 tbsp. 26.0
farina, 1 tbsp. 8.5
farina, prepared with water, 1 cup 24.7
farina, cinnamon *(Quaker)*, ¼ cup 33.0
farina, creamy *(Quaker)*, ¼ cup 34.0
maple brown sugar *(Cream of Wheat* Instant), 1 pkt. 30.0
whole *(Quaker* Natural), ½ cup 30.0
whole, prepared with water, 1 cup 33.2
wheat and oats, peachberry *(Fantastic Foods* Cup), 1.8 oz.........42.0

Cereal bar, see "Granola and cereal bar"
Cereal beverage, see "Coffee substitute"
Cereal snack, see "Snack mix"
Chapati, see "tortilla"
Chayote:
raw, 5¾"-diam, 7.2 oz. 9.1
raw, 1" pieces, 1 cup 6.0
boiled, drained, 1" pieces, 1 cup 8.1
Cheese (see also "Cheese food" and "Cheese product"):
American, processed:
   (Boar's Head), 1 oz. 1.0
   (Healthy Choice Singles), ¾-oz. slice 2.0
   (Kraft Deluxe), 1 oz. ....<1.0
   (Kraft Deluxe Singles), ⅔-, ¾- or 1-oz. slice ....<1.0
   (Kraft 2% Reduced Fat Singles), ¾-oz. slice 2.0
   (Kraft Free Singles), ⅔-oz. slice 3.0
   (Kraft Free Singles), ¾-oz. slice 2.0
   (Kraft Free Singles White), ¾-oz. slice 3.0
   (Land O Lakes Loaf/Reduced Salt), 1 oz. ....<1.0
   (Land O Lakes Reduced Fat Light), 1 oz. 2.0
   (Land O Lakes Sliced), ¾-oz. slice 1.0
   (Land O Lakes Sliced Deli), .67-oz. slice ....<1.0
   (Light n' Lively Singles), ¾-oz. slice 2.0
   (Sara Lee), 1 oz. 0
   diced, 1 cup 2.2
   melted, 1 cup 3.9
   sharp *(Kraft* Old English), 1 oz. ....<1.0
   sharp *(Land O Lakes* Loaf), 1 oz. ....<1.0

Cheese, American, processed *(cont.)*

    sharp *(Land O Lakes* Sliced), 2 slices, 1 oz.............1.0
    jalapeño *(Land O Lakes)*, .67-oz. slice.................1.0
American and Swiss *(Land O Lakes* Loaf), 1 oz...............0
blue, 1" cube 4
blue, 1 oz. 7
brick:
    (Land O Lakes), 1 oz. ....<1.0
    1 oz. 8
    diced, 1 cup...3.7
    shredded, 1 cup or 4 oz..................................3.1
Brie:
    1 oz. 1
    sliced, 1 cup 6
    melted, 1 cup..1.0
Camembert:
    1 oz. 1
    1 cup 1.1
caraway, 1 oz. 9
cheddar:
    (Boar's Head), 1 oz. ....<1.0
    (Boar's Head Canadian), 1 oz. 0
    (Chedarella), 1 oz. 0
    (Land O Lakes), 1 oz. 0
    all varieties *(Cracker Barrel/Kraft* 2% Milk Reduced Fat),
        1 oz...<1.0
    all varieties, except Vermont sharp *(Cracker Barrel)*, 1 oz..........0
    1 oz. 4
    diced, 1 cup...1.7
    melted, 1 cup..3.1
    low-fat or low-sodium, 1 oz. 5
    low-fat or low-sodium, diced, 1 cup.................2.5
    low-fat or low-sodium, shredded, 1 cup 2.2
    medium or mild *(Kraft)*, 1 oz...........................<1.0
    medium or mild *(Kraft Off the Block)*, 1 oz. ....<1.0
    medium or mild, processed *(Kraft* Cheddary Melts), 1 oz.......2.0
    mild *(Sara Lee)*, 1 oz.....................................1.0
    mild *(Sara Lee* Deli), .8-oz. slice 0
    mild or medium, processed, shredded *(Kraft*
        Cheddary Melts), ¼ cup 2.0
    mild or sharp *(Kraft Marbled)*, 1 oz...................<1.0

mild or sharp, finely shredded *(Kraft* 2% Milk
    Reduced Fat), ⅓ cup 1.0
mild or sharp, shredded *(Kraft* 2% Mild Reduced Fat),
    ¼ cup ....<1.0
sharp *(Healthy Choice* Singles), ¾-oz., slice 2.0
sharp, extra *(Land O Lakes* Loaf), 1 oz. ....<1.0
sharp, processed *(Kraft Free* Singles), ⅔-oz. slice 3.0
sharp, Vermont *(Cracker Barrel),* 1 oz. ....<1.0
sharp or extra sharp *(Kraft),* 1 oz. 0
sharp or extra sharp *(Kraft Off the Block),* 1 oz. 0
shredded *(Healthy Choice* Fancy Shreds), ¼ cup 1.0
shredded *(Kraft Free),* ¼ cup 1.0
shredded, medium, mild, or sharp *(Kraft),* ¼ cup ....<1.0
cheddar and Monterey jack:
    (Kraft Marbled), 1 oz. ....<1.0
    shredded *(Kraft),* ¼ cup ....<1.0
    with jalapeños, shredded *(Kraft* Mexican Style), ⅓ cup ....<1.0
cheddar and mozzarella, whole-milk *(Kraft Marbled),* 1 oz. ....<1.0
cheddar and mozzarella, shredded *(Kraft* Pizza 2% Milk
    Reduced Fat), ⅓ cup 1.0
Cheshire, 1 oz. 1.4
Colby:
    (Boar's Head Longhorn), 1 oz. ....<1.0
    (Kraft), 1 oz. ....<1.0
    (Kraft Slices), 1.6-oz. slice ....<1.0
    (Kraft 2% Milk Reduced Fat), 1 oz. 0
    (Land O Lakes), 1 oz. ....<1.0
    (Sara Lee Longhorn), 1-oz. cube..1.0
    (Sara Lee Longhorn), 1-oz. slice ....<1.0
    1 oz. 7
    diced, 1 cup..3.4
    shredded, 1 cup or 4 oz. 2.9
    low-fat or low-sodium, 1 oz. 5
    low-fat or low-sodium, diced, 1 cup......................................2.5
    low-fat or low-sodium, shredded, 1 cup 2.2
Colby jack/Monterey jack:
    (Kraft/Kraft Marbled/Off the Block), 1 oz. 0
    (Land O Lakes), 1 oz. ....<1.0
    (Sara Lee Longhorn), 1 oz..0
    shredded *(Kraft* 2% Milk Reduced Fat), ¼ cup ....<1.0

Cheese *(cont.)*

cottage, ½ cup, except as noted:

4% *(Breakstone's)*	5.0
4% *(Breakstone's* Snack Size), 4 oz.	4.0
4% *(Friendship)*	4.0
4% *(Friendship* California Style)	3.0
4% *(Knudsen)*	4.0
4%, pineapple *(Friendship)*	14.0
2% *(Breakstone's)*	4.0
2% *(Knudsen)*	5.0
2% *(Light n' Lively)*	5.0
1.5%, peach, pineapple, strawberry, or tropical fruit *(Knudsen On the Go!)*, 4 oz.	13.0
1.5%, pineapple *(Knudsen)*	14.0
1% *(Friendship)*	5.0
1% *(Friendship* Low Fat/Pot Style)	3.0
1%, garden salad *(Light n' Lively)*	5.0
1%, peach and pineapple *(Light n' Lively)*	15.0
1%, pineapple *(Friendship)*	16.0

cottage, dry curd *(Breakstone's)*, ¼ cup ... 3.0

cottage, nonfat, ½ cup, except as noted:

(Breakstone's Free)	6.0
(Friendship)	4.0
(Knudsen Free)	4.0
(Knudsen On the Go! Free), 4 oz.	4.0
(Light n' Lively Free)	6.0
peach *(Friendship)*	15.0
pineapple *(Friendship)*	16.0

cream cheese, 2 tbsp., except as noted:

(Boar's Head)	2.0
(Friendship)	1.0
(Healthy Choice Fat Free)	2.0
(Organic Valley), 1 oz.	1.0
(Philadelphia), 1 oz.	<1.0
(Philadelphia Free), 1 oz.	2.0
(Philadelphia Light)	2.0
chive *(Philadelphia)*, 1 oz.	<1.0
garden vegetable *(Philadelphia Free)*	2.0
garlic and herb *(Healthy Choice* Fat Free)	2.0
jalapeño or roasted garlic *(Philly Flavors* Light)	2.0
raspberry *(Philly Flavors* Light)	6.0

strawberry *(Healthy Choice* Fat Free) 5.0
cream cheese, soft, 2 tbsp.:
   (Friendship) 1.0
   (Philadelphia) 1.0
   apple cinnamon or strawberry *(Philly Flavors)*..............5.0
   cheesecake *(Philly Flavors)* 4.0
   chive and onion *(Philly Flavors)* 2.0
   garden vegetable or salmon *(Philly Flavors)* 1.0
   honey-nut or pineapple *(Philly Flavors)*....................4.0
   strawberry *(Philadelphia Free)*, 2 tbsp. 6.0
cream cheese, whipped, 2 tbsp.:
   (Breakstone's Temp-Tee) ....<1.0
   plain or chive *(Philadelphia)* ....<1.0
   salmon *(Philadelphia)*...1.0
Edam, 1 oz. 4
farmer cheese *(Friendship/Friendship* No Salt/Hoop), 1 oz..............0
feta:
   (Krinos), 1 oz...0
   1 oz. 1.2
   crumbled, 1 cup..6.1
fontina:
   1 oz. 5
   diced, 1 cup..2.0
   shredded, 1 cup..1.7
Gjetost *(Ski Queen)*, 1 oz. 11.0
Gjetost, 1 oz..12.1
goat:
   (Chavrie Mild), 1.1 oz. 1.0
   hard type, 1 oz. 6
   semisoft type, 1 oz. 7
   soft type, 1 oz. 3
   with basil and roasted garlic *(Chavrie)*, 1.1 oz. 1.0
   garlic and herbs or four peppers *(Montchevré)*, 1 oz...........1.0
Gouda, 1 oz..6
grated *(Kraft Free)*, 2 tsp...3.0
grated, garlic herb or zesty red pepper *(Kraft Parm Plus!)*,
   2 tsp. 2.0
Gruyère:
   1 oz. 1
   diced, 1 cup..5
   shredded, 1 cup 4

Cheese *(cont.)*

havarti *(Sara Lee)*, 1 oz. 0

havarti, plain, dill, or jalapeño *(Boar's Head)*, 1 oz. 0

Italian style, shredded:

    (Healthy Choice Fancy Shreds), ¼ cup 1.0

    garlic or hearty *(Kraft)*, ⅓ cup 2.0

    garlic and herb or sun-dried tomato *(Healthy Choice* Garlic

        Lovers' Fancy Shreds), ¼ cup 1.0

jalapeño *(Healthy Choice* Singles), ¾-oz. slice 3.0

jalapeño *(Land O Lakes* 50% Reduced Fat Light), 1 oz. 1.0

Limburger:

    (Knirps), 1 oz. 0

    1 oz. 1

    1 cup 7

mascarpone *(Bel Gioioso)*, 1 oz. 5.0

Mexican/Mexican style:

    four-cheese, shredded *(Kraft* Mexican Style), ⅓ cup ....<1.0

    queso anejo, 1 oz. 1.3

    queso anejo, crumbled, 1 cup 6.1

    queso asadero, 1 oz. 8

    queso asadero, shredded, 1 cup 3.2

    queso chihuahua, 1 oz. 1.6

    queso chihuahua, shredded, 1 cup 6.3

Monterey jack:

    (Kraft 2% Milk Reduced Fat), 1 oz. ....<1.0

    (Kraft/Kraft Off the Block), 1 oz. 0

    (Sara Lee), 1 oz. 0

    1 oz. 1.0

    diced, 1 cup 9

    shredded *(Kraft)*, ¼ cup ....<1.0

    shredded, 1 cup or 4 oz. 8

    hot pepper *(Land O Lakes)*, 1 oz. ....<1.0

    jalapeño *(Kraft)*, 1 oz. ....<1.0

    jalapeño *(Land O Lakes* Loaf), 1 oz. ....<1.0

    jalapeño *(Sara Lee* Deli), .8-oz. slice 0

    plain or jalapeño *(Boar's Head)*, 1 oz. 0

mozzarella, whole milk, low moisture:

    (Boar's Head), 1 oz. ....<1.0

    1 oz. 7

    1" cube 4

mozzarella, part skim, low moisture:
  (Kraft Slices), 1.5-oz. slice ....<1.0
  (Kraft/Kraft Off the Block), 1 oz. ....<1.0
  (Land O Lakes), 1 oz. ....<1.0
  (Sara Lee), 1 oz. 1.0
  (Sara Lee Deli), .8-oz. slice ....<1.0
  1 oz. 9
  diced, 1 cup...4.1
mozzarella, shredded:
  (Healthy Choice Fancy Shreds), ¼ cup 1.0
  (Kraft 2% Milk Reduced Fat), ⅓ cup.................<1.0
  (Kraft Free), ¼ cup 2.0
  whole-milk, 1 cup 2.4
  whole-milk, low moisture *(Kraft)*, ⅓ cup 1.0
  part-skim, low moisture *(Kraft)*, ⅓ cup...........<1.0
  part-skim, low moisture, 1 cup 3.5
mozzarella ball *(Healthy Choice)*, 1 oz. 1.0
mozzarella and cheddar, shredded *(Kraft* Pizza), ⅓ cup 1.0
mozzarella and Parmesan *(Kraft* Italian Style), ⅓ cup 1.0
mozzarella and provolone *(Kraft* Pizza), ¼ cup ....<1.0
Muenster:
  (Boar's Head/Boar's Head Low Sodium), 1 oz. 0
  (Land O Lakes), 1 oz. 0
  (Sara Lee), 1 oz. 0
  1 oz. 3
  diced, 1 cup...1.5
  shredded, 1 cup...1.3
Neufchâtel:
  (Organic Valley), 1 oz. 1.0
  (Philadelphia), 1 oz...<1.0
  1 oz. 8
Parmesan:
  1 oz. 9
  1" cube 3
  grated *(Land O Lakes)*, 1 tbsp. 0
  grated, 1 oz. 1.1
  grated, 1 cup...3.7
  grated, 1 tbsp. 2
  grated or shredded *(Di Giorno)*, 2 tsp. 0
  grated or shredded *(Kraft)*, 2 tsp.....................0
  shredded, 1 oz.. .2

Cheese, Parmesan *(cont.)*

shredded, 1 tbsp. 1.0
Parmesan-Romano, grated, 1 tbsp. 0
pimiento, processed:
  (Kraft Deluxe Singles), 1-oz. slice ....<1.0
  1 oz. 5
  diced, 1 cup...2.4
  melted, 1 cup..4.2
pizza, four-cheese, shredded *(Kraft)*, ¼ cup ....<1.0
pizza, shredded *(Healthy Choice* Fancy Shreds), ¼ cup...............1.0
Port du Salut:
  1 oz. 2
  diced, 1 cup..8
  shredded, 1 cup..6
provolone:
  (Land O Lakes), 1 oz. ....<1.0
  (Sara Lee), 1 oz. 1.0
  1 oz. 6
  diced, 1 cup...2.8
  picante/sharp *(Boar's Head)*, 1 oz. 1.0
  smoke flavor *(Kraft* Slices), 1.5-oz. slice..............<1.0
  smoked *(Sara Lee* Deli), .8-oz. slice 0
ricotta:
  (Breakstone's), ¼ cup 3.0
  whole-milk, ½ cup...3.8
  whole-milk, 1 cup..7.5
  part-skim, 1 cup...12.6
Romano:
  1 oz. 1.0
  grated *(Kraft)*, 2 tsp..0
  grated or shredded *(Di Giorno)*, 2 tsp. 0
  grated or shredded, 1 tbsp. 0
Roquefort, 1 oz. 6
string, cheddar or mozzarella *(Healthy Choice)*, 1-oz. stick........1.0
string, mozzarella, low moisture *(Kraft Handi-Snacks* String),
  1 oz. 0
Swiss:
  (Boar's Head Baby/No Salt), 1 oz. ....<1.0
  (Boar's Head Gold Label Premium Imported), 1 oz.................1.0
  (Boar's Head Lacy), 1 oz. 0
  (Cracker Barrel Baby), 1 oz. 0

(Kraft), 1 oz.	0
(Kraft Slices), .8-oz. slice	0
(Kraft Slices), 1.5-oz. slice	<1.0
(Land O Lakes), 1 oz.	<1.0
(Land O Lakes Baby Loaf), 1 oz.	0
(Land O Lakes Baby Wheel), 1 oz.	<1.0
(Land O Lakes 50% Reduced Fat Light), 1 oz.	<1.0
(Sara Lee/Sara Lee Baby), 1 oz.	1.0
(Sara Lee/Sara Lee Baby), .8-oz. slice	0
1 oz.	1.0
diced, 1 cup	4.5
melted, 1 cup	8.2
shredded *(Kraft)*, ⅓ cup	<1.0
processed *(Healthy Choice* Singles), ¾-oz. slice	2.0
processed *(Kraft* Deluxe Singles), ¾- or 1-oz. slice	0
processed *(Kraft* Free Singles), ¾-oz. slice.	3.0
processed, 1 oz.	.6
processed, diced, 1 cup	2.9
processed, shredded, 1 cup	2.4
taco, shredded *(Kraft)*, ⅓ cup	1.0
Tilsit, 1 oz.	.5
"Cheese," substitute and nondairy, 1 oz., except as noted:	
(HempRella)	3.0
(Smart Beat), ⅔-oz. slice	3.0
all varieties:	
(Rella)	0
(TofuRella)	3.0
(Tofutti Slices), .67-oz. slice	2.0
American *(Smart Beat)*, ⅔-oz. slice	3.0
cheddar:	
creamy *(Smart Balance)*, ⅔-oz. slice	2.0
mellow or sharp *(Smart Beat)*, ⅔-oz. slice	3.0
shredded *(Tofutti Better Than Cheddar)*	2.0
cheddar or mozzarella:	
(AlmondRella)	3.0
(Rella Slices)	1.0
(VeganRella)	10.0
cream, all varieties *(Tofutti Better Than Cream Cheese)*	2.0
mozzarella:	
1 oz.	6.7

"Cheese," substitute and nondairy, mozzarella *(cont.)*
    shredded, 1 cup..26.7
    style, shredded *(Smart Balance)* 0
Cheese dip, 2 tbsp., except as noted:
chili *(Fritos)*..3.0
jalapeño and cheddar *(Frito-Lay)* 4.0
medium or mild *(Cheez Whiz)*..3.0
mild *(Frito-Lay)* 3.0
salsa:
    (Chi-Chi's) 4.0
    (Pace Picante Con Queso)....................................6.0
    (Tostitos Salsa Con Queso), 4 tbsp. 10.0
    (Tostitos Salsa Con Queso Low Fat), 4 tbsp..........8.0
    medium *(D. L. Jardine's* Queso Loco) 4.0
    medium or mild *(Taco Bell Home Originals)* 5.0
    spicy *(D. L. Jardine's* Queso Caliente).................5.0
Cheese entree, frozen, cheddar and chicken bake *(Stouffer's),*
    11.5-oz. pkg. 41.0
Cheese fondue:
1 cup..8.1
½ cup...4.1
Cheese food (see also "Cheese" and "Cheese product")
American, processed:
    (Kraft Singles), 1.2-oz. slice 3.0
    (Kraft Singles), ⅔- or ¾-oz. slice 2.0
    (Land O Lakes Sliced), ¾-oz. slice 2.0
    1 oz. 2.0
    1 cup...8.2
    sharp *(Kraft Old English* Singles), 1-oz. slice ....<1.0
garlic or jalapeño *(Kraft)*, 1 oz. 2.0
Italian herb, jalapeño, onion, or salami *(Land O Lakes)*, 1 oz. ...2.0
Mexican, mild, shredded *(Velveeta)*, ¼ cup 3.0
Mexican style, mild *(Kraft* Singles), ¾-oz. slice..............2.0
Monterey *(Kraft* Singles), ¾-oz. slice...............................2.0
pepperoni *(Land O Lakes)*, 1 oz. 1.0
pimiento *(Kraft* Singles), ¾-oz. slice................................2.0
pimiento *(Kraft* Singles), ⅔-oz. slice................................1.0
sharp *(Kraft* Singles), ¾-oz. slice...................................<1.0
Swiss, processed *(Kraft* Singles), ¾-oz. slice.................1.0
Swiss, processed, 1 oz. 1.3

Cheese pastry, see "Danish pastry"
Cheese pocket, 1 piece:
grilled *(Toaster Breaks* Melts), 2.2 oz...............21.0
steak and, see "Beef sandwich/pocket"
Cheese product (see also "Cheese food"):
(Cheez Whiz Light), 2 tbsp...............6.0
(Velveeta Light), 1 oz. 3.0
Cheese sauce:
(Cheez Whiz), 2 tbsp...............3.0
(Cheez Whiz Squeezable), 2 tbsp. 4.0
four, refrigerated *(Di Giorno),* ¼ cup...............3.0
jalapeño or mild salsa *(Cheez Whiz),* 2 tbsp. 3.0
Cheese sauce, cooking, ¼ cup:
Alfredo, classic *(Ragú Cheese Creations!)*...............3.0
Alfredo, light Parmesan *(Ragú Cheese Creations!)*...............2.0
cheddar, double or four cheese *(Ragú Cheese Creations!)*...........2.0
roasted garlic Parmesan *(Ragú Cheese Creations!)*...............3.0
Romano, creamy tomato *(Ragú Cheese Creations!)*...............7.0
Cheese sauce, mix (see also "Pasta sauce, mix"), dry,
   1.2-oz. pkt. 11.8
Cheese snack combination, 1 unit:
(Kraft Handi-Snacks Nacho Stix'n Cheez), 1.1 oz. 11.0
and breadsticks *(Kraft Handi-Snacks* Cheez'n Breadsticks),
   1.1 oz. 12.0
and crackers *(Kraft Handi-Snacks* Cheez'n Crackers), 1 oz. 9.0
and pretzels *(Kraft Handi-Snacks* Cheez'n Pretzels), 1 oz...........11.0
Cheese spread (see also "Cheese" and "Cheese product"):
all varieties *(Velveeta),* 1 oz...............3.0
American, processed:
   (Easy Cheese), 2 tbsp...............2.0
   (Land O Lakes Golden Velvet), 1 oz. 2.0
   (Nabisco), 2 tbsp...............2.0
   1 oz. 2.5
   diced, 1 cup...............12.2
   sharp *(Kraft Old English),* 2 tbsp...............<1.0
bacon *(Kraft),* 2 tbsp...............<1.0
blue *(Kraft Roka),* 2 tbsp...............2.0
cheddar, all varieties *(Easy Cheese),* 2 tbsp...............3.0
cheddar *(Nabisco),* 2 tbsp...............3.0
cheddar and cream cheese, natural, sharp, extra sharp, or with
   herbs *(Cracker Barrel* Whipped Spreadable), 2 tbsp. ....<1.0

Cheese spread *(cont.)*
feta, with garlic and chives *(Cypress)*, 1 oz. 0
Limburger *(Mohawk Valley)*, 2 tbsp. 0
nacho *(Easy Cheese)*, 2 tbsp. 3.0
pimiento or olive and pimiento *(Kraft)*, 2 tbsp. 3.0
pineapple *(Kraft)*, 2 tbsp. 4.0
Cheeseburger, see "Beef sandwich/pocket"
Cheesecake:
(Entenmann's Deluxe French), ⅕ cake......................................46.0
⅙ of 17-oz. cake, 2.8 oz. 20.4
pineapple *(Entenmann's)*, ⅕ cake 38.0
Cheesecake, frozen or refrigerated:
(Baby Watson), ⅙ cake...16.0
(Carousel New York), 3-oz. cake..16.0
(Jell-O Snacks Original), 1 cont. 23.0
(Sara Lee French), ⅙ cake...24.0
(Sara Lee Original), ¼ cake...39.0
(Sara Lee Reduced Fat), ¼ cake 40.0
cherry *(Sara Lee)*, ¼ cake..55.0
chocolate chip *(Sara Lee)*, ¼ cake 47.0
chocolate-dipped praline pecan *(Sara Lee Cheesecake Bites)*,
    .8-oz. piece...8.0
fudge brownie crumble *(Sara Lee Cheesecake Singles)*,
    3.9-oz. slice..41.0
strawberry:
    (Jell-O Snacks), 1 cont. 26.0
    (Sara Lee), ¼ cake 49.0
    French *(Sara Lee)*, ⅙ cake 43.0
    drizzle *(Sara Lee Cheesecake Singles)*, 3.9-oz. slice 45.0
toasted almond crunch *(Sara Lee Cheesecake Bites)*,
    .8-oz. piece...8.0
Cheesecake, mix, ⅛ cake*, except as noted:
(Betty Crocker Original)..32.0
(Jell-O No Bake Homestyle), ⅙ cake* 50.0
(Jell-O No Bake Real), ⅙ cake* 47.0
(Royal No Bake), ⅙ cake 38.0
cherry *(Jell-O* No Bake)..52.0
chocolate chip *(Betty Crocker)*..34.0
strawberry *(Jell-O* No Bake)..52.0
strawberry swirl *(Betty Crocker)*..33.0
strawberry swirl *(Jell-O* No Bake Fat) 44.0

Cherimoya (see also "Custard apple"), fresh, raw:
(Frieda's), 5 oz. 34.0
trimmed, 1 fruit, 1.2 lbs. 131.3
Cherries, fresh, raw:
(Dole), 1 cup 19.0
sour, red:
    with pits, stems, 1 lb. 49.7
    with pits, 1 cup 12.5
    pitted, 1 cup 18.9
sweet:
    with pits, stems, 1 lb. 67.6
    with pits, 1 cup 19.4
    pitted, 1 cup 24.0
Cherries, candied, red *(S&W)*, 1 piece.......................4.0
Cherries, canned, ½ cup, except as noted:
dark, pitted, in heavy syrup *(Del Monte)*, ½ cup 24.0
sour, red:
    in water, 1 cup..21.8
    in light syrup, 1 cup 48.6
    in heavy syrup, 1 cup 59.6
    in extra heavy syrup, 1 cup 76.3
sweet:
    dark, in heavy syrup *(Oregon)*, ½ cup 24.0
    dark, bing, pitted, in heavy syrup *(Oregon)*, ½ cup 26.0
    dark, sweet, pitted, in heavy syrup *(S&W)*, ½ cup...............34.0
    light, pitted, in heavy syrup *(Oregon* Royal Anne), ½ cup 26.0
    pitted, in water, 1 cup...29.2
    pitted, in juice, 1 cup..34.5
    pitted, in light syrup, 1 cup 43.6
    pitted, in heavy syrup, 1 cup 53.8
    pitted, in extra heavy syrup, 1 cup 68.5
Cherries, dried:
bing *(Frieda's)*, ¼ cup, 1.4 oz. 26.0
bing *(Sonoma)*, ¼ cup, 1.4 oz. 34.0
tart *(Frieda's)*, ⅓ cup, 1.4 oz. 33.0
tart, sweet *(Sonoma)*, ¼ cup, 1.4 oz. 33.0
Cherries, frozen:
sour, red, unsweetened, 18-oz. pkg. 56.2
sour, red, unsweetened, unthawed, 1 cup....................17.1
sweet, sweetened, 10-oz. pkg. 63.5
sweet, sweetened, thawed, 1 cup.................................57.9

Cherries, maraschino, green or red:

with liquid, 1 oz...8.3

with whiskey *(Sable & Rosenfeld Tipsy Cherries),* 1 piece 1.0

Cherry drink, 8 fl. oz., except as noted:

(Kool-Aid Bursts), 1 bottle 25.0

(Kool-Aid Splash)..29.0

cider *(R.W. Knudsen* Aseptic) 31.0

nectar *(Santa Cruz Organic)*..26.0

wild *(Capri Sun All Natural),* 1 pouch....................................30.0

mix* *(Kool-Aid* Sugar Sweetened) 16.0

Cherry drink blend:

lemonade *(R.W. Knudsen),* 8 fl. oz. 29.0

wild cherry *(WhipperSnapple),* 10 fl. oz..................................39.0

Cherry filling, see "Pastry filling" and "Pie filling"

Cherry glacé, see "Cherries, candied"

Cherry juice, 8 fl. oz.:

(Dole Mountain) 38.0

(Eden Organic) 33.0

black *(R.W. Knudsen)* 43.0

cider *(R.W. Knudsen)*..33.0

Cherry juice blend, 8 fl. oz.:

(After the Fall Very Cherry) 26.0

(Mott's) 28.0

Cherry juice concentrate, black *(R.W. Knudsen),* 8 fl. oz.* 31.0

Cherry salsa, see "Salsa"

Cherry syrup, maraschino *(Trader Vic's),* 1 fl. oz. 23.0

Chervil, dried:

1 tbsp.. .9

1 tsp... .3

Chestnut, Chinese:

raw, in shell, 1 lb...187.0

dried, shelled, 1 oz..22.7

boiled or steamed, 1 oz...9.5

roasted, 1 oz. 14.8

Chestnut, European:

raw:

in shell, 1 lb...152.8

shelled, with peel, 1 cup, 13 kernels 66.0

shelled, peeled, 1 oz...12.5

dried, unpeeled, 1 oz...21.9

dried, peeled, 1 oz...22.3

boiled or steamed, 1 oz..7.9
roasted:
    in shell, 1 lb...151.3
    shelled, peeled, 1 oz...15.0
    shelled, peeled, 1 cup, approx. 17 kernels 75.7
Chestnut, European, in jar, whole, roasted *(Minerve),* 4 pieces,
    1 oz. 12.0
Chestnut, Japanese:
raw, 1 oz. 9.9
boiled or steamed, 1 oz..3.6
dried, 1 oz. 23.1
dried, 1 cup 126.2
roasted, 1 oz. 12.8
Chia seeds, dried, 1 oz..13.6
Chicken, fresh:
all classes, without added ingredients, 4 oz.....................................0
broiler or fryer, battered, fried:
    with skin, ½ chicken, without bone, 16.4 oz. 43.9
    with skin, 4 oz. 10.7
    dark meat, with skin, ½ chicken, without bone, 9.8 oz. 26.1
    dark meat, with skin, 4 oz. 10.6
    light meat, with skin, ½ chicken, without bone, 6.6 oz. 17.9
    light meat, with skin, 4 oz. 10.7
    skin only, 1 oz. 6.6
    back, with skin, ½ back, without bone, 4.2 oz. 12.3
    breast, with skin, ½ breast, without bone, 4.9 oz. 12.6
    drumstick, with skin, without bone, 2.5 oz......................... 6.0
    leg, with skin, without bone, 5.6 oz.....................................9.0
    neck, with skin, without bone, 1.8 oz. 4.6
    thigh, with skin, without bone, 3 oz. 7.8
    wing, with skin, without bone, 1.7 oz...................................5.4
broiler or fryer, floured, fried:
    with skin, ½ chicken, without bone, 11.1 oz. 9.9
    with skin, 4 oz. 3.6
    dark meat, with skin, from ½ chicken, without bone, 6.5 oz. .7.5
    dark meat, with skin, 4 oz. 4.6
    light meat with skin, from ½ chicken, without bone, 4.6 oz. ..2.4
    light meat, with skin, 4 oz. 2.1
    skin only, 1 oz. 2.6
    back, with skin, ½ back, without bone, 2.5 oz. 4.7
    breast, with skin, ½ breast, without bone, 3.5 oz. 1.6

Chicken, broiler or fryer, floured, fried *(cont.)*
  drumstick, with skin, without bone, 1.7 oz..............................8
  leg, with skin, without bone, 4 oz.....................................2.8
  neck, with skin, without bone, 1.3 oz. 1.5
  thigh, with skin, without bone, 2.2 oz. 2.0
  wing, with skin, without bone, 1.1 oz..................................8
broiler or fryer, fried:
  meat only, 4 oz. 1.9
  meat only, chopped or diced, 1 cup 2.4
  light meat only, 4 oz..5
  light meat only, 1 cup...6
  back, meat only, ½ back without skin or bone, 2 oz. 3.2
  breast, meat only, ½ breast, without skin or bone, 3 oz. 4
  leg, meat only, without skin or bone, 3.3 oz. 6
  neck, meat only, without skin or bone, .8 oz..........................4
  thigh, meat only, without skin or bone, 1.8 oz. 6
roasting:
  raw, whole, 1 chicken, 3.3 lbs...1.4
  roasted, whole, 1 chicken, 2.4 lbs.....................................5
stewing, raw, whole, 1 chicken, 2 lbs. 1.7
Chicken, canned:
all varieties *(Hormel),* 2 oz..0
breast, in water *(Swanson* Premium), 2 oz.........................<1.0
with broth, 5-oz. can 0
Chicken, freeze-dried, diced *(AlpineAire),* ⅓ cup.............................0
Chicken, frozen or refrigerated:
whole or cut, cooked, white or dark meat *(Perdue),* 3 oz. 0
barbecued, whole *(Empire* Kosher), 5 oz. 1.0
bites *(Country Skillet),* 5 pieces 18.0
breast, bone-in, cooked *(Perdue/Perdue Oven Stuffer),* 3 oz...........0
breast, boneless, seasoned, raw, 4 oz.:
  bleu cheese, Italian *(Chicken By George)* 2.0
  Cajun *(Chicken By George)*...3.0
  Caribbean grill *(Chicken By George)*..................................8.0
  lemon herb or lemon oregano *(Chicken By George)* 3.0
  mesquite barbecue *(Chicken By George)* 5.0
  mustard dill *(Chicken By George)*......................................2.0
  roasted *(Chicken By George)*...0
  teriyaki *(Chicken By George)* 6.0
  tomato herb with basil *(Chicken By George)*..........................5.0
breast, boneless or tenderloins, cooked *(Perdue),* 3 oz..................0

breast, carved, cooked, ½ cup:
   (Perdue Short Cuts Original Roasted) 1.0
   honey-roasted *(Perdue Short Cuts)*.................................2.0
   Italian style *(Perdue Short Cuts)* 0
   lemon pepper or Southwestern *(Perdue Short Cuts)* 1.0
breast, crispy baked, 1 piece:
   (Butterball Original) 16.0
   Italian, lemon pepper, or Parmesan *(Butterball)*....................16.0
   Southwestern *(Butterball)*...13.0
breast, seasoned, cooked, 3 oz.:
   boneless, Italian style *(Perdue)* 3.0
   cutlets, thin-sliced, rosemary garlic thyme or tomato herb
     (Perdue)...1.0
   garlic, roasted, herb *(Perdue)*...3.0
   lemon pepper *(Perdue)*...3.0
   teriyaki *(Perdue)*..3.0
breast cutlets, breaded, cooked *(Perdue)*, 3.5 oz......................14.0
breast quarter, oven-roasted *(Boston Market)*, 6 oz.....................0
breast strips, breaded, 3 oz.:
   (Perdue Kick'n Chicken Original) 14.0
   barbecue *(Perdue Kick'n Chicken)*..................................16.0
   hot and spicy *(Perdue Kick'n Chicken)*.............................13.0
   breast strips, grilled, Italian, Southwestern, or teriyaki
     (Louis Rich Carving Board), 3 oz.............................1.0
breast tenderloins, cooked *(Perdue* Individually Frozen), 3 oz.........0
breast tenderloins, breaded, cooked *(Perdue)*, 3 oz....................13.0
breast tenders:
   (Banquet Fat Free), 3 pieces..16.0
   (Banquet Original), 3 pieces 15.0
   (Country Skillet), 3 pieces 16.0
   baked *(Butterball)*, 3 pieces...15.0
   Southern *(Banquet)*, 3 pieces..16.0
broiler, fryer, or roaster, whole or parts *(Empire* Kosher Chill
   Pack), 4 oz..0
chunks *(Country Skillet)*, 5 pieces 18.0
chunks, Southern-fried *(Country Skillet)*, 5 pieces 17.0
fillets, battered and breaded *(Empire* Kosher), 4 oz. 13.0
fried:
   (Banquet Original), 3 oz..15.0
   (Country Skillet), 3 oz..13.0
   breast, battered and breaded *(Empire* Kosher), 3 oz..............3.0

Chicken, frozen or refrigerated, fried *(cont.)*

country, bone-in *(Banquet)*, 3 oz...................................13.0
cut up, assorted *(Empire* Kosher), 3 oz.....................8.0
drum and thigh *(Empire* Kosher), 3 oz....................7.0
hot and spicy *(Banquet)*, 3 oz. 13.0
skinless *(Banquet)*, 3 oz. 7.0
Southern, bone-in *(Banquet)*, 3 oz. 15.0
honey barbecue, fried skinless, bone-in *(Banquet)*, 3 oz. 9.0
leg and thigh pieces, oven-roasted *(Boston Market)*, 6 oz..............0
nuggets:
(Banquet Original), 6 pieces 12.0
(Country Skillet), 10 pieces 16.0
(Kid Cuisine Munchers Dino Mite), 4 pieces 10.0
battered and breaded *(Empire* Kosher), 5 pieces 12.0
breast *(Banquet)*, 7 pieces......................................13.0
breast, cooked *(Perdue)*, 5 pieces.............................14.0
breast, cooked *(Perdue)* Individually Frozen), 5 pieces 15.0
with cheese *(Kid Cuisine Munchers* Radical Racin'),
    4 pieces 12.0
with cheese, cooked *(Perdue)*, 5 pieces 15.0
mozzarella cheese *(Banquet)*, 6 pieces....................19.0
Southern *(Banquet)*, 5 pieces..................................16.0
patties, 1 piece:
(Banquet Original) 10.0
(Country Skillet) 12.0
(Perdue Homestyle)..12.0
baked breast *(Banquet* Fat Free)..............................15.0
grilled honey barbecue *(Banquet)*................................3.0
grilled honey mustard *(Banquet)*..................................5.0
Italian style *(Perdue)* 11.0
Southern *(Banquet)*..10.0
Southern-fried *(Country Skillet)* 12.0
roasted, toasted garlic *(Perdue)*, 3 oz.........................1.0
tenders, breaded, cooked *(Perdue)*, 3 pieces, 3 oz. 12.0
tenders, grilled, hickory smoke or Oriental *(Butterball)*,
    4 pieces with sauce...12.0
thighs, boneless, cooked:
(Perdue), 3.7 oz..0
fajita *(Perdue)*, 2.4 oz. 1.0
honey mustard *(Perdue)*, 2.4 oz.................................4.0

wings:
barbecue *(Perdue Kick'n Wings)*, 3 oz. 7.0
firehouse big *(Banquet)*, 2 pieces...............................1.0
honey barbecue *(Banquet)*, 4 pieces 15.0
hot and spicy *(Banquet)*, 4 pieces 9.0
hot and spicy *(Perdue Kick'n Wings)*, 3 oz. 4.0
roasted *(Perdue Kick'n Wings)*, 3 oz. 2.0
roasted, herb *(Perdue Kick'n Wings)*, 3 oz................4.0
smokehouse big *(Banquet)*, 2 pieces 4.0
teriyaki *(Perdue Kick'n Wings)*, 3 oz. 3.0
Chicken, ground, without added ingredients, 4 oz. 0
"Chicken," vegetarian:
canned:
(Worthington FriChik), 2 pieces, 3.2 oz....................1.0
(Worthington FriChik Low Fat), 2 pieces, 3 oz. 2.0
diced *(Worthington Chik)*, ¼ cup 1.0
fried, with gravy *(Loma Linda Chik'n)*, 2 pieces, 2.8 oz. 4.0
sliced *(Worthington Chik)*, 3 slices, 3.2 oz................2.0
frozen:
(Worthington Chic-Ketts), 2 slices, ⅜"......................2.0
Buffalo wings *(Morningstar Farms MeatFree)*,
   5 pieces, 3 oz..18.0
nuggets *(Loma Linda Chik)*, 5 pieces, 3 oz. 13.0
nuggets *(Morningstar Farms Chik)*, 4 pieces, 3 oz................17.0
patties *(Morningstar Farms Chik)*, 2.5-oz. patty.....................15.0
patties *(Worthington Crispy Chik)*, 2.5-oz. patty 15.0
sliced or roll *(Worthington)*, 2 slices, 2 oz. 1.0
sticks *(Worthington Chik Stiks)*, 1.7-oz. piece 3.0
mix *(Loma Linda* Chicken Supreme), ⅓ cup 6.0
Chicken dinner, frozen, 1 pkg.:
Alfredo broccoli *(Healthy Choice* Meal), 11.5 oz. 34.0
boneless, white meat, mashed potatoes *(Swanson)*, 11 oz. 49.0
boneless, white meat, mashed potatoes *(Swanson
   Hungry-Man)*, 13¾ oz. 72.0
breaded, country *(Healthy Choice* Meal), 10.25 oz. 51.0
Cantonese *(Healthy Choice* Meal), 10.75 oz................34.0
Dijon *(Healthy Choice* Meal), 11 oz. 33.0
fried *(Banquet Extra Helping)*, 14.7 oz. 70.0
fried, boneless, white meat *(Banquet Extra Helping)*, 13 oz........40.0
herb, country *(Healthy Choice* Meal), 12.15 oz...........44.0
honey-glazed *(Healthy Choice* Meal), 10 oz. 32.0

Chicken dinner, frozen *(cont.)*
mesquite barbecue *(Healthy Choice* Meal), 10.5 oz. 48.0
nuggets, white meat, sweet and sour sauce *(Swanson)*,
   10 oz. 71.0
parmigiana *(Healthy Choice* Meal), 11.5 oz..............................46.0
roasted *(Healthy Choice* Meal), 11 oz. 23.0
sesame *(Healthy Choice* Meal), 10.8 oz. 54.0
sweet and sour *(Healthy Choice* Meal), 11 oz. 53.0
teriyaki *(Healthy Choice* Meal), 11 oz.......................................37.0
and vegetable stir-fry, Oriental *(Healthy Choice* Meal), 11.9 oz...57.0
Chicken entree, canned or packaged:
chow mein:
   (Chun King Bi-Pack), 1 cup..12.0
   (La Choy), 1 cup..6.0
   (La Choy Bi-Pack), 1 cup..11.0
and dumplings *(Dinty Moore)*, 7.5-oz. can 21.0
and dumplings *(Dinty Moore* Microwave), 1 cup......................21.0
and noodles *(Dinty Moore American Classics)*, 1 bowl 28.0
with potatoes *(Dinty Moore American Classics)*, 1 bowl 25.0
stew *(Dinty Moore)*, 1 cup 16.0
stew, and dumpling *(Dinty Moore)*, 1 cup 30.0
sweet and sour *(Chun King* Bi-Pack), 1 cup 29.0
sweet and sour *(La Choy* Bi-Pack), 1 cup 28.0
teriyaki *(La Choy* Bi-Pack), 1 cup...15.0
Chicken entree, dried:
almond *(AlpineAire)*, 1¼ cups 53.0
breast, lemon herb, with rice *(AlpineAire)*, 9 oz.......................44.0
brown rice and vegetables *(AlpineAire)*, 1½ cups 55.0
gumbo *(AlpineAire)*, 1¼ cups 102.0
kung fu *(AlpineAire)*, 1½ cups 68.0
pasta Parmesan *(AlpineAire)*, 12 oz...39.0
pasta primavera *(AlpineAire)*, 1⅛ cups....................................44.0
rotelle *(AlpineAire)*, 1 cup...44.0
Sierra *(AlpineAire)*, 1 cup..53.0
summer *(AlpineAire)*, 1½ cups 38.0
Chicken entree, frozen (see also "Chicken, frozen or refrigerated,"
   and "Chicken entree, mix, frozen"), 1 pkg., except as noted:
à la king:
   (Freezer Queen Cook-in-Pouch), 4 oz.....................................5.0
   (Stouffer's), 11.5 oz...47.0
   with noodles *(Michelina's)*, 8 oz...39.0

à l'orange *(Lean Cuisine Cafe Classics)*, 9 oz................33.0
Alfredo:
    (Green Giant Complete Skillet Meal!), 8 oz. 35.0
    (Green Giant Complete Skillet Meal!), 1¼ cups with milk.....37.0
    (Lean Cuisine Skillet Sensations), ½ of 24-oz. pkg...............36.0
    (Marie Callender's Skillet Meals), ½ of 23-oz. pkg................32.0
    (Marie Callender's Skillet Meals), ¼ of 37-oz. pkg. 26.0
    (Stouffer's Skillet Sensations), ½ of 25-oz. pkg...................51.0
    broccoli *(Banquet* Family Size), 1 cup........................28.0
and almonds, with rice *(Michelina's Yu Sing)*, 9 oz. 49.0
bake, country *(Healthy Choice* Bowl), 9.5 oz. 22.0
baked *(Lean Cuisine Cafe Classics)*, 8⅝ oz. 33.0
and barbecue sauce *(Lean Cuisine Hearty Portions Meal)*,
    13⅞ oz..60.0
with basil cream sauce *(Lean Cuisine Cafe Classics)*, 8.5 oz. 33.0
and biscuits *(Freezer Queen* Deluxe Family Entree), 1 cup 28.0
bow ties and, see "Bow tie pasta entree"
breaded strips, with macaroni and cheese *(Healthy Choice)*,
    8 oz. 34.0
breast:
    baked *(Stouffer's* Homestyle), 8⅞ oz. 18.0
    in barbecue sauce *(Stouffer's* Homestyle), 10 oz. 56.0
    fried *(Stouffer's* Homestyle), 8⅞ oz. 41.0
    fried *(Stouffer's* Hearty Portions), 15⅛ oz. 60.0
    glazed, country *(Healthy Choice* Entree), 8.5 oz................31.0
    with mushroom gravy *(Stouffer's* Homestyle), 10 oz. 32.0
    strips, with macaroni and cheese *(Healthy Choice* Entree),
        8 oz...34.0
broccoli, creamy, cheese and rice *(Banquet* Family Size),
    1 cup..25.0
and broccoli pasta bake *(Stouffer's)*, ⅕ of 40-oz. pkg.............28.0
burrito, see "Burrito"
cacciatore *(Michelina's)*, 8 oz......................................38.0
calzone, Thai peanut *(Sara Lee)*, ½ pkg., 5.5 oz................51.0
carbonara *(Lean Cuisine Cafe Classics)*, 9 oz. 36.0
cheese, three *(Lean Cuisine Skillet Sensations)*, ½ of
    24-oz. pkg. 45.0
and cheesy pasta *(Green Giant Complete Skillet Meal!)*, 8 oz.....37.0
and cheesy pasta *(Green Giant Complete Skillet Meal!)*,
    1¼ cups with milk...39.0
chow mein *(Lean Cuisine Everyday Favorites)*, 9 oz. 37.0

Chicken entree, frozen *(cont.)*

chow mein, with rice *(Michelina's Yu Sing)*, 8.75 oz. 43.0
Cordon Bleu *(Marie Callender's Meals)*, 13 oz. 58.0
creamed *(Stouffer's)*, 6.5 oz. 11.0
croquettes, breaded, gravy and *(Freezer Queen*
    Family Entree), 1 croquette and gravy 14.0
and dumplings:
    (Marie Callender's Meals), 14 oz. 34.0
    (Stouffer's Homestyle), 10 oz. 33.0
    country style *(Banquet* Family Size), 1 cup 30.0
enchilada, see "Enchilada"
escalloped, and noodles *(Stouffer's)*, 10 oz. 36.0
escalloped, and noodles *(Stouffer's* 40 oz.), 1 cup 25.0
fajita:
    bake *(Ortega* Family Fiesta), 10 oz., ¼ pkg. 36.0
    fiesta *(Healthy Choice)*, 7 oz. 36.0
    filling *(El Torito)*, 3 oz. 5.0
fettuccine (see also "Fettuccine entree"):
    (Lean Cuisine Everyday Favorites), 9.25 oz. 33.0
    (Stouffer's Homestyle), 10.5 oz. 34.0
    (Stouffer's Hearty Portions), 16.75 oz. 67.0
    Alfredo *(Healthy Choice* Entree), 8.5 oz. 30.0
    with broccoli *(Lean Cuisine Hearty Portions Meal)*,
        13⅝ oz. 48.0
fiesta *(Healthy Choice* Bowl), 9.5 oz. 34.0
fiesta *(Lean Cuisine Cafe Classics)*, 9.25 oz. 40.0
fingers *(Banquet)*, 7.1 oz. 67.0
fingers, with barbecue sauce, mashed potatoes, and corn
    (Freezer Queen Meal), 9 oz. 39.0
Florentine *(Lean Cuisine Everyday Favorites)*, 8 oz. 32.0
Florentine *(Lean Cuisine Hearty Portions Meal)*, 13.25 oz. 53.0
fried:
    (Banquet Original), 9 oz. 35.0
    (Morton), 9 oz. 30.0
    country, and gravy *(Marie Callender's* Meals), 16 oz. 63.0
    country, and gravy, with mashed potatoes *(Marie Callender's*
        Family), 1 patty with gravy, ½ cup potatoes 48.0
    white meat *(Banquet)*, 8.75 oz. 40.0
    white meat, boneless *(Banquet)*, 8.25 oz. 41.0
fried rice, see "Rice dish, frozen"

garlic:
    (Lean Cuisine Skillet Sensations), ½ of 24-oz. pkg................56.0
    lemon, with rice *(Healthy Choice* Bowl), 9.5 oz.....................48.0
    Milano *(Healthy Choice* Entree), 9.5 oz. 34.0
    pasta *(Green Giant Complete Skillet Meal!)*, 8 oz. 30.0
    with rice *(Michelina's Yu Sing)*, 8 oz. 42.0
    roasted, with potatoes, vegetables, sauce *(Stouffer's Oven*
      Sensations), ½ of 24-oz. pkg. 39.0
ginger, with rice *(Michelina's Yu Sing)*, 8 oz. 41.0
glazed:
    (Lean Cuisine Cafe Classics), 8½ oz. 25.0
    (Lean Cuisine Hearty Portions Meal), 13 oz. 34.0
    (Marie Callender's Meals), 13 oz. 40.0
    country *(Healthy Choice)*, 8.5 oz. 30.0
    Oriental *(Lean Cuisine Hearty Portions Meal)*, 14 oz. 66.0
    with rice *(Michelina's)*, 8 oz...43.0
    with rice *(Michelina's)*, 9.5 oz..49.0
grilled:
    (Banquet), 9.9 oz...37.0
    (Lean Cuisine Cafe Classics), 9⅜ oz. 29.0
    Alfredo, with broccoli *(Michelina's)*, 10 oz. 37.0
    barbecue glaze, garlic dill potatoes *(Boston Market)*,
      15.1 oz..50.0
    breast, and rice pilaf *(Marie Callender's* Meals), 11.75 oz.....38.0
    with mashed potatoes *(Healthy Choice* Entree), 8 oz. 18.0
    with mashed potatoes *(Marie Callender's* Meals), 10 oz. 20.0
    in mushroom sauce *(Marie Callender's* Meals), 14 oz...........54.0
    and penne pasta *(Lean Cuisine Hearty Portions Meal)*,
      14 oz...51.0
    Sonoma *(Healthy Choice* Entree), 9 oz. 30.0
    Southwestern style *(Marie Callender's* Meals), 14 oz. 43.0
    with vegetables *(Stouffer's Skillet Sensations)*, ½ of
      25-oz. pkg...62.0
herb *(Marie Callender's* Skillet Meals), ½ of 24-oz. pkg. 42.0
herb, and roasted potatoes *(Lean Cuisine Skillet Sensations)*,
    ½ of 24-oz. pkg...39.0
herb-roasted:
    (Lean Cuisine Cafe Classics), 8 oz...................................22.0
    (Michelina's), 10 oz. 34.0
    and mashed potatoes *(Marie Callender's* Meals), 14 oz. 26.0
home style *(Stouffer's Skillet Sensations)*, ½ of 25-oz. pkg.......47.0

Chicken entree, frozen *(cont.)*

honey barbecue, with rice *(Michelina's)*, 8.5 oz. 56.0
honey mustard *(Healthy Choice Entree)*, 9.5 oz. 38.0
honey mustard *(Lean Cuisine Cafe Classics)*, 8 oz. 40.0
honey-roasted *(Lean Cuisine Cafe Classics)*, 8.5 oz. 41.0
honey-roasted *(Marie Callender's Meals)*, 14 oz. 27.0
imperial, with rice *(Freezer Queen Homestyle)*, 8.5 oz. 39.0
Italiano *(Michelina's)*, 7.5 oz. 30.0
lasagna, see "Lasagna, frozen"
lo mein *(Green Giant Complete Skillet Meal!)*, 8 oz. 30.0
lo mein *(Michelina's Yu Sing)*, 8.5 oz. 34.0
mandarin:
    (Healthy Choice Entree), 10 oz. 44.0
    (Lean Cuisine Everyday Favorites), 9 oz. 38.0
    with rice *(Michelina's Yu Sing)*, 8 oz. 57.0
Marsala, with garlic mashed potatoes *(Michelina's)*, 8.5 oz. 22.0
medallions, with creamy cheese sauce *(Lean Cuisine Cafe
    Classics)*, 9⅜ oz. 40.0
Mediterranean *(Lean Cuisine Cafe Classics)*, 10.5 oz. 38.0
Mexicali bake *(Ortega Family Fiesta)*, 10 oz., ¼ pkg. 38.0
(Michelina's Littles), 5.5 oz. 29.0
noodle, creamy *(Green Giant Complete Skillet Meal!)*, 8 oz. 42.0
noodle, creamy *(Green Giant Complete Skillet Meal!)*,
    1¼ cups with milk 45.0
and noodles *(Marie Callender's Meals)*, 13 oz. 42.0
noodles with, see "Noodle entree, frozen"
nuggets:
    (Banquet), 6.75 oz. 42.0
    (Freezer Queen Family Entree), 6 pieces, 3 oz. 16.0
    (Freezer Queen Meal), 6 oz. 27.0
    (Morton), 7 oz. 31.0
Oriental *(Lean Cuisine Skillet Sensations)*, ¼ of 40-oz. pkg. 46.0
Oriental *(Stouffer's)*, 10⅝ oz. 38.0
Parmesan *(Lean Cuisine Cafe Classics)*, 10⅞ oz. 41.0
parmigiana:
    (Banquet), 9.5 oz. 29.0
    (Stouffer's Homestyle), 12 oz. 54.0
    breaded *(Marie Callender's Meals)*, 16 oz. 63.0
    breaded *(Michelina's)*, 10 oz. 48.0
pasta *(Empire Kosher)*, 1 cup 17.0
and pasta, home style *(Healthy Choice Entree)*, 9 oz. 32.0

and pasta, Southwestern (Healthy Choice Bowl), 9.5 oz............39.0
pasta primavera (Banquet), 9.5 oz. 40.0
patties, breaded (Morton), 6.75 oz...............................24.0
patties, with mashed potatoes and corn (Freezer Queen
    Meal), 7.5 oz...36.0
in peanut sauce (Lean Cuisine Cafe Classics), 9 oz. 32.0
pesto, with penne (Michelina's), 8 oz............................36.0
piccata (Lean Cuisine Cafe Classics), 9 oz. 41.0
piccata, with rice (Michelina's), 9 oz. 40.0
pie/potpie:
    (Banquet), 7 oz...36.0
    (Empire Kosher), 1 pie 41.0
    (Healthy Choice Bowl Colonial), 9.5 oz.....................40.0
    (Lean Cuisine Everyday Favorites), 9.5 oz.................38.0
    (Marie Callender's), 9.5 oz...................................53.0
    (Marie Callender's), ½ of 16.5-oz. pkg.....................44.0
    (Stouffer's), 10 oz..38.0
    (Stouffer's 16 oz.), 1 cup...................................40.0
    (Stouffer's Hearty Portions), ½ of 16-oz. pkg. 49.0
    (Swanson), 7 oz...43.0
    au gratin (Marie Callender's), 9.5 oz......................50.0
    au gratin (Marie Callender's), ½ of 16.5-oz. pkg..........46.0
    and broccoli (Banquet), 7 oz. 32.0
    and broccoli (Marie Callender's), 9.5 oz. 54.0
    and broccoli (Marie Callender's), ½ of 16.5-oz. pkg. 41.0
    hearty (Banquet Family Size), 1 cup 39.0
    potato-topped (Swanson), 12 oz. 51.0
primavera (Lean Cuisine Skillet Sensations), ½ of 24-oz. pkg. ..50.0
primavera, with spirals (Michelina's), 8 oz....................34.0
and rice:
    with broccoli and cheese (Marie Callender's Skillet Meals),
      ½ of 25-oz. pkg. 47.0
    savory (Stouffer's Skillet Sensations), ¼ of 40-oz. pkg. 51.0
    spicy sauce and (Michelina's), 8 oz. 44.0
roasted:
    (Lean Cuisine Everyday Favorites), 8⅛ oz.................34.0
    with mushrooms (Lean Cuisine Healthy Portions),
      12.5 oz..49.0
    and vegetables (Marie Callender's Skillet Meals), ½ of
      25-oz. pkg..30.0

Chicken entree, frozen, roasted *(cont.)*
    and vegetables *(Marie Callender's* Skillet Meals),
       ¼ of 40-oz. pkg. 24.0
sandwich, see "Chicken sandwich/pocket"
sesame *(Healthy Choice* Entree), 9.75 oz. 38.0
sliced, gravy and *(Freezer Queen* Cook-in-Pouch), 4 oz. 4.0
Sorrentino, with linguine *(Michelina's),* 8.5 oz. 37.0
sweet and sour:
    (Green Giant Complete Skillet Meal!), 8 oz. 62.0
    (Marie Callender's Meals), 14 oz. 86.0
    with rice *(Freezer Queen* Homestyle), 8.5 oz. 51.0
    with rice *(Michelina's Yu Sing),* 8.5 oz. 66.0
teriyaki:
    (Green Giant Complete Skillet Meal!), 8 oz. 45.0
    (Marie Callender's Meals), 13 oz. 71.0
    (Marie Callender's Skillet Meals), ½ of 24-oz. pkg. 61.0
    (Stouffer's Skillet Sensations), ½ of 25-oz. pkg. 59.0
    with rice *(Healthy Choice* Bowl), 9.5 oz. 41.0
    with rice *(Michelina's),* 8.5 oz. 65.0
tetrazzini *(Michelina's),* 8 oz. 35.0
vegetable and, stir-fry *(Michelina's),* 8 oz. 30.0
and vegetables:
    (Lean Cuisine Cafe Classics), 10.5 oz. 30.0
    in cheese sauce with pasta *(Freezer Queen* Deluxe Family
       Entree), 1 cup 30.0
    with linguine *(Freezer Queen* Deluxe Family Entree), 1 cup...30.0
    Marsala *(Healthy Choice* Entree), 11.5 oz. 32.0
    with noodles *(Freezer Queen* Homestyle), 8 oz. 27.0
    rice bake *(Stouffer's* Grandma's 36 oz.), 1 cup 36.0
in wine sauce *(Lean Cuisine Cafe Classics),* 8⅛ oz. 23.0
Chicken entree, mix, dry, 1 cup*, except as noted:
cheddar and broccoli *(Chicken Helper)* 29.0
cheddar and mozzarella *(Chicken Helper Oven Favorites)*...........34.0
cheese, four *(Chicken Helper)* 27.0
creamy roasted garlic *(Chicken Helper)* 29.0
fettuccine Alfredo *(Chicken Helper)* 28.0
fried rice *(Chicken Helper)* 23.0
and herb rice *(Chicken Helper)* 24.0
Parmesan pasta *(Chicken Helper)* 30.0
and penne, Alfredo, three-cheese *(Lipton Sizzle & Stir),* ⅙ pkg. ...27.0
potatoes au gratin *(Chicken Helper Oven Favorites)* 29.0

and rice, creamy *(Chicken Helper Oven Favorites)*.......................30.0
and rice, lemon garlic *(Lipton Sizzle & Stir)*, 1/6 pkg. 33.0
and rice, teriyaki stir-fry *(Lipton Sizzle & Stir)*, 1/6 pkg...............34.0
Southwestern *(Chicken Helper)*......................................27.0
stuffing, home style, and gravy *(Chicken Helper Oven*
    Favorites)...31.0
and stuffing *(Chicken Helper)* 28.0
Chicken entree, mix*, frozen:
Alfredo *(Birds Eye Chicken Voila!)*, 1 cup 26.0
Alfredo pasta *(Green Giant Create A Meal!)*, 1¼ cups 36.0
cheese, three *(Birds Eye Chicken Voila!)*, 1 cup....................24.0
garden herb *(Birds Eye Chicken Voila!)*, 1 cup 28.0
garlic, zesty *(Birds Eye Chicken Voila!)*, 1 cup 28.0
garlic and ginger stir-fry *(Green Giant Create a Meal!)*,
    1½ cups..25.0
garlic herb, oven-roasted *(Green Giant Create a Meal!)*,
    1¾ cups..35.0
grilled salsa, with rice *(Birds Eye Chicken Voila!)*, 1 cup 35.0
herb, garden, pasta *(Green Giant Create a Meal!)*, 1¼ cups.......30.0
lemon pepper, oven-roasted *(Green Giant Create a Meal!)*,
    1⅔ cups..30.0
lo mein stir-fry *(Green Giant Create a Meal!)*, 1¼ cups 33.0
mushroom wine pasta *(Green Giant Create a Meal!)*,
    1¼ cups..31.0
Parmesan herb, oven-roasted *(Green Giant Create a Meal!)*,
    1¾ cups..29.0
pesto, Italian *(Birds Eye Chicken Voila!)*, 1 cup 24.0
Romano herb, with roasted potatoes *(Birds Eye*
    Chicken Voila!), 1 cup 22.0
sweet and sour stir-fry *(Green Giant Create a Meal!)*,
    1¼ cups..43.0
teriyaki *(Birds Eye Chicken Voila!)*, 1 cup 26.0
teriyaki stir-fry *(Green Giant Create a Meal!)*, 1¼ cups.............18.0
Chicken fat:
1 oz. 0
rendered *(Empire* Kosher), 1 tbsp...............................<1.0
Chicken frankfurter, see "Frankfurter"
Chicken giblet gravy, see "Chicken gravy"
Chicken giblets:
broiler or fryer:
    raw, 2.6 oz..1.3

Chicken giblets *(cont.)*
fried, chopped or diced, 1 cup	6.3
simmered, chopped or diced, 1 cup	1.4
capon, see "Capon giblets"	
roasting, raw, 4 oz.	1.3
roasting, simmered, chopped, or diced, 1 cup	1.2
stewing, raw, 2.9 oz.	1.7
stewing, simmered, chopped, or diced, 1 cup	.2

Chicken gizzard, see "Gizzard"

Chicken gravy, ¼ cup, except as noted:
(Boston Market Roasted)	3.0
(Franco-American Regular/Fat Free)	3.0
(Franco-American Slow Roasted)	3.0
(Franco-American Slow Roasted Fat Free)	4.0
(Heinz Classic Home/Classic Style Fat Free)	3.0
giblet *(Franco-American)*	3.0

Chicken gravy mix, roasted *(Knorr* Gravy Classics), 1 tbsp.,
¼ cup*	3.0

"Chicken" gravy mix, vegetarian, dry:
(Hain), 2 tsp.	6.0
(Loma Linda Gravy Quik), 1 tbsp.	3.0

Chicken heart, see "Heart"

Chicken liver, see "Liver"

Chicken liver paté, see "Paté"

Chicken lunch meat, 2 oz., except as noted:
(Carl Buddig Lean), 2.5-oz. pkg.	1.0
(Carl Buddig Lean), 9 slices, 2 oz.	1.0
breast:	
barbecue *(Black Bear)*	1.0
barbecue-sauce-basted *(Boar's Head)*	3.0
browned *(Healthy Choice)*	0
grilled *(Louis Rich Carving Board),* 2 slices, 1.6 oz.	1.0
oven-roasted *(Boar's Head)*	<1.0
oven-roasted *(Carl Buddig* Premium Lean Slices), 2.5-oz. pkg.	1.0
oven-roasted *(Healthy Choice)*	1.0
oven-roasted *(Healthy Choice)* 1-oz. slice	2.0
oven-roasted *(Healthy Choice* 10 oz.), 1-oz. slice	1.0
oven-roasted *(Healthy Choice Deli Traditions),* 6 slices, 1.9 oz.	3.0
oven-roasted *(Louis Rich),* 1-oz. slice	1.0

oven-roasted *(Louis Rich Variety-Pak Fat Free)*, 4 slices,
   2 oz..1.0
oven-roasted *(Sara Lee)*..1.0
oven-roasted *(Sara Lee)*, 3 slices, 1.6 oz.........................1.0
oven-roasted, rotisserie-flavored *(Sara Lee)* 1.0
rotisserie-seasoned *(Healthy Choice* Hearty Deli Flavor)*,
   3 slices, 2 oz..2.0
skinless *(Healthy Choice)* 0
breast, smoked:
   (Healthy Choice), 1-oz. slice..2.0
   (Healthy Choice Deli Traditions), 6 slices, 1.9 oz. 1.0
   hickory *(Boar's Head)* ....<1.0
   honey *(Carl Buddig* Premium Lean Slices)*, 2.5-oz. pkg....3.0
   honey roast *(Healthy Choice Savory Selections)*, 6 slices,
      1.9 oz..4.0
   mesquite *(Healthy Choice)* 0
roll, light meat..1.4
Chicken pie, see "Chicken entree, frozen"
Chicken salad:
with crackers *(Bumble Bee)*, 1 cont. 25.0
without crackers *(Bumble Bee)*, 1 cont..........................10.0
Chicken sandwich/pocket, 1 piece:
(Mrs. Patterson's Aussie Pie/Mrs. Patterson's Aussie Pie Low
   Fat)*, 5.5 oz. 44.0
breaded *(Hormel Quick Meal)*, 4.3 oz..............................40.0
and broccoli:
   (Healthy Choice Hearty Handfuls), 6.1 oz.......................51.0
   (Healthy Choice Meals to Go Bread Stuffs)*, 6.1 oz. 50.0
   and cheddar *(Croissant Pockets)*, 4.5 oz.........................41.0
   supreme *(Lean Pockets)*, 4.5 oz......................................42.0
and cheddar with broccoli *(Hot Pockets)*, 4.5 oz. 40.0
fajita *(Lean Pockets)*, 4.5 oz..39.0
grilled *(Hormel Quick Meal)*, 4.7 oz.................................36.0
Parmesan *(Lean Pockets)*, 4.5 oz. 44.0
Chicken sauce, 2 tbsp.:
Dijon *(Lawry's* Weekday Gourmet)....................................5.0
fajita *(Lawry's* Weekday Gourmet) 3.0
orange glaze liquid *(Lawry's* Weekday Gourmet) 6.0
teriyaki *(Lawry's* Weekday Gourmet)...............................10.0
Chicken sauce, cooking, ½ cup:
cacciatore *(Chicken Tonight)*..10.0

Chicken sauce, cooking *(cont.)*
French, country *(Chicken Tonight)* 6.0
honey mustard *(Chicken Tonight)* 13.0
mushroom, creamy *(Chicken Tonight)* 5.0
sweet and sour *(Chicken Tonight)* 34.0
Chicken seasoning mix:
citrus, California *(Lawry's Spices & Seasonings)*, 1 tsp. 1.0
Dijonne *(Knorr Recipe Classics)*, 1 tbsp. 5.0
fajita, see "Fajita seasoning mix"
marinade, see "Marinade seasoning mix"
and rice dinner *(A Taste of Thai)*, ¼ pkt. 3.0
taco, see "Taco seasoning mix"
Chicken seasoning and coating mix, ⅛ pkt., except as noted:
(Don's Chuck Wagon Baking Mix), ¼ cup 21.0
(Shake 'n Bake Original Recipe) 7.0
barbecue, honey mustard, or tangy honey *(Shake 'n Bake*
    Glazes) 9.0
Buffalo wings *(Shake 'n Bake)*, ⅒ pkt. 8.0
extra crispy *(Oven Fry)* 10.0
flour recipe *(Oven Fry Home Style)* 7.0
hot and spicy *(Shake 'n Bake)* 7.0
Italian, classic *(Shake 'n Bake)* 7.0
Chicken spread, canned, 1 tbsp. 7
Chickpeas, see "Garbanzo beans"
Chickpea flour, 1 cup 53.2
Chick-fil-A, 1 serving:
chicken soup, hearty breast of 10.0
chicken dishes:
    Chick-fil-A chargrilled chicken garden salad...............12.0
    Chick-fil-A chicken Caesar salad.................................5.0
    Chick-fil-A chicken nuggets (8 pieces) 12.0
    Chick-fil-A Chick-n-Strips (4 pieces) 10.0
    Chick-fil-A Chick-n-Strips salad.................................21.0
Chick-fil-A chargrilled chicken sandwich..............................36.0
Chick-fil-A chargrilled chicken club sandwich.......................38.0
Chick-fil-A chicken salad sandwich 42.0
Chick-fil-A chicken sandwich 29.0
side items:
    carrot and raisin salad, cup 28.0
    Chick-fil-A waffle potato fries 49.0
    coleslaw, cup 11.0

tossed salad 6.0
dipping sauces:
    barbecue sauce...11.0
    honey mustard sauce 11.0
    Dijon honey mustard sauce 2.0
    Polynesian sauce.......................................13.0
salad dressings:
    basil vinaigrette 5.0
    blue cheese...2.0
    buttermilk ranch 2.0
    Dijon honey mustard, fat-free...................17.0
    house..9.0
    Italian, light..2.0
    spicy 2.0
    Thousand Island 6.0
desserts:
    Chick-fil-A cheesecake, plain 23.0
    Chick-fil-A lemon pie 19.0
    fudge nut brownie 41.0
    Icedream, 1 cone......................................16.0
Chicory, witloof, fresh, raw:
(Frieda's Endive), 2 cups, 3 oz. 3.0
1 head, 1.9 oz. 2.1
½ cup...1.8
Chicory greens, fresh, raw, chopped, 1 cup................8.5
Chicory root, fresh, raw:
2.1-oz. root 10.5
1" pieces, ½ cup 7.9
Chili, canned or packaged, 1 cup, except as noted:
with beans:
    (Bearitos Original Low Fat).....................36.0
    (Castleberry's)...26.0
    (Hormel)...34.0
    (Hormel), 7.5-oz. can 29.0
    (Hormel Microcup Meals)........................27.0
    (Gebhardt), ½ cup 16.0
    (Just Rite)..31.0
    (Stagg Chili Laredo) 27.0
    (Stagg Chunkero) 26.0
    (Stagg Classic) 28.0
    (Stagg Country Brand) 29.0

Chili, canned or packaged, with beans *(cont.)*
    (Stagg Silverado)..33.0
    (Wolf) 23.0
    black bean *(Bearitos Premium Low Fat)*....................29.0
    black bean *(Health Valley Chili-in-a-Cup)*, ¾ cup 21.0
    black bean, mild or spicy *(Health Valley Fat Free)*.....28.0
    burrito, enchilada, or fajita flavor *(Health Valley Fat Free)*.....30.0
    chicken *(Greene's Farm)*..29.0
    chunky *(Wolf)*..31.0
    chunky or hot *(Hormel)*...34.0
    hot *(Hormel)*, 7.5-oz. can.......................................29.0
    hot *(Hormel Microcup Meals)* 27.0
    hot *(Stagg Dynamite Hot)*...30.0
    lean *(Wolf)*..19.0
    spicy *(Bearitos Premium Low Fat)* 36.0
    spicy, Texas style *(Health Valley Chili-in-a-Cup)*, ¾ cup........21.0
    three-bean, mild *(Health Valley Fat Free)*................28.0
without beans:
    (Hormel)...17.0
    (Hormel Microcup Meals)...15.0
    (Gebhardt), ½ cup...11.0
    (Stagg Double Barrel Beef)......................................19.0
    (Stagg Steak House)..16.0
    (Wolf) 22.0
    (Wolf Micro) 15.0
    chunky *(Wolf)*..21.0
    chunky, steak-cut *(Wolf)* 17.0
    hot *(Hormel)*...17.0
    lean *(Wolf)*..15.0
chicken *(Stagg Ranch House)*.......................................32.0
chicken, without beans *(Stagg Chicken Grande)*...........17.0
with macaroni *(Chef Boyardee Chili Mac)*, ½ of 15-oz. can........30.0
with macaroni *(Hormel Microcup Meals)*........................17.0
turkey:
    (Health Valley 99% Fat Free) 34.0
    (Hormel)...26.0
    (Stagg Turkey Ranchero)..31.0
    without beans *(Hormel)*...17.0
    without beans *(Wolf)*...17.0
vegetable/vegetarian:
    (Hormel Vegetarian) 38.0

(Natural Touch)..21.0
(Stagg Vegetable Garden)...........................37.0
(Wolf)...27.0
(Worthington/Worthington Low Fat)..............21.0
lentil (Health Valley/Health Valley No Salt)..............28.0
medium (Amy's Organic)................................29.0
medium or spicy (Amy's Organic)...............26.0
mild or spicy (Health Valley/Health Valley No Salt)..............30.0
regular or spicy (Shari Ann's Organic)..............45.0
three-bean (Greene's Farm Vegetarian)..............33.0

Chili, dried:
beef and beans (AlpineAire Black Bart), 1¼ cups..............39.0
meatless (AlpineAire Mountain), 1¼ cups..............48.0
turkey, with beans (AlpineAire), 12 oz..............43.0

Chili, frozen, vegetarian (Tabatchnick), 7.5 oz............28.0

Chili beans, canned, ½ cup:
(Eden Organic)..21.0
(Westbrae Natural).......................................15.0
Mexican (Allens/Brown Beauty)..................22.0
spicy (Green Giant)......................................20.0
spicy (Joan of Arc)......................................20.0
in zesty sauce (Campbell's)........................21.0

Chili dinner, frozen, and cornbread (Amy's), 10.5 oz............59.0

Chili dip (see also "Cheese dip"):
(Fritos), 6 oz..16.0
(La Victoria), 2 tbsp...0

Chili dish, mix:
black bean, with corn (Fantastic Foods Chili Olé! Cup), 2.4 oz.....47.0
macaroni, with ziti pasta (Fantastic Foods Chili Olé! Cup),
   2.5 oz..48.0
nacho, with tortilla (Fantastic Foods Chili Olé! Cup), 2.5 oz......50.0
white bean, spicy (Fantastic Foods Chili Olé! Cup), 2.3 oz.........46.0

Chili entree, frozen, 1 pkg., except as noted:
bean, three, with rice (Lean Cuisine Everyday Favorites),
   10 oz..37.0
with beans (Stouffer's), 8.75 oz..................29.0
black bean, with green tomatoes (Michelina's), 8 oz..............58.0
black bean, with rice (Michelina's), 10 oz..............76.0
and corn bread (Healthy Choice Bowl), 9.5 oz..............49.0
and corn bread (Marie Callender's Meals), 16 oz..............67.0
with macaroni (Michelina's Chili-Mac), 8 oz..............37.0

Chili pepper, see "Pepper, chili"
Chili pepper paste *(A Taste of Thai)*, 1 tsp..................................2.0
Chili powder:
1 tbsp..4.1
1 tsp..1.4
Chili relish, Indian *(Patak's)*, 1 tbsp..0
Chili sauce (see also "Curry sauce" and "Hot sauce"):
(Bennetts), 1 tbsp. 4.0
(Del Monte), 1 tbsp. 5.0
(Gebhardt Hot Dog), ¼ cup 8.0
(Just Rite Hot Dog), 1 oz. 3.0
(Heinz), 1 tbsp. 4.0
(Wolf Hot Dog), ¼ cup..7.0
curry, see "Curry sauce"
sweet, green or red *(A Taste of Thai)*, 1 tsp..............................2.0
Chili seasoning mix, dry:
(Adolph's Meal Makers), 1 tbsp. 5.0
(Bearitos), 4 tsp. 5.0
(D.L. Jardine's Bag of Texas/Texas Works), 3 tbsp. 9.0
(Gebhardt Chili Quik), 2 tbsp. 8.0
(Hain), 1⅓ tbsp...7.0
(Shotgun Willie's Texas), 3 tbsp...8.0
Chimichanga entree, frozen *(Banquet)*, 9.5-oz. pkg. 56.0
Chitterlings, pork, raw, without refuse, 12¾ oz. (yield from
   1 lb. raw with refuse) 1.2
Chives:
fresh, raw, chopped, 1 tbsp. 1
fresh, raw, chopped, 1 tsp. 0
freeze-dried, ¼ cup 5
freeze-dried, 1 tbsp. 1
Chocolate, see "Candy"
Chocolate, baking (see also specific listings):
(Nestlé Choco Bake), .5 oz...4.0
bar:
   bittersweet *(Baker's)*, ½ square, .5 oz......................................7.0
   semisweet *(Baker's)*, ½ square, .5 oz. 8.0
   semisweet *(Hershey's)*, ½ bar, .5 oz. 9.0
   semisweet *(Nestlé)*, .5 oz...9.0
   sweet *(Baker's German's)*, 2 squares, .5 oz............................8.0
   unsweetened *(Baker's)*, ½ square. .5 oz. 4.0

unsweetened *(Hershey's)*, ½ bar, .5 oz. 4.0
unsweetened *(Nestlé)*, .5 oz. 5.0
white *(Baker's)*, ½ square, .5 oz. 8.0
white *(Nestlé Premier)*, .5 oz. 8.0
white, 3-oz. bar...50.4
1-oz. square...8.0
1 cup, grated 37.4
chips or morsels:
   milk *(Hershey's* Real), 1 tbsp. 9.0
   milk *(Hershey's* Bake Shoppe Reduced Fat Chips), 1 tbsp. 11.0
   milk *(Nestlé* Morsels), 1 tbsp. 9.0
   milk or semisweet *(Baker's* Real), 1 tbsp. 9.0
   mint *(Hershey's)*, 1 tbsp. 10.0
   mint *(Nestlé* Morsels), 1 tbsp. 9.0
   semisweet *(Baker's)*, 1 tbsp. 10.0
   semisweet *(Hershey's* Real), 1 tbsp. 10.0
   semisweet *(Nestlé* Morsels), 1 tbsp. 9.0
   semisweet, 6-oz. pkg., 1 cup...106.0
   semisweet, large, 1 cup..114.8
   semisweet, mini *(Hershey's* Real), 1 tbsp. 10.0
   semisweet, mini *(Nestlé* Morsels), 1 tbsp. 9.0
   peanut butter, see "Peanut butter baking chips"
   raspberry *(Hershey's)*, 1 tbsp..10.0
   toffee, see "Toffee baking bits"
   white *(Hershey's Premier)*, 1 tbsp. 9.0
   white *(Nestlé* Premier Morsels), 1 tbsp...............................9.0
chunks, semisweet *(Nestlé)*, 1 tbsp. 8.0
Mexican, .7-oz. tablet..15.5
Chocolate drink:
(Hershey's), 1 cup or 1 box 28.0
(Yoo-hoo), 9 fl. oz. 33.0
(Yoo-hoo), 8-fl.-oz. box...29.0
(Yoo-hoo Lite), 9 fl. oz. 15.0
Chocolate drink mix, powder:
(Nesquik), 2 tbsp. 19.0
(Nesquik No Sugar), 2 tbsp. 7.0
2–3 heaping tsp., ¾ oz. 19.5
prepared with milk, 8 fl. oz. 30.9
low-calorie, ¾-oz. pkt. 10.7
low-calorie, prepared with water, 6 fl. oz. 10.6

Chocolate malt syrup, see "Chocolate syrup"
Chocolate milk (see also "Chocolate shake"), 1 cup:
(Hershey's), 1 cup...28.0
(Hershey's Fat Free) 29.0
(Hershey's Reduced Fat) 30.0
(Nesquik) 33.0
(Nesquik Fat Free) 31.0
Chocolate shake *(Hershey's),* 1 container 41.0
Chocolate sprinkles, 2 tbsp.:
mint *(Hershey's York Chocolate Shoppe)*...........................21.0
peanut butter *(Hershey's Reese's Chocolate Shoppe)*................17.0
peanut butter, candy-coated *(Hershey's Reese's Chocolate
    Shoppe)*...19.0
Chocolate syrup, 2 tbsp.:
(Fox's U-Bet) 29.0
(Hershey's), 2-oz. pouch 36.0
(Hershey's Flavored Lite) 12.0
(Hershey's Special Dark) 26.0
(Nesquik) 23.0
(Smucker's Sundae) 25.0
cherries jubilee *(Hershey's Chocolate Shoppe)*....................26.0
flavored *(Estee)*...5.0
malt *(Hershey's)*...36.0
mint *(Hershey's Chocolate Shoppe Fat Free)* 26.0
Chocolate topping, dessert, 2 tbsp.:
(Hershey's Chocolate Shoppe Apple Pie à la Mode) 25.0
(Hershey's Shell) 16.0
(Krackel Shell) 14.0
(Kraft)..26.0
(Smucker's Magic Shell) 13.0
cookie dough crunch *(Smucker's Magic Shell)*....................13.0
fudge:
    (Hershey's) 19.0
    (Hershey's Shell) 15.0
    (Smucker's Microwave Squeeze).......................................28.0
    (Smucker's Spoonable) 28.0
    (Smucker's Magic Shell)..13.0
    dark *(Mrs. Richardson's)*...20.0
    double *(Hershey's)* 24.0
fudge, hot:
    (Hershey's) 20.0

(Hershey's Chocolate Shoppe Fat Free) 23.0
(Kraft) 24.0
(Mrs. Richardson's) 20.0
(Mrs. Richardson's Fat Free) 25.0
(Smucker's Microwave Squeeze) 24.0
(Smucker's Microwave Squeeze Fat Free) 26.0
(Smucker's Special Recipe) 22.0
(Smucker's Spoonable) 24.0
(Smucker's Spoonable Light) 23.0
peanut (Hershey's Shell) 17.0
toffee (Hershey's Heath Shell) 17.0
white, with cookies (Hershey's Shell) 14.0

Chorizo:
(Fiorucci Cantimpalo), 1 oz. 1.0
beef, raw (Aidells Mexican), 3.5-oz. link 3.0
pork and beef, 2.1-oz. link 1.1

Chow chow relish (Crosse & Blackwell), 1 tbsp. 1.0

Chrysanthemum garland:
raw, untrimmed, 1 lb. 19.0
raw, 1" pieces, 1 cup 1.1
boiled, drained, 1" pieces, 1 cup 4.3

Chrysanthemum leaves, raw, chopped, 1 cup 1.5

Churro, cinnamon:
(Bearitos), ½ cup, 1 oz. 20.0
(Tio Pepe's), 1-oz. piece 14.0

Chutney, 1 tbsp., except as noted:
(Trader Vic's Calcutta), 2 tbsp. 11.0
apple curry (Crosse & Blackwell) 7.0
cranberry (Crosse & Blackwell) 10.0
Major Grey:
(Crosse & Blackwell) 14.0
(Patak's) 12.0
mango (Bombay Brand), 2 tbsp. 25.0
mango:
ginger (Bombay Brand), 2 tbsp. 23.0
hot (Crosse & Blackwell) 14.0
regular, hot, or mango and lime (Patak's) 12.0
sweet (Patak's) 13.0
tomato, dried (Sonoma) 9.0

Cilantro, fresh:
raw, 1 cup 2.0

Cilantro *(cont.)*

raw, 1 tsp. 1

Cinnamon, ground:

1 tbsp. 5.4

1 tsp. 1.8

Cinnamon bun or roll, see "Bun, sweet"

Cisco, without added ingredients 0

Citronella, see "Lemongrass"

Citrus drink blend, see "Fruit juice drink blend"

Clams, fresh, meat only:

raw:

     4 oz. 2.9

     9 large or 20 small, 6.3 oz. 4.6

     1 large, .7 oz. 5

     1 cup with liquid 5.8

boiled, poached, or steamed, 4 oz. 5.8

boiled, poached or steamed, 20 small, 6.7 oz. 9.7

breaded, fried, 20 small, 6.6 oz. 19.4

Clams, canned:

baby *(Bumble Bee)*, 2 oz. 2.0

chopped or minced *(Neptune* Fancy Atlantic Surf)*, ¼ cup 1.0

ocean, chopped *(Chincoteague)*, ¼ cup 1.0

ocean, chopped or minced *(Neptune* Atlantic)*, ¼ cup 2.0

sea, chopped *(Chincoteague)*, ¼ cup 0

Clam chowder, see "Soup"

Clam dip, 2 tbsp.:

(Breakstone's Chesapeake) 1.0

(Kraft) 3.0

(Kraft Premium Sour Cream) 1.0

Clam entree, frozen:

breaded, fried:

     (Chincoteague), 3 oz. 24.0

     (Howard Johnson's), 5-oz. pkg. 36.0

     (Mrs. Paul's/Van de Kamp's), 18 pieces 26.0

on half shell *(Chincoteague)*, 2 pieces, 1 oz. 1.0

stuffed *(Chincoteague)*, 1 piece, 2 oz. 9.0

Clam juice:

ocean *(Chincoteague)*, ½ cup 1.0

sea *(Chincoteague)*, ½ cup 0

Clam sauce, canned, ½ cup:

red *(Olde Cape Cod)* 12.0

red *(Progresso)*...8.0
white:
    (Chincoteague Premium)..9.0
    (Colavita) 3.0
    (Progresso) 5.0
    creamy *(Progresso)*..8.0
    with garlic and herbs *(Progresso)*......................5.0
Clover sprouts, 1 cup:
(Jonathan's) 3.0
with broccoli sprouts *(Jonathan's)*.................................4.0
Cloves, ground:
1 tbsp...4.0
1 tsp...1.3
Coating mix, see "Seasoning and coating mix"
Cobbler, dried, apple-blueberry *(AlpineAire),* ½ cup 38.0
Cobbler, frozen:
apple:
    (Marie Callender's), ¼ of 17-oz. pkg. 45.0
    (Mrs. Smith's 80 oz.), 1/18 pkg., 4.4 oz..............42.0
    (Mrs. Smith's 32 oz.), ⅛ pkg., 4 oz....................43.0
berry *(Marie Callender's),* ¼ of 17-oz. pkg. 41.0
blackberry *(Mrs. Smith's* 32 oz.), ⅛ pkg., 4 oz..............43.0
blackberry *(Mrs. Smith's* 80 oz.), 1/18 pkg., 4.4 oz..................41.0
cherry:
    (Marie Callender's), ¼ of 17-oz. pkg. 50.0
    (Mrs. Smith's 80 oz.), 1/18 pkg., 4.4 oz..............47.0
    (Mrs. Smith's 32 oz.), ⅛ pkg., 4 oz....................46.0
peach:
    (Marie Callender's), ¼ of 17-oz. pkg. 47.0
    (Mrs. Smith's 80 oz.), 1/18 pkg., 4.4 oz..............40.0
    (Mrs. Smith's 32 oz.), ⅛ pkg., 4 oz....................42.0
Cocktail sauce, see "Seafood sauce"
Cocoa, 1 tbsp.:
(Hershey's/Hershey's Breakfast/European Style)............................3.0
(Nestlé Baking), 1 tbsp...3.0
baking, unsweetened..2.9
Cocoa mix, dry:
(Hershey's Classic), 1-oz. pkg.....................................24.0
(Hershey's Goodnight Hugs/Kisses), 1.2-oz. pkg.........27.0
(Swiss Miss Cocoa and Cream), 1.2-oz. pkt. 25.0
(Swiss Miss Diet), .25-oz. pkt.......................................4.0

Cocoa mix *(cont.)*
(Swiss Miss Fat Free), .5-oz. pkt...9.0
(Swiss Miss Lite), .75-oz. pkt. 17.0
(Swiss Miss No Sugar), .5-oz. pkt. 10.0
chocolate:
   (Swiss Miss Chocolate Sensation), 1.2-oz. pkt. 27.0
   all varieties, except amaretto, mocha, or black cherry
     (Land O Lakes Cocoa Classics), 1 pouch 25.0
   almond, Dutch, mint, or raspberry *(Hershey's Hot Cocoa*
     Collection), 1.2-oz. pkg...27.0
   amaretto, mocha, or black cherry *(Land O Lakes Cocoa*
     Classics), 1 pouch 24.0
   dark *(Nestlé Homemade Classics),* 1⅔ tbsp. 21.0
   double *(Carnation* Meltdown), 1.23-oz. pkg. 29.0
   Dutch *(Hershey's Hot Cocoa Collection* Fat Free),
     .5-oz. pkg...10.0
   milk *(Nestlé Homemade Classics),* 1⅔ tbsp. 23.0
   milk *(Swiss Miss),* 1-oz. pkt...22.0
   milk or rich *(Carnation),* 3 tbsp., 1-oz. pkg. 23.0
   milk, with mini marshmallows *(Swiss Miss),* 1-oz. pkt........22.0
   rich *(Carnation* Fat Free), .3-oz. pkg..................................4.0
   rich *(Carnation* No Sugar), 3 tbsp., .5-oz. pkg. 9.0
   rich *(Swiss Miss),* 1-oz. pkt..23.0
   rich, with mini marshmallows *(Carnation),* 3 tbsp.,
     1-oz. pkg...23.0
   toffee, English *(Swiss Miss),* 1.25-oz. pkt. 28.0
Irish creme *(Hershey's Hot Cocoa Collection),* 1.2-oz. pkg.........27.0
with marshmallows:
   (Carnation Fat Free), .4-oz. pkg...8.0
   (Carnation Marshmallow Madness), 1.55-oz. pkg...............36.0
   (Swiss Miss Marshmallow Lovers), 1.25-oz. pkg. 27.0
   (Swiss Miss Marshmallow Lovers Fat Free), 1.2-oz. pkt.......12.5
   (Swiss Miss No Sugar), .5-oz. pkt.....................................10.0
vanilla, French:
   (Carnation), 1-oz. pkg..22.0
   (Hershey's Hot Cocoa Collection), 1.2-oz. pkg. 28.0
   (Hershey's Hot Cocoa Collection Fat Free), .5-oz. pkg............11.0
   (Swiss Miss), 1-oz. pkt..21.0
   (Swiss Miss Fat Free), .5-oz. pkt..8.0
Cocoa coffee mix *(Trader Vic's* Kafe-La-Te), 2 rounded tsp.,
   .5 oz. 13.0

Coconut, fresh, shelled:
(Frieda's White or Young), ¼ cup, 1.4 oz.................................6.0
1 medium, 14 oz. 60.5
shredded or grated, 1 cup not packed 12.2
Coconut, canned or packaged:
dried:
    unsweetened, 1 oz..6.9
    creamed, 1 oz..6.1
    toasted, 1 oz..12.6
flaked *(Angel Flake* Bag or Can), 2 tbsp. 6.0
flaked, sweetened, 1 cup 35.2
shredded:
    (Baker's Premium), 2 tbsp..6.0
    sweetened, 7-oz. pkg..94.9
    sweetened, 1 cup...44.3
Coconut cooking sauce, see "Curry sauce"
Coconut cream[1], fresh:
1 cup...16.0
1 tbsp..1.0
Coconut cream, canned:
1 cup...24.7
1 tbsp..1.6
sweetened *(Goya* Coco Cream of Coconut), 2 tbsp. 22.0
Coconut milk[2], fresh:
1 cup...13.3
1 tbsp..8
Coconut milk, canned:
(Goya), 1 tbsp..1.0
(A Taste of Thai), ¼ cup...2.0
(A Taste of Thai Lite), ⅓ cup...3.0
1 cup...6.4
1 tbsp..4
Coconut milk, frozen:
1 cup...13.4
1 tbsp..8
Coconut nectar *(R.W. Knudsen),* 8 fl. oz. 26.0
Cod, Atlantic or Pacific, without added ingredients 0

[1] *Liquid expressed from grated coconut.*
[2] *Liquid expressed from mixture of grated coconut and water.*

Cod entree, frozen:
au gratin *(Oven Poppers),* ½ pkg., 5 oz. 5.0
fillet, breaded *(Mrs. Paul's* Premium), 1 piece 17.0
fillet, breaded *(Van de Kamp's* Premium), 1 piece 19.0
nuggets *(Bunch O Crunch),* 6 pieces, 3 oz. 17.0
stuffed with broccoli and cheese *(Oven Poppers),* ½ pkg.,
   5 oz. 4.0
Cod liver oil 0
Coffee:
brewed, 6 fl. oz. 9
instant:
   regular, 1 rounded tsp. 7
   decaffeinated, 1 rounded tsp. 8
   with chicory, 1 rounded tsp. 1.3
Coffee, flavored, mix, regular or decaffeinated, 8 fl. oz.*,
   except as noted:
all varieties *(General Foods International Coffees*
   Sugar/Fat Free) 5.0
amaretto *(Maxwell House Cafe)* 19.0
café Français *(General Foods International Coffees)* 7.0
café Vienna *(General Foods International Coffees)* 11.0
café Vienna *(General Foods International Coffees* Sugar Free) 3.0
cappuccino:
   all varieties *(Land O Lakes Cappuccino Classics),*
      1 pouch..23.0
   amaretto or caramel *(Nescafé Frothé),* 3 tbsp. 16.0
   French vanilla *(Nescafé Frothé),* 3 tbsp. 15.0
   iced, all varieties *(Land O Lakes Downtown Café),*
      1 pouch..14.0
   latté *(Nescafé Frothé),* 3 tbsp. 14.0
   orange *(General Foods International Coffees)* 11.0
chocolate mocha, regular, hazelnut, mint, or raspberry *(Nescafé*
   Frothé), 3 tbsp. 16.0
French vanilla café *(General Foods International Coffees)* 10.0
hazelnut Belgian café *(General Foods International Coffees)* 12.0
Irish cream *(Maxwell House Cafe)* 19.0
Irish cream café *(General Foods International Coffees)* 10.0
Kahlua Café (General Foods International Coffees)......................10.0
mocha *(Maxwell House Cafe)* 17.0
mocha or vanilla *(Maxwell House Cafe* Sugar Free) 7.0
Suisse mocha *(General Foods International Coffees)* 9.0

vanilla *(Maxwell House Cafe)*...19.0
Viennese chocolate café *(General Foods International
    Coffees)*..10.0
Coffee, iced, 8 fl. oz.:
café mocha *(Blue Luna Café Lite)*......................................10.0
café latte *(Blue Luna Café)*...24.0
cappuccino, mix* *(Maxwell House)*......................................27.0
latte supreme or mocha latte *(AriZona)*............................21.0
Coffee creamer, see "Creamer, nondairy"
Coffee liqueur:
63 proof, 1.5-oz. jigger..16.7
53 proof, 1.5-oz. jigger..24.3
with cream, 34 proof, 1.5-oz. jigger..9.8
Coffee substitute, cereal grain:
1 tsp..1.9
prepared with water, 8 fl. oz..2.4
prepared with milk, 6 fl. oz..10.4
Cold cuts, see specific listings
Coleslaw (see also "Salad blend"), prepared, refrigerated:
(Blue Ridge Farms), 4 oz..20.0
(Chef's Express), 4 oz..15.0
Coleslaw dressing, see "Salad dressing"
Collard greens, fresh:
raw, 1 oz..2.0
raw, chopped, ½ cup..1.3
boiled, drained, chopped, ½ cup..3.9
Collard greens, canned, ½ cup:
(Allens/Sunshine)..5.0
(Stubb's Harvest)...5.0
seasoned *(Sylvia's)*..8.0
Collard greens, frozen, chopped:
(Birds Eye Southern), 1 cup..2.0
(McKenzie's), 1 cup..2.0
unprepared, 10-oz. pkg...18.3
boiled, drained, 1 cup..12.1
Cookie:
all varieties *(Health Valley* Cobbler Bites), 2 pieces, .8 oz............21.0
almond:
    (Stella D'oro Breakfast Treats), .8-oz. piece 16.0
    (Stella D'oro Chinese Dessert), 1 piece.................................21.0
    (Stella D'oro Almond Toast), 2 pieces, 1 oz. 21.0

Cookie, almond *(cont.)*

Chinese *(Frieda's)*, 2 pieces, 1 oz. 19.0

animal cookie:

(Grandma's Tiny Bites), 11 pieces.....................................42.0

(Hain), 9 pieces, 1 oz. 16.0

(Keebler Ernie's), 1 box...41.0

(Nabisco Barnum's Animals), 10 pieces.........................23.0

chocolate chip *(Barbara's Snackimals)*, 8 pieces, 1.1 oz. 18.0

chocolate chip *(Keebler)*, 7 pieces, 1 oz. 22.0

frosted *(Keebler)*, 6 pieces, 1 oz. 18.0

graham cracker, chocolate *(Hain)*, 15 pieces, 1.1 oz. 21.0

graham cracker, honey *(Hain)*, 15 pieces, 1 oz. 12.0

graham cracker, peanut butter *(Hain)*, 15 pieces, 1.1 oz. 20.0

iced or sprinkled *(Keebler)*, 6 pieces, 1.1 oz. 24.0

oatmeal, wheat-free *(Barbara's Snackimals)*, 8 pieces,

1.1 oz. 19.0

vanilla *(Barbara's)*, 8 pieces, 1 oz. 20.0

vanilla *(Barbara's Snackimals)*, 8 pieces, 1.1 oz. 19.0

anise *(Stella D'oro Anisette Sponge)*, 2 pieces, 1 oz. 19.0

anise *(Stella D'oro Anisette Toast)*, 3 pieces, 1.2 oz. 27.0

apple:

(Fig Newtons Fat Free), 2 pieces, 1 oz. 21.0

cinnamon *(Newtons Cobblers)*, .8-oz. piece.........................17.0

raisin *(Health Valley* Jumbo Fat Free), .9-oz. piece...............19.0

spice *(Health Valley* Fat Free), 3 pieces, 1.2 oz. 24.0

anisette sponge, .5-oz. piece...7.8

apricot *(Health Valley* Delight Fat Free), 3 pieces, 1.2 oz. 24.0

apricot glazed pastry puff *(Real Torino)*, 3 pieces, 1.1 oz. 18.0

arrowroot *(Nabisco National)*, .2-oz. piece.....................................4.0

(Bahlsen Nuss Dessert), 3 pieces, 1.1 oz...................................17.0

banana sandwich, chocolate-filled *(Delicious Chiquita Banana*

Ramas), 2 pieces, .9 oz. 17.0

banana split wafer *(Estee)*, 5 pieces..22.0

biscotti:

(Almondina Choconut), 4 pieces, 1.1 oz. 20.0

(Real Torino Amaretti), 6 pieces, 1.1 oz. 27.0

almond, mini *(Real Torino)*, 4 pieces, 1.1 oz. 22.0

amaretto or chocolate *(Health Valley)*, 2 pieces, 1.1 oz. 23.0

cashews *(Stella D'oro)*, 1 piece 13.0

chocolate *(Nonni's* Decadence), 1.2-oz. piece 19.0

chocolate *(Real Torino)*, 1.1-oz. piece.....................................21.0

chocolate *(Stella D'oro)*, .8-oz. piece.................................15.0
chocolate-almond *(Stella D'oro)*, 1 piece 15.0
chocolate with almond *(Real Torino)*, 1.1-oz. piece 21.0
chocolate with almond, mini *(Real Torino)*, 4 pieces,
    1.1 oz..22.0
chocolate chunk or French vanilla *(Stella D'oro)*,
    .8-oz. piece 16.0
fudge-dipped, almond, chocolate chunk, or
    French vanilla *(Stella D'oro)*, 1 piece 18.0
hazelnut *(Stella D'oro)*, .8-oz. piece...........................15.0
raisin, mini *(Real Torino)*, 4 pieces, 1.1 oz...........................21.0
butter:
    (Keebler), 5 pieces, 1.1 oz.....................................22.0
    (Keebler Danish Wedding), 4 pieces, 1 oz.................20.0
    (Keebler Cookie Stix), 5 pieces, 1.2 oz.....................22.0
    (Pepperidge Farm Chessmen), 3 pieces, .9 oz. 18.0
    .2-oz. piece 3.4
    waffles *(Jules Destrooper)*, 2 pieces, .9 oz. 16.0
butter flavor sandwich, fudge-filled *(E. L. Fudge)*,
    2 pieces, .9 oz. 17.0
cappuccino chocolate pastry puff *(Ferrara)*, 5 pieces, 1.1 oz......18.0
cappuccino crisp *(Murray* Sugar Free), 4 pieces, 1.1 oz.............23.0
cappuccino sandwich *(Café Cremes)*, 2 pieces...........................22.0
caramel *(SnackWell's* Delights), .6-oz. piece..........................13.0
caramel bar *(Little Debbie)*, 1.2-oz. piece 22.0
(Carr's Biscuits for Tea), 2 pieces, 1 oz...................................20.0
(Carr's Chococcines), 3 pieces, 1 oz. 16.0
Chinese, see "almond," above and "fortune," below
chocolate:
    (Frito-Lay Emperador), 2 pieces, .9 oz. 18.0
    (Stella D'oro Breakfast Treats), .8-oz. piece 15.0
    (Stella D'oro Castelets), 2 pieces, 1 oz..................19.0
    creme wafer *(Real Torino)*, 2 pieces, .9 oz. 16.0
    crisps *(SnackWell's)*, 18 pieces...............................25.0
    double Dutch *(Barbara's* Crisp), .6-oz. piece 10.0
    peanut butter/caramel wafer *(Estee)*, 5 pieces 22.0
    wafer *(Estee)*, 5 pieces...19.0
    wafer *(Nabisco Famous)*, 5 pieces, 1.1 oz.................24.0
    wafer *(Nilla* Reduced Fat), 8 pieces, 1 oz. 23.0
    walnut *(Estee* Smart Treats), 3 pieces, 1 oz. 22.0

Cookie *(cont.)*

chocolate chip/chunk:

(Barbara's Crisp), .6-oz. piece	10.0
(Chips Ahoy!), 1.4-oz. pkg.	27.0
(Chips Ahoy!), 3 pieces, 1.1 oz.	21.0
(Chips Ahoy! Chewy), 3 pieces, 1.3 oz.	24.0
(Chips Ahoy! Chunky), .6-oz. piece	10.0
(Chips Ahoy! Mini), 1.5-oz. pkg.	29.0
(Chips Ahoy! Mini), 5 pieces, 1.1 oz.	20.0
(Chips Ahoy! Reduced Fat), 3 pieces	22.0
(Estee), 4 pieces, 1 oz.	21.0
(Estee Smart Treats), 3 pieces, 1 oz.	22.0
(Grandma's Big Homestyle), 1.4-oz. piece	25.0
(Grandma's Rich N' Chewy), 1 pkg.	39.0
(Grandma's Tiny Bites), 12 pieces	38.0
(Health Valley Wheat/Dairy Free), .8-oz. piece	14.0
(Health Valley Healthy Chips Fat Free), 3 pieces, 1.2 oz.	24.0
(Keebler Chips Deluxe), .5-oz. piece	9.0
(Keebler Chips Deluxe Chocolate Lovers/Soft 'n Chewy), .6-oz. piece	11.0
(Keebler Cookie Stix), 4 pieces, 1 oz.	19.0
(Keebler Soft Batch Homestyle), .6-oz. piece	10.0
(Little Debbie Singles), 1.3 oz.	24.0
(Murray Sugar Free), 3 pieces, 1.1 oz.	20.0
(SnackWell's Bite Size), 13 pieces, 1 oz.	22.0
(Tofutti), 1 piece	19.0
chunk *(Keebler Soft Batch* Homestyle), .9-oz. piece	17.0
crisp *(SnackWell's),* 18 pieces	27.0
dark chocolate *(Pepperidge Farm Nantucket),* .9-oz. piece	16.0
dark chocolate, with pecans *(Pepperidge Farm Chesapeake),* .8-oz. piece	15.0
double *(Chips Ahoy!),* 3 pieces	23.0
double *(SnackWell's),* 13 pieces, 1.1 oz.	22.0
double chocolate *(Health Valley Healthy Chips* Fat Free), 3 pieces, 1.2 oz.	24.0
double chocolate chunk *(Keebler Soft Batch* Homestyle), .9-oz. piece	17.0
fudge *(Grandma's* Big Homestyle), 1.4-oz. piece	26.0
milk chocolate, with macadamias *(Pepperidge Farm Sausalito),* .9-oz. piece	16.0

milk chocolate, with walnuts *(Pepperidge Farm Montauk),*
.9-oz. piece 17.0

with pecans *(Chips Ahoy!* Mini), 5 pieces 19.0

rainbow *(Keebler Chips Deluxe),* .6-oz. piece 10.0

regular, chocolate, or pecan *(Westbrae Natural),*
.9-oz. piece 18.0

walnut *(Westbrae Natural),* .9-oz. piece 17.0

walnut, crunchy *(Keebler Chips Deluxe),* .6-oz. piece 9.0

chocolate mocha *(Pepperidge Farm Salzburg),* 2 pieces,
1 oz. 21.0

chocolate sandwich:

  (Droxies), 3 pieces, 1.1 oz. 21.0

  (Droxies Reduced Fat), 3 pieces, 1.1 oz. 23.0

  (Estee), 3 pieces, 1.1 oz. 24.0

  (Murray Sugar Free), 3 pieces, 1 oz. 19.0

  (Oreo), 2-oz. pkg. 40.0

  (Oreo), 3 pieces, 1.2 oz. 23.0

  (Oreo Minis), 1.5-oz. pkg. 31.0

  (Oreo Minis), 9 pieces 21.0

  (Oreo Reduced Fat), 3 pieces 25.0

  (Oreo Double Stuf), 2 pieces, 1 oz. 19.0

  (Pepperidge Farm Brussels), 3 pieces, 1.1 oz. 20.0

  (Pepperidge Farm Milano/Milano Endless Chocolate),
  3 pieces, 1.2 oz. 21.0

  (SnackWell's), 2 pieces 20.0

  (SnackWell's Creme), 1.7-oz. pkg. 38.0

  (SnackWell's Creme), 2 pieces, .9 oz. 20.0

  chocolate-covered *(Pepperidge Farm Milano* Enrobed),
  .6-oz. piece 10.0

  double chocolate *(Pepperidge Farm Milano),* 2 pieces,
  1 oz. 17.0

  fudge-covered *(Oreo),* .75-oz. piece 14.0

  mint *(Pepperidge Farm Milano),* 2 pieces, .9 oz. 16.0

chocolate-topped:

  dark *(Carr's* Biscuits for Tea), 2 pieces, .9 oz. 17.0

  dark *(Carr's Imperials),* 2 pieces, 1 oz. 19.0

  dark *(Pepperidge Farm Geneva),* 3 pieces, .9 oz. 19.0

  milk *(Carr's* Biscuits for Tea), 2 pieces, .9 oz. 16.0

  milk *(Carr's Imperials),* 2 pieces, 1 oz. 18.0

Cookie *(cont.)*

cinnamon, Viennese *(Stella D'oro* Breakfast Treats),
.8-oz. piece 17.0

coconut:

    (Estee), 4 pieces, 1 oz. 19.0

    (Estee Smart Treats), 3 pieces, 1 oz. 22.0

    (Keebler Chips Deluxe), .6-oz. piece 10.0

    almond, cocoa-coated *(Barbara's Nature's Choice),*
        1.1-oz. bar 20.0

    creme *(SnackWell's),* 2 pieces 19.0

coffee creme sandwich *(Peek Freans),* 2 pieces, 1.1 oz. 21.0

cranberry *(Fig Newtons* Fat Free), 2 pieces, 1 oz. 22.0

cranberry biscuits *(Keebler Golden Fruit),* .7-oz. piece 14.0

creme sandwich *(SnackWell's),* 2 pieces, .9 oz. 20.0

date *(Health Valley* Delight Fat Free), 3 pieces, 1.2 oz. 24.0

(Delicious Heath), 3 pieces, 1.3 oz. 21.0

(Delicious Nestlé Butterfinger), 3 pieces, 1 oz. 18.0

devil's food:

    (SnackWell's), 1.1-oz. pkg. 22.0

    (SnackWell's Fat Free), 1 piece 10.0

    golden *(SnackWell's),* .6-oz. piece 11.0

egg:

    (Stella D'oro Jumbo), 2 pieces, .8 oz. 18.0

    (Stella D'oro Roman Egg Biscuits), 1.2-oz. piece 21.0

    kichel *(American Hearth Bakeries* Bowties), 2 pieces,
        1 oz. 12.0

espresso bean, cocoa-coated *(Barbara's Nature's Choice),*
    1.1-oz. bar 22.0

fig bar:

    (Barbara's Fat Free), .7-oz. bar 15.0

    (Barbara's Low Fat Traditional), .7-oz. bar 14.0

    (Estee), 2 bars, 1 oz. 23.0

    (Fig Newtons), 2 pieces, 1.1 oz. 22.0

    (Fig Newtons Fat Free), 2.1-oz. pkg. 23.0

    (Little Debbie), 1.5 oz. 31.0

    (Tofutti), 2 bars 21.0

    apple cinnamon *(Barbara's* Fat Free), .7-oz. bar 14.0

    blueberry *(Barbara's* Low Fat Traditional), .7-oz. bar 14.0

    raspberry *(Barbara's* Fat Free), .7-oz. bar 15.0

    whole-wheat *(Barbara's* Fat Free), .7-oz. bar 16.0

fortune:
  (Frieda's), 4 pieces, 1 oz..23.0
  (La Choy), 4 pieces, 1.1 oz...27.0
  .3-oz. piece...6.7
frosted pastry puff, plain or chocolate *(Real Torino)*,
  2 pieces, .8 oz. 12.0
fruit, Hawaiian *(Health Valley* Fat Free), 3 pieces, 1.2 oz. 24.0
fruit-filled *(Bahlsen* Deloba Biscuits), 4 pieces, 1 oz..................19.0
fudge:
  (Estee), 4 pieces, 1 oz. 19.0
  (Grandma's Mini), 9 pieces 21.0
  cake type, ¾-oz. piece..16.4
  chocolate, creme-filled *(Keebler Classic Collection)*,
    .6-oz. piece 12.0
  double *(Murray* Sugar Free), 3 pieces, 1.2 oz. 21.0
  double, caramel *(Keebler Fudge Shoppe)*, 2 pieces, 1.1 oz. ...20.0
  mint *(Keebler Fudge Shoppe* Grasshoppers), 4 pieces,
    1.1 oz...20.0
  stick *(Keebler Fudge Shoppe)*, 3 pieces, 1 oz......................20.0
  stripe *(Fudge Favorites)*, 3 pieces, 1.1 oz. 21.0
  stripe *(Keebler Fudge Shoppe)*, 3 pieces, 1 oz.....................21.0
  Swiss *(Stella D'oro)*, 2 pieces, .9 oz....................................16.0
fudge sandwich:
  (Grandma's Value Line), 3 pieces 31.0
  fudge-creme-filled *(E. L. Fudge)*, 2 pieces, .9 oz. 17.0
  peanut-butter-filled *(E. L. Fudge)*, 2 pieces, .9 oz...............16.0
ginger *(Little Debbie)*, .7 oz..15.0
ginger-lemon creme *(Carr's)*, 2 pieces, 1 oz. 19.0
gingersnap:
  (Keebler), 5 pieces, 1.2 oz..24.0
  (Murray Sugar Free), 6 pieces, 1 oz.....................................21.0
  (Nabisco), 4 pieces, 1 oz..22.0
  (Westbrae Natural), 3 pieces, 1 oz. 18.0
  ¼-oz. piece...5.4
golden bar *(Stella D'oro Golden Bars)*, 1-oz. piece 16.0
graham cracker:
  (Estee Old Fashioned), 2 pieces 17.0
  (Honey Maid), 2 pieces, 8 sections, 1 oz. 22.0
  (Honey Maid Low Fat), 2 pieces, 8 sections, 1 oz.................23.0
  (Keebler Grahams), 8 pieces, 1 oz. 22.0
  (Nabisco), 4 pieces, 1 oz..22.0

Cookie, graham cracker *(cont.)*

(New Morning Ginger Grahams), 2 pieces, 1.1 oz. 26.0

amaranth or oat bran *(Health Valley* Low Fat), 6 pieces,
    1 oz. 3.0

animal, see "animal cookie," above

chocolate *(Estee)*, 2 pieces 27.0

chocolate *(Hain)*, 2 pieces, 1.1 oz. 21.0

chocolate *(Honey Maid)*, 2 pieces, 8 sections 22.0

chocolate *(Keebler Grahams)*, 8 pieces, 1.1 oz. 23.0

chocolate *(New Morning* Chocolate Grahams),
    2 pieces, 1.1 oz. 21.0

chocolate *(Sweet Crispers)*, 18 pieces, 1.1 oz. 25.0

chocolate *(Teddy Grahams)*, 24 pieces, 1.1 oz. 23.0

chocolate-coated *(Keebler Fudge Shoppe* Deluxe),
    3 pieces, 1 oz. 19.0

chocolate- or vanilla-frosted *(Teddy Grahams Dizzy Grizzly)*,
    8 pieces, 1.1 oz. 24.0

chocolatey chip *(Teddy Grahams)*, 23 pieces, 1.1 oz. 22.0

cinnamon *(Estee)*, 2 pieces 18.0

cinnamon *(Honey Maid)*, 2 pieces, 8 sections 23.0

cinnamon *(Keebler Cinnamon Crisp)*, 8 pieces, 1.1 oz. 23.0

cinnamon *(Keebler Snackin' Grahams)*, 21 pieces, 1 oz. 23.0

cinnamon *(New Morning* Cinnamon Grahams),
    2 pieces, 1.1 oz. 20.0

cinnamon *(New Morning* Cinnamon Grahams Mini-Bites),
    15 pieces, 1.1 oz. 24.0

cinnamon or honey *(Hain)*, 2 pieces, 1 oz. 12.0

cinnamon or honey *(Sweet Crispers)*, 18 pieces, 1.1 oz. 26.0

cinnamon or honey *(Teddy Grahams)*, 24 pieces, 1.1 oz. 22.0

cinnamon sugar *(Elf Grahams)*, 16 pieces, 1.1 oz. 22.0

frosted, chocolate or vanilla, with sprinkles *(Teddy Grahams
    Dizzy Grizzlies)*, 8 pieces 24.0

fudge-covered *(Fudge Favorites)*, 3 pieces, 1 oz. 18.0

honey *(Elf Grahams)*, 16 pieces, 1.1 oz. 23.0

honey *(Keebler Grahams)*, 8 pieces, 1.1 oz. 23.0

honey *(Keebler Grahams* Low Fat), 9 pieces, 1.1 oz. 25.0

honey *(New Morning* Honey Grahams), 2 pieces, 1.1 oz. 21.0

honey *(New Morning* Honey Grahams Mini-Bites),
    15 pieces, 1.1 oz. 24.0

honey *(Teddy Grahams)*, 24 pieces, 1.1 oz. 23.0

lemon *(New Morning* Lemon Grahams Mini-Bites),
   15 pieces, 1.1 oz...23.0
   oatmeal crunch *(Honey Maid),* 2 pieces, 8 sections.............23.0
   vanilla, French *(Hain),* 2 pieces, 1.1 oz..................................16.0
hazelnut *(Bahlsen* Kipferl), 4 pieces, 1 oz. 16.0
holiday *(Stella D'oro* Rings and Stars), 3 pieces, 1.2 oz. 22.0
holiday *(Stella D'oro* Trinkets), 4 pieces, 1.1 oz.........................20.0
honey almond *(Westbrae Natural),* .9-oz. piece 17.0
kichel, see "egg," above
lady finger *(Real Torino),* 3 pieces, 1 oz....................................23.0
lemon:
   (Estee Smart Treats), 3 pieces, 1 oz....................................22.0
   (Frito-Lay Piruetas), 3 pieces, 1.1 oz...................................21.0
   (Keebler Lemon Coolers), 5 pieces, 1.1 oz............................21.0
   (Pepperidge Farm Spritzers), 5 pieces, 1.1 oz.......................21.0
   cream wafer *(Estee),* 5 pieces 22.0
   crisp *(Murray* Sugar Free), 4 pieces, 1.1 oz. 22.0
   nut *(Pepperidge Farm),* 3 pieces, 1.1 oz. 19.0
   snap *(Westbrae Natural),* 3 pieces, 1.1 oz.............................20.0
   thin *(Estee),* 4 pieces, 1 oz...19.0
   yogurt-coated *(Barbara's Nature's Choice),* 1.1-oz. bar.........22.0
lemon sandwich *(Murray* Sugar Free), 3 pieces, 1 oz.................20.0
lemon sandwich *(Vienna Fingers),* 2 pieces, 1 oz. 21.0
lime *(Peek Freans* Calypso), 2 pieces..20.0
lime, Key *(Pepperidge Farm Spritzers),* 5 pieces, 1.1 oz.............21.0
marshmallow, chocolate-coated *(Mallomars),* 2 pieces, .9 oz. ...17.0
marshmallow, chocolate-coated *(Pinwheels),* 1 piece 21.0
meringue, coconut *(Miss Meringue),* 4 pieces, 1.25 oz...............23.0
meringue, lemon or strawberry *(Miss Meringue),* 4 pieces,
   1.25 oz. 24.0
mint creme *(SnackWell's),* 2 pieces, .9 oz. 19.0
mint sandwich, chocolate-covered *(Mystic Mint),* .6-oz. piece.....11.0
molasses:
   (Grandma's Big Homestyle), 1.4-oz. piece 29.0
   3½"–4"-diam. piece, 1.1 oz...23.6
oat graham *(Carr's Hob Nobs),* 2 pieces, 1 oz. 19.0
oatmeal:
   (Barbara's Crisp Old Fashioned), .6-oz. piece.......................11.0
   (Keebler Country Style), 2 pieces, .8 oz. 17.0
   (Murray Sugar Free), 3 pieces, 1.1 oz. 20.0
   plain or iced *(Nabisco* Family Favorites), .6-oz. piece 12.0

Cookie, oatmeal *(cont.)*
 snap *(Westbrae Natural)*, 3 pieces, 1.1 oz.............................20.0
oatmeal raisin:
 (Estee), 4 pieces, 1 oz. 19.0
 (Grandma's Big Homestyle), 1.4-oz. piece 26.0
 (Grandma's Tiny Bites), 12 pieces.....................................39.0
 (Health Valley Fat Free), 3 pieces, 1.2 oz..........................24.0
 (Keebler Soft Batch), .6-oz. piece.....................................10.0
 (Keebler Soft Batch Homestyle), .9-oz. piece 20.0
 (Little Debbie Singles), 1.3 oz. 25.0
 (Pepperidge Farm Soft Baked), .9-oz. piece 17.0
 (Tofutti), 1 piece 20.0
 (Westbrae Natural), .9-oz. piece 18.0
orange creme wafer *(Real Torino)*, 2 pieces, .9 oz......................16.0
pastry puff, see specific cookie listings
peach-apricot *(Newtons Cobblers)*, .8-oz. piece 17.0
peanut *(Health Valley* Wheat/Dairy Free), .8-oz. piece 14.0
peanut caramel cluster, fudge *(Keebler Fudge Shoppe)*,
 .7-oz. piece 12.0
peanut, roasted, cocoa-coated *(Barbara's Nature's Choice)*,
 1.1-oz. bar 20.0
peanut butter:
 (Grandma's Big Homestyle), 1.4-oz. piece 22.0
 (Grandma's Mini), 9 pieces 21.0
 (Hain Cookie Jar Bits), 17 pieces, .5 oz...............................12.0
 (Murray Sugar Free), 8 pieces, 1 oz. 20.0
 (Tofutti), 1 piece 18.0
 chip *(SnackWell's* Bite Size), 13 pieces, 1 oz. 20.0
 chocolate chip *(Grandma's* Big Homestyle), 1.4-oz. piece 23.0
 cream wafer *(Estee)*, 5 pieces 22.0
 cup *(Keebler Chips Deluxe)*, .6-oz. piece................................9.0
 fudge stick *(Keebler Fudge Shoppe)*, 3 pieces, 1 oz.............18.0
 nut *(Westbrae)*, .9-oz. piece 17.0
 patty *(Nutter Butter)*, 5 pieces 17.0
peanut butter sandwich:
 (Estee), 3 pieces, 1.1 oz..22.0
 (Grandma's), 5 pieces 28.0
 (Nutter Butter), 2 pieces, 1 oz. 19.0
 (Nutter Butter Bites), 10 pieces 20.0
 .5-oz. piece 9.2
 chocolate *(Nutter Butter)*, 2 pieces, 1 oz..............................18.0

(Peek Freans Nice), 4 pieces, 1.2 oz. 25.0
pfeffernuss *(Stella D'oro)*, 3 pieces, 1 oz. 21.0
rainbow *(Beigel's)*, 1.2-oz. piece 15.0
raisin, soft type, .5-oz. piece 10.2
raisin biscuit *(Keebler Golden Fruit)*, .7-oz. piece 15.0
raspberry:
    (Fig Newtons Fat Free), 2 pieces, 1 oz. 23.0
    (Health Valley Jumbo Fat Free), .9-oz. piece 19.0
    (Pepperidge Farm Spritzers), 5 pieces, 1.1 oz. 21.0
    vanilla *(Westbrae Natural)*, .9-oz. piece 17.0
sandwich (see also specific listings):
    (Estee Original), 3 pieces, 1.1 oz. 24.0
    (Frito-Lay Merengue), 3 pieces, 1 oz. 21.0
    (Frito-Lay Suplex), 3 pieces, 1.1 oz. 22.0
shortbread:
    (Barbara's Crisp Traditional), .6-oz. piece 10.0
    (Estee), 4 pieces, 1 oz. 22.0
    (Lorna Doone), 4 pieces, 1 oz. 19.0
    (Murray Sugar Free), 8 pieces, 1 oz. 20.0
    (Sandies Reduced Fat), .6-oz. piece 11.0
    (Sandies Simply Shortbread), .5-oz. piece 9.0
    (Walkers), .7-oz. piece 19.0
    (Walkers Triangles), 2 pieces, .7 oz. 12.0
    (Westbrae Natural Original), 3 pieces, 1.1 oz. 19.0
    .3-oz. piece 5.2
    almond *(Crookes & Hanson* English), .9-oz. piece ...13.0
    chocolate *(Westbrae)*, 4 pieces, 1.1 oz. 18.0
    with dark chocolate *(Walkers* Royal), 2 pieces, .9 oz. ...15.0
    fudge-striped *(Fudge Favorites)*, 3 pieces 21.0
    pecan *(Pecanz)*, .6-oz. piece 9.0
    pecan *(Sandies)*, .6-oz. piece 9.0
S'mores *(Hain* Cookie Jar Bits), 17 pieces, .5 oz. 12.0
S'mores *(Keebler Fudge Shoppe)*, 3 pieces, 1.2 oz. ...22.0
(Social Tea Biscuits), 6 pieces, 1 oz. 22.0
(Stella D'oro Continental Collection), 1 oz. 20.0
(Stella D'oro Angel Wings), 2 pieces, .9 oz. 13.0
(Stella D'oro Anginetti), 4 pieces, 1.1 oz. 23.0
(Stella D'oro Lady Stella Assortment), 3 pieces, 1 oz. ...19.0
(Stella D'oro Margherite Combination), 2 pieces, 1.1 oz. ...22.0
strawberry *(Fig Newtons* Fat Free), 2 pieces, 1 oz. 23.0

Cookie *(cont.)*
sugar:
   (Grandma's Tiny Bites), 12 pieces.................................38.0
   .5-oz. piece..10.2
   rainbow *(Keebler Cookie Stix),* 5 pieces, 1.2 oz. 23.0
sugar wafer:
   chocolate creme *(Keebler),* 3 pieces, 1.1 oz.......................18.0
   creme-filled *(Bisco),* 8 pieces, 1 oz. 21.0
   creme-filled or lemon *(Keebler),* 3 pieces, .9 oz..................19.0
   peanut butter creme *(Keebler),* 4 pieces, 1.1 oz.................18.0
   plain, lemon, strawberry, or vanilla *(Murray* Sugar Free),
      6 pieces, 1.1 oz...21.0
   strawberry or vanilla *(Grandma's),* 3 pieces......................23.0
strawberry *(Frito-Lay Piruetas),* 3 pieces, 1.1 oz. 22.0
tropical creme *(Peek Freans),* 2 pieces 20.0
tropical strawberry-kiwi *(Newtons),* 2 pieces......................19.0
vanilla:
   (Frito-Lay Emperador), 2 pieces, .9 oz. 18.0
   (Grandma's Mini), 9 pieces 22.0
   creme wafer *(Real Torino),* 2 pieces, .9 oz. 16.0
   strawberry wafer *(Estee),* 5 pieces 22.0
   thin *(Estee),* 4 pieces, 1 oz. 19.0
   wafer *(Estee),* 5 pieces 21.0
   wafer *(Murray* Sugar Free), 9 pieces, 1.1 oz. 23.0
   wafer *(Nilla),* 8 pieces, 1.1 oz. 21.0
   wafer *(Nilla* Reduced Fat), 8 pieces, 1 oz. 24.0
   wafer, chocolate *(Nilla* Reduced Fat), 8 pieces, 1 oz. 23.0
   wafer, golden *(Keebler),* 8 pieces, 1.1 oz........................20.0
   wafer, golden *(Keebler* Reduced Fat), 8 pieces, 1.1 oz. 25.0
   wafer, rainbow *(Keebler),* 8 pieces 20.0
vanilla sandwich:
   (Estee), 3 pieces, 1.1 oz. 25.0
   (Café Cremes), 2 pieces 22.0
   (Cameo), 1.9-oz. pkg...40.0
   (Cameo), 2 pieces, 1 oz. 21.0
   (Grandma's), 5 pieces 30.0
   (Grandma's Value Line), 3 pieces 32.0
   (Murray Sugar Free), 3 pieces, 1 oz. 21.0
   (Vienna Fingers), 2 pieces, 1 oz. 21.0
   (Vienna Fingers Reduced Fat), 2 pieces, 1 oz...................22.0
   creme-filled, .5-oz. piece..10.8

fudge *(Café Cremes)*, 2 pieces 27.0
fudge *(Grandma's* Value Line), 3 pieces 21.0
waffle sandwich, apricot-filled *(Carr's Petits Bijoux)*, 4 pieces,
1.1 oz. 21.0

Cookie, frozen or refrigerated:
(Pillsbury M&M's), ⅟₁₈ pkg..18.0
chocolate chip:
   (Nestlé Toll House/Nestlé Toll House Big Batch), 2 tbsp.,
    1.1-oz. piece 20.0
   (Nestlé Toll House 50% Reduced Fat), 2 tbsp.,
    1.2-oz. piece 23.0
   (Pillsbury), ⅟₁₈ pkg. 17.0
   (Pillsbury Ready-to-Bake Tray), ⅟₂₀ pkg. 15.0
   (Pillsbury One Step), ⅟₁₀ pkg..20.0
   .4-oz. piece* 8.2
   bar *(Nestlé Toll House)*, .9-oz. piece..............................16.0
   bar, walnut *(Nestlé Toll House)*, .9-oz. piece 14.0
   with walnuts *(Pillsbury)*, ⅟₁₈ pkg. 16.0
   and white fudge *(Nestlé Toll House)*, 2 tbsp.,
    1.2-oz. piece 21.0
chocolate chunk *(Nestlé Toll House)*, 2 tbsp., 1.2-oz. piece 22.0
oatmeal, .4-oz. piece* 7.9
peanut butter, .4-oz. piece* 6.9
peanut butter chocolate chip *(Nestlé Toll House)*, 2 tbsp.,
   1.2-oz. piece 19.0
rugalach *(Tofutti Better Than Cream Cheese)*, .75-oz. piece 14.0
sugar *(Pillsbury)*, 2 slices, ¼" 19.0
sugar, .4-oz. piece* 7.9
sugar bar *(Nestlé Toll House)*, .9-oz. piece 15.0
Cookie, mix, 2 pieces*, except as noted:
brownie, see "Brownie mix"
chocolate chip *(Arrowhead Mills/Arrowhead Mills* Wheat Free),
   1 piece* 16.0
chocolate chip *(Betty Crocker* Pouch).................................21.0
chocolate chunk, double *(Betty Crocker* Pouch) 21.0
chocolate peanut butter *(Betty Crocker* Pouch) 20.0
oatmeal *(Betty Crocker* Pouch) 22.0
oatmeal chocolate chip *(Betty Crocker* Pouch) 21.0
oatmeal raisin *(Arrowhead Mills)*, 1 piece* 16.0
peanut butter *(Betty Crocker* Pouch)...................................20.0
sugar *(Betty Crocker* Pouch)..22.0

Cookie crumbs (see also "Pie crust"):
chocolate:

    cookie *(Oreo)*, 2 tbsp..............................13.0

    cookie *(Oreo Crunchies)*, 2 tbsp.....................8.0

    wafer, 1 cup, 4 oz. 81.1

graham cracker:

    (Keebler), 3 tbsp..............................13.0

    (Nabisco), 2½ tbsp. 12.0

    1 cup, 3 oz...................................64.5

vanilla wafer, lower fat, 1 cup, 2.8 oz.....................6.1

Cookie topping, see "Chocolate topping"

Cookies and fruit spread *(Kraft Handi-Snacks Cookie Jammers),*

    1 unit, 1.3 oz................................26.0

Cooking sauce, see specific listings

Conch, see "Scungilli"

Coriander, fresh, raw:

9 plants 5

¼ cup..1

Coriander, dried:

leaf, 1 tbsp. 9

leaf, 1 tsp. 3

seed, 1 tbsp. 2.7

seed, 1 tsp. 1.0

Corkscrew pasta, plain, see "Pasta"

Corkscrew pasta dish, mix, about 1 cup*:

four-cheese sauce *(Pasta Roni)*.........................50.0

garlic sauce, creamy *(Pasta Roni)* 41.0

Corn, fresh, sweet:

golden:

    raw *(Dole)*, 1 medium ear, 3.2 oz......................18.0

    raw, untrimmed, 1 lb. 31.1

    boiled, drained, 1 baby ear, .3 oz....................2.0

    boiled, drained, kernels from 3.2-oz. ear...............17.1

    boiled, drained, kernels, 1 cup 41.2

white:

    raw, 1 large ear, 7¾"–9" long.......................27.2

    raw, 1 cup....................................29.3

    boiled, drained, kernels from 1 ear...................19.3

    boiled, drained, kernels, ½ cup.....................20.6

Corn, canned (see also "Hominy"):
kernels, golden:
    (Del Monte), ½ cup 18.0
    (Del Monte Supersweet No Sugar/No Salt), ½ cup 11.0
    (Del Monte Supersweet Vacuum Pack), ½ cup 13.0
    (Green Giant), ½ cup 18.0
    (Green Giant Niblets), ⅓ cup 16.0
    (Greene's Farm), ½ cup 15.0
    (Hain), ½ cup 14.0
    (S&W), ½ cup 14.0
    ½ cup 19.7
    vacuum pack, ½ cup 20.4
kernels, golden and white *(Del Monte* Supersweet), ½ cup 18.0
kernels, white:
    (Del Monte), ½ cup 11.0
    (Green Giant Shoepeg), ⅓ cup 16.0
    ½ cup 19.7
    vacuum pack, ½ cup 20.4
cream style:
    (Green Giant 8.5 oz.*,* ½ cup 21.0
    (Green Giant 14.75 oz.)*,* ½ cup 19.0
    golden *(Del Monte/Del Monte* No Salt), ½ cup 20.0
    golden *(Del Monte* Supersweet), ½ cup 14.0
    golden or white, 17-oz. can 87.4
    golden or white, 1 cup 46.4
    white *(Del Monte)*, ½ cup 21.0
with red and green peppers:
    (Del Monte Fiesta), ½ cup 12.0
    (Green Giant Mexicorn), ⅓ cup 14.0
    1 cup 41.2
Corn, freeze-dried *(AlpineAire)*, ½ cup 16.0
Corn, frozen:
on cob, sweet, white or yellow:
    (Freshlike 6/8/12/24 Ear Pkg.), 1 ear 18.0
    (Freshlike 3/4 Ear Pkg.), 1 ear 34.0
    (Green Giant Extra Sweet), 1 ear 22.0
    (Green Giant Nibblers), 2.15-oz. ear 14.0
    (Green Giant Niblets), 5-oz. ear 32.0
    (John Cope's), 1 ear 34.0
    (John Cope's Mini), 1 ear 18.0
    (Seneca), 4.4-oz. ear 29.0

Corn, frozen, on cob, sweet, white or yellow *(cont.)*

unprepared, kernels from 4.4-oz. ear	29.4
boiled, drained, kernels from 2.2-oz. ear	14.1

kernels, baby:

gold and white *(Birds Eye)*, ⅔ cup	15.0
white *(Birds Eye)*, ⅔ cup	22.0

kernels, golden:

(Birds Eye Sweet), ⅓ cup	17.0
(Birds Eye Tender Sweet), ⅓ cup	14.0
(Freshlike), ⅔ cup	19.0
(Green Giant Niblets), ⅔ cup	17.0
(Seabrook Farms), ⅔ cup	19.0
(Seneca), ⅔ cup	20.0

kernels, gold and white *(Freshlike)*, ⅔ cup 15.0

kernels, sweet, golden or white:

unprepared, 10-oz. pkg.	59.1
unprepared, ½ cup	17.1
boiled, drained, 10-oz. pkg.	55.3
boiled, drained, ½ cup	16.0

kernels, white *(Freshlike)*, ⅔ cup	14.0
kernels, white *(Green Giant* Shoepeg), ½ cup	14.0

in butter sauce:

(Birds Eye), ½ cup	23.0
(Green Giant Niblets), ⅔ cup	23.0
white *(Green Giant)*, ¾ cup	21.0

cream style *(Green Giant)*, ½ cup	23.0
in herb sauce *(Boston Market)*, 10-oz. pkg.	49.0

Corn, frozen, combination:

bean *(Birds Eye* Baby Corn Blend), 3 oz.	12.0
broccoli, carrots *(Birds Eye/Freshlike* Baby Corn Blend), ⅔ cup	11.0

Corn, pickled, in jar, baby, whole *(Haddon House)*,

3 pieces, 1 oz.	1.0

Corn bran, crude:

1 oz.	24.3
1 cup	65.1

Corn bread, see "Bread mix"

Corn chips, puffs, and similar snacks, 1 oz., except as noted:

(Barbara's Thangs Major Corn)	22.0
(Bugles Original), 1⅓ cups, 1.1 oz.	18.0
(Bugles Original Baked), 1½ cups, 1.1 oz.	23.0
(Corn Nuts Original), 1.7-oz. pkg.	34.0

(Corn Nuts Original), ⅓ cup..20.0
(Corn Nuts Original), .8-oz. pkg. 16.0
(Fritos King Size/Scoops).......................................16.0
(Fritos Original) 15.0
(Fritos Racerz Original) 14.0
(Funyuns)..18.0
(Little Bear Original)...15.0
(Little Bear Reduced Fat)..18.0
(Munchos) 16.0
barbecue:
    (Bugles Smokin BBQ), 1⅓ cups, 1.1 oz. 19.0
    (Corn Nuts), 1.7-oz. pkg...................................34.0
    (Corn Nuts), 1.3 cup...20.0
    (Fritos)..16.0
    honey *(Fritos* Texas Grill)..................................17.0
    honey *(Fritos Racerz)*..14.0
cheese:
    (Chee•tos X's & O's)..15.0
    (Chee•tos Zig Zags)...17.0
    (Little Bear Crunchitos), 1 cup, 1 oz. 17.0
    balls *(Planters Cheez Mania),* 1.75-oz. pkg. 23.0
    balls, puffed *(Chee•tos)*......................................15.0
    balls, white cheddar *(Planters Cheez Mania)*.........14.0
    chili *(Fritos)*...15.0
    curls *(Planters Cheez Mania)*.............................15.0
    curls *(Weight Watchers),* 1 pkg..........................10.0
    curls or crunchy *(Chee•tos)* 15.0
    hot *(Chee•tos* Flamin' Hot) 16.0
    hot *(Chee•tos* Hot Puff Rods)..............................15.0
    puffs *(Chee•tos)* 15.0
    puffs *(Chee•tos* Jumbo) 13.0
    puffs *(Barbara's* Bakes), 1½ cups, 1 oz. 13.0
    puffs *(Barbara's* Original), ¾ cup, 1 oz. 16.0
    puffs *(Boston's Cheez Bopps)* 17.0
    puffs *(Little Bear* Baked), 2 cups, 1.1 oz. 16.0
    puffs, cheddar *(Bearitos),* 2 cups, 1.1 oz. 16.0
    puffs, cheddar *(Bearitos* Lite), 2 cups, 1.1 oz. 22.0
    puffs, cheddar *(Little Bear* Lite), ¾ oz. 16.0
    puffs, cheddar *(Little Bear* Lite), 2 cups, 1.1 oz. 22.0
    jalapeño *(Barbara's),* ¾ cup, 1 oz...........................15.0
    onion *(Barbara's Onion Zings)*..............................17.0

Corn chips, puffs, and similar snacks *(cont.)*

chili and cheese *(Little Bear)*...15.0
chili con queso or nacho cheese *(Bugles)*, 1⅓ cups, 1.1 oz.......18.0
chili picante *(Corn Nuts)*, ⅓ cup...19.0
guacamole *(Harry's Rio Grande)*..20.0
hot *(Fritos Sabrositas* Flamin' Hot).....................................15.0
lime and chili *(Fritos Sabrositas)*..17.0
nacho cheese *(Corn Nuts)*, ⅓ cup...19.0
nacho cheese *(Fritos Racerz)*..14.0
nacho cheesy *(Little Bear* Reduced Fat)..................................17.0
pepperoni pizza *(Corn Nuts)*, 1.7-oz. pkg................................33.0
pepperoni pizza *(Corn Nuts)*, ⅓ cup.....................................20.0
ranch:
    (Bugles), 1⅓ cups, 1.1 oz..18.0
    (Corn Nuts), 1.7-oz. pkg...33.0
    (Corn Nuts), ⅓ cup..19.0
    onion *(Barbara's Onion Zings)*.....................................18.0
    wild *(Barbara's Thangs)*..21.0
salsa, sassy *(Barbara's Thangs)*...21.0
sour cream and onion *(Corn Nuts)*, ⅓ cup...............................19.0
tortilla:
    (Air Crisps Original)...20.0
    (Doritos Taco Supreme/Toasted Corn)..........................18.0
    (Garden of Eatin' White/Yellow Chips/Mini Corns)..............19.0
    (Harry's Rio Grande)..19.0
    (Little Bear)...18.0
    (Santitas Restaurant Style/100% White Corn)...................19.0
    (Tostitos Baked Original/Bite Size)..............................24.0
    (Tostitos Bite Size)...17.0
    (Tostitos Crispy Rounds)...18.0
    (Tostitos Restaurant Style).......................................19.0
    (Tostitos Santa Fe Gold)..19.0
    (Tostitos Wow Original)...20.0
    baked:
        (Boston's), 13 chips, 1.1 oz................................23.0
        regular, hot and smoky chipotle, or yogurt and green onion
            (Garden of Eatin' California Bakes)...................23.0
        roasted sesame *(Garden of Eatin' California Bakes)*..........20.0
        salsa *(Garden of Eatin' California Bakes Sunny Salsa)*......21.0
    barbecue *(Doritos* Smoky Red)..................................21.0
    black bean, regular or with jalapeño *(Garden of Eatin')*.........18.0

blue corn *(Barbara's/Barbara's No Salt)*, 1.1 oz....................16.0
blue corn *(Garden of Eatin'/Garden of Eatin' Red Hot
    Blues)* 18.0
blue corn *(Garden of Eatin' Little Soy Blues)* 18.0
blue corn *(Harry's Rio Grande)* 19.0
blue corn *(Little Bear)*...15.0
blue corn, sesame or sunflower *(Garden of Eatin' Sesame
    Blues/Sunny Blues)*...16.0
blue, white, or yellow corn *(Bearitos/Bearitos Unsalted)*.......18.0
cheddar quesadilla *(Tostitos Baked Bite Size)* 22.0
chili and lime *(Garden of Eatin')*...20.0
hot *(Doritos Flamin' Hot)*..17.0
jalapeño cheddar *(Doritos 3D's)*...20.0
multigrain *(Garden of Eatin' Garden Grains)* 18.0
nacho cheese *(Air Crisps)*...21.0
nacho cheese *(Doritos/Doritos 3D's Cheesier)* 17.0
nacho cheese, spicy *(Doritos)*..18.0
ranch *(Doritos/Doritos 3D's Cooler Ranch)*.............................18.0
red corn *(Garden of Eatin' Red Chips)* 18.0
red corn, salsa *(Garden of Eatin' Salsa Reds)* 17.0
picante *(Doritos Baja)*...18.0
salsa *(Barbara's Pinta)*...19.0
salsa *(Doritos Salsa Verde)* 20.0
salsa and cream cheese *(Tostitos Baked Bite Size)* 21.0
sour cream *(Doritos Sonic)*...17.0

Corn chips and dip:
chili dip *(Fritos)*, ½ kit 36.0
sloppy Joe dip *(Fritos)*, ½ kit 38.0
tortillas, salsa con queso dip *(Tostitos)*, 1 pkg. 45.0
tortillas, salsa dip *(Tostitos)*, 1 pkg. 43.0
Corn flake crumbs *(Kellogg's)*, 2 tbsp. 9.0
Corn flour:
whole-grain, white or yellow, 1 oz. 21.8
whole-grain, white or yellow, 1 cup 89.9
masa, white or yellow, 1 oz...21.6
masa, white or yellow, 1 cup 86.9
Corn fritter, frozen *(Mrs. Paul's)*, 1 piece 15.0
Corn fritter mix *(Casbah Perfect)*, 2 fritters* 25.0
Corn grits, dry:
(Quaker Instant), 1 pkt. 22.0
white *(Arrowhead Mills)*, ¼ cup..30.0

Corn grits *(cont.)*
white or yellow, quick:
  (Quaker Quick Hominy Grits), ¼ cup 29.0
  1 cup 124.2
  1 tbsp. 7.7
  prepared with water, 1 cup 31.5
  prepared with water, ¾ cup 23.7
yellow *(Arrowhead Mills)*, ¼ cup 29.0
bacon bits, imitation *(Quaker* Instant), 1-oz. pkt. 22.0
bacon bits, imitation, and cheddar flavor *(Quaker* Instant),
  1-oz. pkt. 20.0
butter flavor, American cheese flavor, imitation ham bits, or
  cheese flavor with imitation sausage bits *(Quaker* Instant),
  1-oz. pkt. 21.0
Corn relish *(Green Giant)*, 1 tbsp. 5.0
Corn soufflé, frozen *(Stouffer's)*, ½ cup 21.0
Corn syrup, dark or light:
(Karo), 2 tbsp. 31.0
1 cup 251.2
1 tbsp. 15.3
Cornichon, see "Pickle"
Cornish hen, without added ingredients 0
Cornmeal (see also "Corn flour" and "Polenta"):
(Goya Fine), 3 tbsp. 23.0
blue *(Arrowhead Mills)*, ¼ cup 25.0
masa harina *(Quaker)*, ¼ cup 24.0
white:
  (Hodgson Mill), scant ¼ cup 22.0
  buttermilk, self-rising *(Aunt Jemima* Mix), 3 tbsp. 18.0
  self-rising *(Aunt Jemima)*, 3 tbsp. 20.0
  self-rising *(Aunt Jemima* Mix Bolted), 3 tbsp. 19.0
white or yellow, self-rising, 1 cup 85.7
white or yellow, whole-grain, 1 cup 93.8
yellow:
  (Arrowhead Mills), ¼ cup 27.0
  (Hodgson Mill), scant ¼ cup 28.0
  (Hodgson Mill Organic), ¼ cup 22.0
  self-rising *(Aunt Jemima* Mix), 3 tbsp. 19.0
  self-rising *(Hodgson Mill)*, ¼ cup 21.0
Cornstarch:
(Argo/Kingsford), 1 tbsp. 7.0

(Hodgson Mill), 2 tsp. 9.0
Cottonseed flour:
partially defatted, 1 cup...38.1
partially defatted, 1 tbsp...2.0
lowfat, 1 oz. 10.2
Cottonseed kernels:
roasted, 1 cup 32.6
roasted, 1 tbsp...2.2
Cottonseed meal, partially defatted, 1 oz. 10.9
Country gravy mix *(Loma Linda Gravy Quik),* 1 tbsp. 4.0
Couscous:
dry:
   (Arrowhead Mills), ¼ cup.......................................35.0
   (Fantastic Foods), ¼ cup.......................................43.0
   (Frieda's), ¼ cup 43.0
   (Marrakesh Express), 2 scoops, 2.2 oz. 45.0
   (Near East), ⅓ cup 46.0
   1 cup 134.0
   whole-wheat *(Fantastic Foods),* ¼ cup.................45.0
cooked, 1 cup 122.6
cooked, dried, regular or whole-wheat *(AlpineAire),* ½ cup........20.0
Couscous dish, mix:
almondine *(Nile Spice),* 1 cont. 37.0
broccoli *(Near East),* 2 oz. 42.0
cranberry *(Marrakesh Express* Calypso), ⅓ cup, 1 cup* 42.0
garlic:
   and olive oil *(Near East),* 2 oz. 41.0
   with red pepper *(Fantastic Foods* Healthy Complements),
    ⅓ cup 42.0
   roasted, and olive oil *(Casbah),* ¼ cup, about 1 cup* 38.0
   roasted, and olive oil *(Near East),* 1 cont. 59.0
   roasted, and olive oil *(Nile Spice* Chef Express), 1 cont........59.0
lemon-spinach *(Casbah),* ¼ cup, about 1 cup* 40.0
lentil curry *(Marrakesh Express),* ⅓ cup, 1 cup* 35.0
lentil curry *(Nile Spice),* 1 cont. 36.0
mango salsa *(Marrakesh Express),* ⅓ cup, 1 cup* 40.0
minestrone *(Nile Spice),* 1 cont. 34.0
mushroom, wild *(Marrakesh Express),* ⅓ cup, 1 cup* 38.0
mushroom, wild forest *(Casbah),* ¼ cup, about 1 cup* 35.0
nutted, with currants and spice *(Casbah),* ¼ cup, about 1 cup* 42.0
olive-garlic *(Marrakesh Express),* ⅓ cup, 1 cup* 34.0

Couscous dish, mix *(cont.)*
Parmesan *(Near East),* 2 oz. 41.0
Parmesan *(Nile Spice),* 1 cont. 34.0
sesame-ginger *(Marrakesh Express),* ⅓ cup, 1 cup* 36.0
Thai *(Fantastic Foods* Healthy Complements Royal), ⅓ cup.......41.0
tomato, sun-dried *(Marrakesh Express),* ⅓ cup, 1 cup* 36.0
tomato lentil *(Near East),* 2 oz. 42.0
toasted:
   garlic, roasted *(Marrakesh Express* Grande), ½ pkg.,
     1 cup*...51.0
   onion, toasted *(Marrakesh Express* Grande), ½ pkg.,
     1 cup*...52.0
   red pepper, roasted *(Marrakesh Express* Grande), ½ pkg.,
     1 cup*...52.0
   tomato, sun-dried *(Marrakesh Express* Grande), ½ pkg.,
     1 cup*...51.0
vegetable *(Marrakesh Express* Lucky 7), ⅓ cup, 1 cup* 38.0
Couscous salad *(Cedarlane),* ½ cup.................................21.0
Couscous wrap, see "Vegetable pocket/wrap"
Cowpeas:
(Frieda's Black-Eyed Peas), ⅓ cup, 3 oz. 21.0
immature:
   raw, 1 cup..27.4
   boiled, drained, 1 cup...33.5
young pods, with seeds:
   raw, 1 pod 1.1
   raw, 1 cup..8.9
   boiled, drained, 1 cup...6.7
leafy tips:
   raw, 1 leaf..1
   raw, chopped, 1 cup...1.7
   boiled, drained, chopped, 1 cup...1.5
mature:
   raw, 1 cup..99.6
   boiled, 1 cup..34.7
   common, raw, 1 cup 100.3
   common, raw, 1 tbsp. 6.3
   common, boiled, 1 cup...35.7
Cowpeas, canned, see "Black-eyed peas"
Cowpeas, frozen:
unprepared, 10-oz. pkg..71.4

unprepared, 1 cup...40.2
boiled, drained, 1 cup 40.4
Cowpeas, catjang, see "Catjang"
Crab, meat only, 4 oz.:
Alaska king, without added ingredients...0
blue, without added ingredients 0
Dungeness, raw, 5¾-oz. crab 1.2
Dungeness, boiled, poached or steamed, 4.5 oz...................1.2
Crab, canned:
(Orleans Fancy White), 2 oz. 1.0
(Reese), ½ cup 0
"Crab," imitation, frozen or refrigerated:
  from surimi, 1 oz..2.9
Crab cake, see "Crab entree"
Crab entree, frozen:
cake:
  (Chincoteague Maryland Style), 4-oz. cake 28.0
  (Van de Kamp's), 1 cake...20.0
  deviled *(Mrs. Paul's),* 1 cake 17.0
  mini *(Mrs. Paul's),* 6 cakes...22.0
  mini *(Van de Kamp's,* 4 pieces 31.0
  unbreaded *(Chincoteague* Maryland Style), 1 cake, 1 oz........8.0
cheese and *(Mrs. Paul's* Poppers), 4 pieces.........................27.0
cheese and *(Van de Kamp's* Bites), 4 pieces........................27.0
nuggets, breaded *(Chincoteague* Cocktail), 3 oz. 21.0
nuggets, unbreaded *(Chincoteague* Cocktail), 6 pieces, 3 oz.......8.0
Crabapple, fresh:
(Frieda's), 5 oz..28.0
with peel, sliced, 1 cup 21.9
Cracker:
animal, see "Cookie"
bacon *(Flavor Crisps),* 15 pieces..19.0
baked *(Munch 'ems* Original), 35 pieces, 1.1 oz.....................21.0
baked, seasoned *(Snax Stix),* 21 pieces, 1 oz. 18.0
butter/butter flavor:
  (Harvest Bakery Country), 2 pieces, .6 oz. 9.0
  (Hi Ho), 4 pieces, .5 oz...8.0
  (Hi Ho Reduced Fat), 5 pieces, .5 oz. 10.0
  (Keebler Club), 4 pieces, .5 oz...9.0
  (Keebler Club Reduced Fat), 5 pieces, .6 oz. 12.0
  (Keebler Club Reduced Sodium), 4 pieces, .5 oz. 9.0

Cracker, butter, butter flavor *(cont.)*

   (Ritz Original/Low Sodium), 5 pieces, .6 oz. 10.0
   (Ritz Reduced Fat/Whole Wheat), 5 pieces 11.0
   (Ritz Air Crisps), 24 pieces, 1.1 oz. 22.0
   (Toasteds Butter Crisp), 5 pieces, .6 oz. 10.0
   (Town House), 5 pieces, .6 oz. 9.0
   (Town House Reduced Fat), 6 pieces, .5 oz. 11.0
   (Town House Reduced Sodium), 5 pieces, .6 oz. 10.0
  (Carr's Distinctive Flavor Assortment), 3 pieces, .5 oz. 10.0
  (Carr's Cocktail Croissants), 22 pieces, 1.1 oz. 21.0
  (Carr's Croissant), 3 pieces, .5 oz. 10.0
  cheese:
   (Barbara's Bites), 26 pieces, 1.1 oz. 24.0
   (The Big Cheez-It), 13 pieces, 1.1 oz. 16.0
   (Cheese Nips), 1.1 oz. 18.0
   (Cheese Nips Reduced Fat), 31 pieces, 1.1 oz. 21.0
   (Cheese Nips Air Crisps Original), 32 pieces, 1.1 oz. 21.0
   (Cheez-It Big Crunch), ¾ cup, 1.1 oz. 20.0
   (Cheez-It Original), 27 pieces, 1.1 oz. 16.0
   (Cheez-It Reduced Fat), 29 pieces, 1.1 oz. 20.0
   (Cheez-It Chip-Its), 29 pieces, 1.1 oz. 18.0
   (Tid-Bit), 32 pieces, 1.1 oz. 16.0
   baked *(Cheez-It),* ½ cup, 1.1 oz. 21.0
   baked, double cheese *(Cheez-It),* ¾ cup, 1.1 oz. 19.0
   bite-size, 1 cup, 2.2 oz. 36.1
   cheddar *(Better Cheddars* Reduced Fat), 24 pieces,
    1.1 oz. 19.0
   cheddar *(Better Cheddars/Better Cheddars* Low Sodium),
    22 pieces, 1.1 oz. 18.0
   cheddar *(Carr's),* 3 pieces, .5 oz. 8.0
   cheddar *(Cheese Nips),* 1.65-oz. pkg. 29.0
   cheddar *(Cheese Nips),* 29 pieces 18.0
   cheddar *(Pepperidge Farm Goldfish),* 55 pieces, 1.1 oz. 19.0
   cheddar *(Pepperidge Farm Goldfish* 30% Less Sodium),
    60 pieces, 1.1 oz. 18.0
   cheddar *(Sportz),* 40 pieces 19.0
   cheddar, baked *(Munch 'ems),* 39 pieces, 1.1 oz. 19.0
   cheddar, baked, zesty *(Snax Stix),* 20 pieces, 1.1 oz. 17.0
   cheddar, extra, or pizza *(Cheese Nips),* 27 pieces 19.0
   cheddar, white *(Cheez-It),* 26 pieces, 1.1 oz. 18.0
   hot and spicy *(Cheez-It),* 26 pieces, 1.1 oz. 17.0

nacho *(Cheez-It)*, 1.5-oz. pkg. 26.0
Parmesan *(Pepperidge Farm Goldfish)*, 60 pieces, 1.1 oz.....19.0
sesame *(Twigs)*, 15 pieces, 1.1 oz. 17.0
Swiss *(Flavor Crisps Swiss Cheese)*, 15 pieces 18.0
Swiss *(Nabisco)*, 15 pieces, 1 oz. 18.0
zesty *(SnackWell's)*, 38 pieces, 1.1 oz.............................23.0
cheese sandwich:
    (Ritz), 1.4-oz. pkg...22.0
    (Ritz Bits), 1.75-oz. pkg..28.0
    (Ritz Bits), 14 pieces, 1.1 oz...................................17.0
    bacon cheddar *(Chee•tos)*, 1 pkg. 25.0
    cheese on cheese *(Little Debbie)*, .9 oz. 15.0
    cheese on cheese *(Little Debbie Singles)*, 1.4 oz. 21.0
    cheddar *(Carr's Cocktail Cheddars)*, 22 pieces, 1.1 oz. 17.0
    cheddar *(Chee•tos)*, 1 pkg...................................23.0
    cheddar *(Combos)*, 1.7-oz. bag.............................31.0
    cheddar *(Keebler Club)*, 1.3-oz. pkg........................20.0
    cheddar, real *(Cheese Nips)*, 1.4-oz. pkg.................22.0
    cheddar, white or golden, bites *(Hain)*, 22 pieces, 1.1 oz......23.0
    jalapeño *(Doritos)*, 1 pkg....................................26.0
    nacho *(Doritos Cheesier)*, 1 pkg..........................25.0
    peanut butter *(Cheese Nips)*, 1.4-oz. pkg................23.0
    peanut butter *(Keebler)*, 1.4-oz. pkg......................22.0
    peanut butter *(Little Debbie)*, .9 oz........................16.0
    peanut butter *(Little Debbie Singles)*, 1.4 oz. 22.0
    peanut butter *(Nabisco)*, 1.4-oz. pkg......................22.0
    peanut butter *(Peter Pan)*, 1 pkg. 23.0
    peanut butter, ¼-oz. piece.....................................4.0
    toast *(Nabisco)*, 1.4-oz. pkg. 23.0
(Chicken in a Biskit), 12 pieces, 1.1 oz. 17.0
corn bread *(Harvest Bakery)*, 2 pieces, .6 oz. 11.0
cracked pepper *(Estee)*, 18 pieces, 1 oz. 24.0
cracked pepper *(Health Valley Low Fat)*, 5 pieces, .5 oz. 10.0
cream cheese and chive *(Little Debbie)*, .9 oz.................17.0
crispbread, rye, .4-oz. piece...8.2
flatbread:
    (Real Torino Classical), 2 pieces, .9 oz....................16.0
    all varieties *(Tofutti Soy Lavasch)*, .5 oz...................10.0
    rosemary *(Real Torino)*, 2 pieces, .9 oz....................19.0
    sesame or crushed pepper *(Real Torino)*, 2 pieces, .9 oz. 18.0
garlic, roasted *(Health Valley Low Fat)*, 10 pieces, .5 oz.............10.0

Cracker *(cont.)*

garlic, roasted, and herb *(Barbara's* Wafer Crisps), 3 pieces,
  .5 oz. 12.0
garlic, sesame, or seeds and spice *(Burns & Ricker* Crispini),
  5 pieces, 1.1 oz. 20.0
golden *(Estee)*, 10 pieces, 1 oz. 28.0
graham, see "Cookie"
herb:
  (Hain), 11 pieces, 1.1 oz. 23.0
  garden *(Health Valley* Low Fat), 6 pieces, .5 oz. 10.0
  Italian *(Harvest Crisp)*, 15 pieces, 1.1 oz. 22.0
lavasch, see "flatbread," above
matzo:
  1 oz. 23.7
  egg, 1 oz. 22.3
  egg and onion, 1 oz. 21.9
  whole-wheat, 1 oz. 22.4
melba:
  rounds, 1 cup, 1.2 oz. 25.3
  rounds, salt-free, 1 cup, 1.2 oz. 23.0
  rye or pumpernickel, .2-oz. piece 3.9
  wheat, .2-oz. piece 3.8
milk, .4-oz. piece 7.7
multigrain:
  (Harvest Bakery), 2 pieces, .6 oz. 10.0
  (Wheat Thins), 17 pieces, 1.1 oz. 21.0
  five-grain *(Harvest Crisp)*, 13 pieces, 1.1 oz. 23.0
  seven-grain *(Wheatables)*, 12 pieces, 1.1 oz. 20.0
nori maki *(Eden)*, 15 pieces, 1.1 oz. 24.0
oat, baked *(Nabisco* Thins), 1.1 oz. 20.0
onion:
  (Toasteds), 5 pieces, .6 oz. 10.0
  French *(Barbara's* Wafer Crisps), 3 pieces, .5 oz. 12.0
  French *(Health Valley* Low Fat), 6 pieces, .5 oz. 10.0
  French *(SnackWell's)*, 38 pieces, 1.1 oz. 23.0
  French *(Triscuit* Thin Crisps), 14 pieces, 1 oz. 20.0
oyster/soup:
  (Hain), 36 pieces, .5 oz. 13.0
  1 cup, 1.6 oz. 32.2
peanut butter sandwich (see also "cheese sandwich," above):
  (Ritz), 1.4-oz. pkg. 24.0

(Ritz Bits), 1.75-oz. pkg....................................29.0
(Ritz Bits), 14 pieces, 1.1 oz. 18.0
toast *(Chee•tos* Golden Toast), 1 pkg............25.0
toast *(Keebler),* 1.4-oz. pkg............................23.0
toast *(Little Debbie* Singles), .9 oz. 16.0
toast *(Peter Pan),* 1 pkg................................23.0
(Pepperidge Farm Goldfish Original), 55 pieces, 1.1 oz. 19.0
pizza *(Pepperidge Farm Goldfish),* 55 pieces, 1.1 oz.............19.0
pizza *(Sportz),* 39 pieces 19.0
ranch *(SnackWell's),* 38 pieces, 1.1 oz. 28.0
ranch, baked *(Munch 'ems),* 33 pieces, 1 oz....................21.0
rice, brown:
   (Eden), 5 pieces, 1.1 oz............................22.0
   sesame *(San-J),* 5 pieces, 1 oz. 19.0
   sesame, black *(San-J),* 5 pieces, 1 oz. 17.0
   tamari *(San-J),* 6 pieces, 1.1 oz. 26.0
   wafers, all varieties *(Westbrae),* 7 pieces, .5 oz. 11.0
rich *(Hain),* 11 pieces, 1.1 oz.........................18.0
rusk, .4-oz. piece...7.2
rye *(Triscuit* Deli-Style), 7 pieces 22.0
rye sandwich, with cheese, ¼-oz. piece............4.3
rye wafer, .4-oz. piece...................................8.8
saltine:
   (Hain), 5 pieces, .5 oz. 13.0
   (Krispy Fat Free), 5 pieces, .5 oz. 11.0
   (Krispy/Krispy Unsalted Tops), 5 pieces, .5 oz. 10.0
   (Premium Fat Free), 5 pieces, .5 oz............12.0
   (Premium Original/Unsalted Tops/Low Sodium/Multi-grain),
     5 pieces, .5 oz...................................10.0
   (Zesta), 5 pieces, .5 oz. 10.0
   (Zesta Fat Free/Reduced Sodium), 5 pieces, .5 oz. 11.0
   (Zesta Unsalted Tops), 5 pieces, .5 oz. 10.0
   cheddar, mild *(Krispy),* 5 pieces, .5 oz.......10.0
   multigrain *(Premium),* 5 pieces, .5 oz.........10.0
   whole-wheat *(Krispy),* 5 pieces, .5 oz.........10.0
sesame:
   (Hain), 11 pieces, 1.1 oz. 19.0
   (Health Valley Low Fat), 5 pieces, .5 oz. 10.0
   (Toasteds), 5 pieces, .6 oz......................10.0
   toasted *(Barbara's* Wafer Crisps), 3 pieces, .5 oz. 11.0
sesame cheese stick *(Flavor Crisps Twigs),* 15 pieces................17.0

Cracker *(cont.)*

sesame and onion *(Carr's Monterey)*, 3 pieces, .5 oz. 9.0

sesame spring vegetable *(Carr's Cocktail Croissants)*, 22 pieces,
1.1 oz. 17.0

(Sociables), 7 pieces, .5 oz. 9.0

soda/water:

    (Carr's Assorted Biscuits for Cheese), 3 pieces, .6 oz. 12.0

    (Carr's Table Water), 5 pieces, .6 oz. 13.0

    (Crown Pilot), .6-oz. piece 13.0

    (Royal Lunch), .4-oz. piece 8.0

    (Zesta Export), 3 pieces, .5 oz. 10.0

    cracked pepper *(SnackWell's)*, 5 pieces, .5 oz. 10.0

    cracked pepper, garlic and herb, or toasted sesame *(Carr's*
      Table Water), 5 pieces, .6 oz. 13.0

    poppy and sesame seed *(Carr's)*, 4 pieces, .6 oz. 9.0

soup and oyster:

    (Krispy), 17 pieces, .5 oz. 11.0

    (Premium), 23 pieces, .5 oz. 11.0

    (Zesta), 45 pieces, .5 oz. 9.0

sour cream and onion *(Ritz Air Crisps)*, 23 pieces, 1.1 oz. 22.0

sour cream and onion, baked *(Munch 'ems)*, 28 pieces,
1.1 oz. 19.0

tomato, sun-dried, and basil *(Barbara's* Wafer Crisps), 3 pieces,
.5 oz. 12.0

(Uneeda), 2 pieces, .5 oz. 11.0

vegetable:

    (Flavor Crisps Vegetable Thins), 14 pieces, 1.1 oz. 19.0

    (Hain), 11 pieces, 1.1 oz. 19.0

    (Health Valley Bruschetta Low Fat), 6 pieces, .5 oz. 10.0

    garden *(Harvest Crisp)*, 15 pieces, 1.1 oz. 22.0

    roasted *(Carr's Monterey)*, 3 pieces, .5 oz. 10.0

wheat:

    (Barbara's Lite Rite Rounds), 5 pieces, .5 oz. 12.0

    (Carr's Wheatolo English Biscuits), .5-oz. piece 10.0

    (Estee), 17 pieces, 1 oz. 18.0

    (SnackWell's), 5 pieces, .5 oz. 11.0

    (Toasteds), 5 pieces, .6 oz. 11.0

    (Toasteds Reduced Fat), 5 pieces, .5 oz. 10.0

    (Triscuit Original/Low Sodium), 7 pieces, 1.1 oz. 22.0

    (Triscuit Reduced Fat), 8 pieces, 1.2 oz. 24.0

    (Triscuit Thin Crisps), 15 pieces, 1.1 oz. 21.0

(Waverly), 5 pieces, .5 oz. 10.0
(Wheat Thins Big), 11 pieces, 1.1 oz. 20.0
(Wheat Thins Low Sodium), 16 pieces, 1 oz. 20.0
(Wheat Thins Original), 16 pieces, .8 oz. 19.0
(Wheat Thins Reduced Fat), 18 pieces, 1 oz. 21.0
(Wheat Thins Air Crisps Original), 24 pieces, 1 oz. 21.0
(Wheatables Original), 12 pieces, 1.1 oz. 19.0
(Wheatables Reduced Fat), 13 pieces, 1 oz. 21.0
(Wheatsworth), 5 pieces, .6 oz. 10.0
all flavors *(Barbara's Wheatines)*, ½"-square, .5 oz. 10.0
baked, hearty *(Snax Stix)*, 20 pieces, 1.1 oz. 18.0
hearty or savory *(Carr's Monterey)*, 3 pieces, .5 oz. 9.0
herb, garden *(Triscuit)*, 6 pieces, 1 oz. 20.0
honey *(Wheatables)*, 12 pieces, 1.1 oz. 20.0
ranch *(Wheat Thins)*, 14 pieces 19.0
ranch *(Wheat Thins Air Crisps)*, 23 pieces, 1 oz. 21.0
savory *(Monterey)*, 3 pieces, .5 oz. 9.0
stoned *(Health Valley* Low Fat), 5 pieces, .5 oz. 10.0
whole *(Carr's)*, 2 pieces, .6 oz. 11.0
whole *(Hain)*, 11 pieces, 1.1 oz. 24.0
whole *(Health Valley* Low Fat), 6 pieces, .5 oz. 10.0
wheat sandwich:
   cheddar *(Keebler)*, 1.3-oz. pkg. 18.0
   cheese, ¼-oz. piece 4.1
   peanut butter, ¼-oz. piece 3.8
zweiback *(Nabisco)*, .3-oz. piece 6.0
Cracker crumbs and meal:
crushed:
   butter flavor, 1 cup 43.9
   cheese, 1 cup 41.9
   crispbread, rye, 1 cup 45.2
   rye wafer, 1 cup 49.0
   saltine or oyster, 1 cup 50.1
   wheat, 1 cup 53.9
graham cracker, see "Cookie crumbs"
meal *(Nabisco)*, ¼ cup 22.0
meal, 1 cup 93.0
Cranberries, fresh:
whole:
   (Dole), ½ cup 6.0
   (Ocean Spray), ½ cup 7.0

Cranberries, whole *(cont.)*
1 cup	12.0
chopped, 1 cup	13.9

Cranberries, canned:
whole *(Ocean Spray)*, ¼ cup	28.0
jellied *(Ocean Spray)*, ¼ cup	27.0
jellied *(S&W)*, ¼ cup	26.0
sauce *(R.W. Knudsen* Natural), 1 tbsp.	6.0

Cranberries, dried:
(Frieda's), ⅓ cup, 1.4 oz.	28.0
(Sonoma), ⅓ cup, 1.4 oz.	29.0
sweetened *(Craisins)*, ⅓ cup	33.0
sweetened *(Sunsweet Cranberry Fruitlings)*, ⅓ cup, 1.4 oz.	34.0

Cranberry beans:
mature, raw, 1 cup	117.1
mature, boiled, 1 cup	43.3
canned, with liquid, 1 cup	39.3

Cranberry chutney, see "Chutney"

Cranberry juice, 8 fl. oz.:
(After the Fall Cape Cod)	24.0
(R.W. Knudsen Just Cranberry)	14.0
concentrate* *(R.W. Knudsen)*	13.0
nectar *(R.W. Knudsen)*	38.0

Cranberry juice blend, 8 fl. oz., except as noted:
(Rocket Juice Cranberry Echinacea), 16 fl. oz.	57.0
apple:	
(Dole)	30.0
(Juicy Juice)	30.0
(Ocean Spray Granny Smith)	32.0
(Snapple), 12 fl. oz.	51.0
grape, Concord *(Ocean Spray)*	39.0
grapefruit *(After the Fall* Ruby of the Cape)	29.0
kiwi *(After the Fall* Ruby of the Cape)	26.0
lime, Key *(Ocean Spray)*	35.0
orange *(After the Fall* Ruby of the Cape)	28.0
raspberry *(After the Fall* Cranberry Meets Raspberry)	23.0
raspberry, Pacific *(Ocean Spray)*	34.0
strawberry *(After the Fall* Ruby of the Cape)	26.0

Cranberry juice concentrate *(R.W. Knudsen)*, 8 fl. oz.* | 13.0

Cranberry juice drink, 8 fl. oz.:
(Crystal Light Cranberry Breeze)	0

cocktail:
   (Mott's)..37.0
   (Ocean Spray)................................34.0
   (Ocean Spray Plus).........................41.0
   (Ocean Spray Light) 10.0
   frozen*...35.0
mix* *(Crystal Light Cranberry Breeze)* 0
nectar *(Santa Cruz Organic)*....................27.0
Cranberry juice drink blend, 8 fl. oz.:
(Mott's) 43.0
apple *(Cranapple)*................................41.0
cherry *(Ocean Spray Cran•Cherry)*............39.0
currant *(Ocean Spray Cran•Currant)* 33.0
grape *(Ocean Spray Cran•Grape)* 41.0
grape *(Ocean Spray Cran•Grape Light)* 10.0
hibiscus tea *(R. W. Knudsen)*...................30.0
lemonade *(R. W. Knudsen)*......................29.0
mango *(Ocean Spray Cran•Mango)*.............33.0
mango *(Ocean Spray Cran•Mango Light)* 10.0
punch *(Tropicana Twister)*, 10 fl. oz............43.0
raspberry:
   (Ocean Spray Cran•Raspberry) 36.0
   (Ocean Spray Cran•Raspberry Light) 10.0
   (R. W. Knudsen).............................36.0
   (Snapple)....................................29.0
   (Snapple Diet)..............................2.0
strawberry *(Ocean Spray Cran•Strawberry)*....36.0
tangerine *(Ocean Spray Cran•Tangerine)* 33.0
Cranberry sauce, see "Cranberries, canned"
Cranberry-orange relish, canned, 1 cup........127.1
Crayfish, without added ingredients...............0
Cream (see also "Crème fraîche"):
half-and-half:
   (Land O Lakes), 2 tbsp. 1.0
   (Parmalat), 2 tbsp. 1.0
   1 cup 10.4
   1 tbsp. 6
light, coffee or table, 1 cup 8.8
light, coffee or table, 1 tbsp. 6
medium (25% fat), 1 cup 8.3
medium (25% fat), 1 tbsp. 5

Cream *(cont.)*

sour, see "Cream, sour"

whipped topping, see "Cream topping"

whipping[1]:

    light, 1 cup 7.1

    light, 1 tbsp. 4

    heavy *(America's Choice)*, 1 tbsp. 1.0

    heavy, 1 cup 6.6

    heavy, 1 tbsp. 4

Cream, double, in jar *(Devon Cream Company English Double*

    Devon), 1 oz. 1.0

Cream, sour, 2 tbsp., except as noted:

(Breakstone's) 1.0

(Friendship) 1.0

(Knudsen Hampshire) 1.0

(Land O Lakes) 2.0

1 cup 9.8

reduced-fat:

    (Breakstone's Reduced Fat) 2.0

    (Friendship Light) 3.0

    (Knudsen Light) 2.0

    (Land O Lakes Light) 4.0

    1 cup 10.3

fat-free:

    (Breakstone's Free) 6.0

    (Friendship) 4.0

    (Knudsen Free) 6.0

    (Land O Lakes) 5.0

nondairy, 1 oz. 1.9

nondairy, 1 cup 15.2

Cream, sour, dressing:

1 cup 11.0

1 tbsp. 6

Cream, sour, flavored, roasted garlic or salsa

    (Friendship), 2 tbsp. 2.0

Cream, sour, powder *(AlpineAire)*, ½ cup 20.0

Cream topping, 2 tbsp., except as noted:

(Cool Whip/Cool Whip Extra Creamy) 2.0

(Cool Whip Free) 3.0

---

[1]*Unwhipped; volume approximately doubled when whipped*

(Cool Whip Lite) 2.0
(Crowley Real) 2.0
(Estee Aspartame), ¾ tsp. 1.0
(Kraft Dairy Whip) ....<1.0
(Kraft Free) 2.0
(Reddi Wip Extra Creamy/Original) ....<1.0
(Reddi Wip Fat Free/Nondairy) 2.0
mix*, nondairy *(Dream Whip)* 2.0
Cream of tartar, 1 tsp. 1.8
Creamer, nondairy:
fluid, 1 tbsp.:
   (Coffee-mate Low Fat) 1.0
   (Coffee-mate/Coffee-mate Fat Free) 2.0
   flavored, all varieties *(Coffee-mate)* 5.0
fluid, soy, 1 tbsp.:
   (WestSoy Creme de la Soy/Lite Original) ...2.0
   amaretto *(WestSoy* Creme de la Soy Original) ...4.0
   vanilla, French *(WestSoy* Creme de la Soy Original) ...3.0
powder, 1 tsp.:
   (Coffee-mate) 1.0
   (Coffee-mate Fat Free/Lite) 2.0
   (Cremora) 1.0
powder, flavored, 4 tsp.:
   amaretto, Irish creme, hazelnut, French vanilla, or mocha
     almond *(Coffee-mate)* 9.0
   chocolate, Swiss *(Coffee-mate/Coffee-mate* Fat Free) ...10.0
   hazelnut or French vanilla *(Coffee-mate* Fat Free) ...11.0
Crème de menthe, 72 proof:
1.5-fl. oz. jigger 20.8
1 fl. oz. 14.0
Crème fraîche *(Allouette),* 2 tbsp. ....<1.0
Crêpe, fresh *(Frieda's),* 2 pieces 9.0
Cress, garden:
raw, 1 cup 2.8
boiled, drained, 1 cup 5.1
Cress, water, see "Watercress"
Croaker, Atlantic:
without added ingredients 0
breaded, fried, 3.1-oz. fillet 6.6
Croissant, 1 piece, except as noted:
(Sara Lee), 1½ oz. 20.0

Croissant *(cont.)*
apple, 2 oz..21.1
butter:
   (Awrey's), 3 oz...29.0
   (Awrey's), 2 oz...19.0
   (Awrey's), 1½ oz..15.0
   (Awrey's), 1 oz...10.0
cheese, 1½ oz..19.7
margarine, sliced:
   (Awrey's Sandwich), 2½ oz...............................24.0
   (Awrey's Sandwich), 2 oz..................................19.0
   (Awrey's Sandwich), 1½ oz...............................15.0
mini *(Sara Lee* Petite), 2 pieces, 2 oz. 26.0
mini, 1 oz. 13.0
Crookneck squash, fresh:
raw, untrimmed, 1 lb..18.2
raw, sliced, 1 cup...5.3
boiled, drained, sliced, 1 cup.....................................7.8
boiled, drained, sliced, ½ cup....................................3.9
baby *(Frieda's)*, ⅔ cup, 3 oz. 3.0
Crookneck squash, canned, drained:
diced, 1 cup 6.2
mashed, 1 cup 7.1
Crookneck squash, frozen:
unprepared, sliced, 1 cup..6.2
boiled, drained, sliced, 1 cup...................................10.6
sliced *(Birds Eye* Deluxe Yellow Squash), ⅔ cup 2.0
Croutons:
(Pepperidge Farm Generous Cut), 6 pieces 5.0
plain, 1 cup, 1.1 oz..22.1
cheese and garlic or seasoned *(Arnold)*, 2 tbsp..........5.0
cheese and garlic or seasoned *(Pepperidge Farm* Classic Cut),
   9 pieces 4.0
classic Caesar or zesty Italian *(Pepperidge Farm* Generous Cut),
   6 pieces 4.0
seasoned, 1 cup, 1.4 oz..25.4
Cubanella chili, see "Pepper, chili"
Cucumber, fresh, raw:
with peel, 8¼" cucumber...8.3
with peel, sliced, ½ cup...1.4
peeled, sliced, 1 cup...3.0

peeled, pared, chopped, 1 cup 3.3
Japanese or hothouse *(Frieda's)*, ⅔ cup, 3 oz. 2.0
Cucumber, pickled, see "Pickle"
Cumin seed, ground:
1 tbsp. 2.7
1 tsp. 9
Cupcake, see "Cake, snack"
Currants, fresh, raw:
black, European, 1 cup 17.2
red or white, 1 cup 15.5
Currants, dried, zante, 1 cup 106.7
Curry base, 1 tsp.:
all varieties, except Panang *(A Taste of Thai)* 1.0
Panang *(A Taste of Thai)* 2.0
Curry paste, concentrate, 2 tbsp.:
balti *(Patak's)* 6.0
biryani *(Patak's)* 3.0
garam Masala *(Patak's)* 4.0
hot or vindaloo *(Patak's)* 4.0
Kasmiri Masala *(Patak's)* ....<1.0
Madras *(Patak's)* 4.0
mild *(Patak's)* 5.0
tikka Masala *(Patak's)* 5.0
Curry sauce, cooking, ½ cup, except as noted:
(A Taste of Thai Lite Mussaman/Panang), 3.5 fl. oz. 7.0
chili, hot:
   with coriander *(Patak's* Vindaloo) 15.0
   with cumin *(Patak's* Madras 15 oz.) 13.0
   with cumin *(Patak's* Madras 10 oz.) 15.0
coconut, rich, creamy, mild *(Patak's* Korma) 11.0
coriander, tangy, and lemon *(Patak's* Tikka Masala) 13.0
green, red, or yellow *(A Taste of Thai* Lite), 3.5 fl. oz. 6.0
sweet peppers and coconut *(Patak's* Jalfrezi) 12.0
tomato, rich, and onion *(Patak's* Dopiaza) 13.0
tomato, spicy, and cardamon *(Patak's* Rogan Josh) 12.0
Curry sauce, marinade, 2 tbsp.:
coriander and ginger *(Patak's* Tikka Marinade & Grill) 4.0
ginger and garlic, spicy *(Patak's* Tandoori Marinade & Grill) 6.0
ginger and garlic, spicy *(Patak's* Tandoori Marinade & Grill No
   Artificial Colorings) 7.0

Curry powder:
1 tbsp. 3.7
1 tsp. 1.2
Curry sauce mix, dry, except as noted:
1¼-oz. pkt. 17.9
8 fl. oz.* 14.3
Cusk, without added ingredients.....................................0
Custard, see "Pudding and pie filling mix"
Custard apple, 1 oz. 7.1
Custard marrow, see "Chayote"
Cuttlefish, meat only:
raw, 4 oz. 9
boiled, poached, or steamed, 4 oz. 1.9

D

FOOD AND MEASURE   **CARBOHYDRATE GRAMS**

Daikon, see "Radish, Oriental"
Daiquiri drink mixer:
6.8-fl.-oz. can 32.5
Hawaiian *(Trader Vic's)*, 4 fl. oz. 42.0
strawberry *(Mr & Mrs T)*, 3.5 fl. oz. 34.0
Dairy Queen/Brazier, 1 serving:
Basket, chicken strip 102.0
Basket, The Great Steakmelt 70.0
burgers:
   DQ Homestyle bacon double cheeseburger 31.0
   DQ Homestyle cheeseburger or double cheeseburger 29.0
   DQ Homestyle hamburger 29.0
   DQ Ultimate burger 29.0
chicken sandwich, breast fillet 37.0
chicken sandwich, grilled 30.0
hot dog 19.0
hot dog, chili 'n' cheese 22.0
sides:
   fries, medium 53.0
   fries, small 42.0
   onion rings 39.0
Blizzard Flavor Treats:
   chocolate chip cookie dough, medium 143.0
   chocolate chip cookie dough, small 99.0
   chocolate sandwich cookie, medium 97.0
   chocolate sandwich cookie, small 79.0
cones:
   chocolate, medium 53.0
   chocolate, small 37.0
   dipped, medium 59.0
   dipped, small 42.0
   DQ chocolate or vanilla soft serve, ½ cup 22.0
   vanilla, large 65.0
   vanilla, medium 53.0

Dairy Queen/Brazier, cones *(cont.)*

vanilla, small	38.0
DQ cake, undecorated, frozen, 8" round, ⅛ cake	56.0
DQ cake, undecorated, layered, 8" round, ⅛ cake	49.0
DQ Treatzza Pizza, Heath, ⅛ pizza	28.0
DQ Treatzza Pizza, M&M's, ⅛ pizza	29.0

malts, shakes, and smoothies:

chocolate malt, medium	153.0
chocolate malt, small	111.0
chocolate shake, medium	130.0
chocolate shake, small	94.0
hot chocolate, frozen	127.0
strawberry-banana *DQ Glacier Smoothy*	128.0
Misty slush, medium	74.0
Misty slush, small	20.0

novelties:

Buster Bar	41.0
chocolate *Dilly* bar	21.0
DQ fudge bar, no sugar added	13.0
DQ sandwich	24.0
DQ vanilla-orange bar, no sugar added	17.0
lemon *DQ Freez'r,* ½ cup	20.0
Starkiss	21.0

Royal Treats:

banana split	96.0
Chocolate Rock treat	87.0
Peanut Buster parfait	99.0
Pecan Mudslide treat	85.0
strawberry shortcake	70.0
sundae, chocolate, medium	71.0
sundae, chocolate, small	49.0

yogurt, frozen:

Breeze, Heath, medium	123.0
Breeze, Heath, small	85.0
Breeze, strawberry, medium	99.0
Breeze, strawberry, small	68.0
cone, medium	56.0
cup, medium	48.0
DQ nonfat, ½ cup	21.0
strawberry sundae, medium	61.0

Dandelion greens:
raw *(Frieda's),* 2 cups, 3 oz...8.0
raw, chopped, 1 cup..5.1
boiled, drained, chopped, 1 cup...6.7
Danish pastry (see also "Bun, sweet"), 1 piece:
almond, raisin-nut, or cinnamon-nut, 2.3 oz......................29.7
apple, strawberry, or cheese:
    (Awrey's), 2.75 oz...38.0
    (Awrey's Grande), 4.5 oz. 51.0
    (Awrey's Petite), 1.5 oz..21.0
cinnamon:
    (Awrey's Grande), 4.5 oz. 68.0
    (Awrey's Homestyle), 3 oz..45.0
    (Awrey's Petite), 1.5 oz..21.0
    large, 5 oz..63.3
    swirl *(Awrey's),* 2.75 oz..42.0
    swirl *(Awrey's* Grande), 3.75 oz................................57.0
cheese, 2.5 oz. 26.4
fruit, large, 5 oz..67.9
pineapple *(Awrey's* Petite), 1.5 oz.......................................21.0
raspberry-cheese swirl *(Awrey's* Grande), 3.75 oz..........44.0
Dasheen, see "Taro"
Date, natural, dry, domestic:
(Sonoma Organic), 5 dates, 1.4 oz. 30.0
pitted *(Dole),* 5–6 dates 31.0
pitted, chopped *(Dole),* 1 oz..33.0
pitted, chopped, 1 cup..130.8
Date filling, see "Pastry filling"
De arbol chili, see "Pepper, chili"
Delicata squash *(Frieda's),* ¾ cup, 3 oz. 7.0
Denny's, general menu, 1 serving:
breakfast dishes:
    All American Slam, 13 oz. 9.0
    Big Texas Chicken Fajita Skillet, 17 oz. 25.0
    chicken-fried steak and eggs, 8 oz. 1.0
    Cinnamon Swirl Slam, 13 oz. 68.0
    Country Slam, 18 oz. 61.0
    eggs Benedict...34.0
    Farmer's Omelette, 14 oz. 17.0
    Farmer's Slam, 19 oz. 82.0
    French Slam, 14 oz...58.0

Denny's, breakfast dishes (cont.)

French toast, plain, 2 pieces 54.0
French toast, cinnamon swirl, 12 oz. 124.0
Grand Slam original, 10 oz. 65.0
ham 'n cheddar omelette, 10 oz. 4.0
hotcakes, plain 95.0
Meat Lover's Skillet, 15 oz. 24.0
Moons Over My Hammy, 12 oz. 46.0
Play It Again Slam, 15 oz. 98.0
potato pancakes, 13 oz. 59.0
Sausage Lover's Slam, 17 oz. 33.0
Sausage Supreme Skillet, 16 oz. 30.0
Scramble Slam, 18 oz. 14.0
sirloin or T-bone steak and eggs 1.0
Slim Slam, without syrup 98.0
Southern Slam, 13 oz. 47.0
Ultimate Omelette, 13 oz. 9.0
veggie-cheese omelette, 12 oz. 9.0
waffle, plain 23.0

breakfast items/à la carte:

bacon, 4 strips 1.0
bacon, peppered, 4 strips 2.0
bagel, dry, 3 oz. 46.0
banana, whole, 4 oz. 29.0
biscuit, buttered, 3 oz. 39.0
biscuit and sausage gravy, 7 oz. 45.0
cantaloupe or honeydew melon, 3 oz. 8.0
cereal, dry *Kellogg's,* 1 oz. 23.0
cream cheese, 1 oz. 1.0
egg, 1 ....1.0
Egg Beaters, 2 oz. 1.0
English muffin, dry, 4-oz. piece 24.0
fruit mix, 3 oz. 9.0
grapefruit, ½ fruit 16.0
grapes, 3 oz. 15.0
grits, 4 oz. 18.0
ham, grilled, 3-oz. slice 2.0
hash browns, covered, 4 oz. 20.0
hash browns, covered and smothered, 8 oz. 26.0
hash browns, double, covered and smothered, 13 oz. 48.0
hotcakes, buttermilk, 3 cakes 95.0

oatmeal, *Quaker,* 4 oz. 18.0
potatoes, country fried, 6 oz. 23.0
sausage, 4 links, 3 oz. 0
sausage, 2 patties, 3 oz. 1.0
sausage gravy, 4 oz. 6.0
strawberry-banana medley, 4 oz. 27.0
syrup, 1.5 oz.:
    blueberry 26.0
    maple 36.0
    maple, sugar-free...9.0
toast, dry, 1-oz. slice 17.0
topping, blueberry or strawberry, 3 oz. 26.0
topping, cherry, 3 oz. 21.0
waffle, 6-oz. piece 23.0
whipped cream, .3-oz. dollop.......................................2.0
burgers:
    bacon cheddar 58.0
    big Texas BBQ 53.0
    buffalo chicken 67.0
    classic 42.0
    classic with cheese 43.0
    double decker 82.0
    garden 75.0
    garlic mushroom Swiss......................................58.0
sandwiches:
    bacon, lettuce, and tomato 37.0
    Charleston Chicken...53.0
    chicken, grilled 64.0
    club 62.0
    ham and Swiss on rye..40.0
    Reuben 37.0
    The Super Bird 48.0
    turkey breast with multigrain...........................39.0
soup, 8 oz.:
    broccoli, cream of 15.0
    cheese 13.0
    chicken noodle 8.0
    clam chowder...22.0
    potato, cream of..23.0
    split pea 18.0
    vegetable beef..11.0

Denny's (cont.)

chili, with cheese topping, 11 oz..21.0

appetizers, without condiments:

    Buffalo wings, 12 wings, 15 oz. 3.0

    cheese fries, chili, 12 oz. 77.0

    cheese fries, smothered, 9 oz....................................69.0

    chicken strips, 5 pieces, 10 oz. 56.0

    chicken strips, Buffalo, 5 pieces, 10 oz. 43.0

    mozzarella sticks, 8 sticks, 8 oz. 49.0

    Sampler, 17 oz...12.0

dinner entree meat/fish/poultry:

    chicken, grilled, 4 oz. 0

    chicken, Charleston, with gravy, 6 oz. 16.0

    chicken strips, 10 oz. 55.0

    fish dinner, 9 oz..48.0

    pot roast, with gravy, 7 oz. 5.0

    salmon, Alaskan, grilled, 6 oz....................................1.0

    shrimp, fried, 8 oz. 49.0

    sirloin steak, 6 oz. 0

    steak, chicken-fried, 7 oz. 24.0

    steak and shrimp, 9 oz. 31.0

    T-bone steak, 12 oz..1.0

    turkey, roast, with stuffing and gravy, 14 oz. 38.0

sides:

    applesauce, *Musselman's,* 3 oz. 15.0

    bread stuffing, plain, 3 oz..19.0

    broccoli in butter sauce, 4 oz......................................7.0

    carrots in honey glaze, 4 oz. 12.0

    corn in butter sauce, 4 oz..19.0

    cottage cheese, 3 oz. 2.0

    fries, seasoned, 4 oz..35.0

    fries, unsalted, 4 oz. 44.0

    gravy, brown, chicken, or country, 1 oz. 2.0

    green beans with bacon, 4 oz......................................6.0

    green peas in butter sauce, 4 oz. 14.0

    mushrooms, grilled, 2 oz. 2.0

    onion rings, 4 oz. 38.0

    potato, baked, plain, 7 oz. 51.0

    potato, mashed, 6 oz. 21.0

    toast, herb, 2 oz. 15.0

    tomatoes, sliced, 3 slices, 2 oz. 3.0

vegetable rice pilaf, 3 oz..16.0
salads, without dressing, except as noted:
  chicken:
    Buffalo, 16 oz...26.0
    fried, 15 oz..26.0
    garden delite, 16 oz. 30.0
    grilled, Caesar, with dressing, 13 oz. 19.0
    grilled, California, 13 oz. 10.0
  side, Caesar, with dressing, 6 oz. 20.0
  side, garden, 7 oz...16.0
condiments and dressings:
  BBQ sauce, 1.5 oz...11.0
  blue cheese or Caesar dressing, 1 oz. 1.0
  French dressing, 1 oz. 3.0
  guacamole, 1.5 oz. 4.0
  honey mustard, fat-free, 1 oz. 9.0
  Italian dressing, low-calorie...........................3.0
  marinara sauce, 1.5 oz....................................7.0
  ranch dressing, 1 oz. 1.0
  salsa, 1.5 oz. 1.0
  sour cream, 1.5 oz. 2.0
  tartar sauce, 1.5 oz..5.0
  Thousand Island dressing, 1 oz......................5.0
desserts:
  banana royale, 10 oz. 80.0
  banana split, 19 oz. 121.0
  Butterfinger Blender Blaster, 13 oz. 97.0
  chocolate layer cake, 3 oz. 42.0
  float, root beer or cola, 12 oz. 47.0
  hot fudge cake, 7 oz. 73.0
pie:
  apple, 7 oz..64.0
  apple, Dutch, 7 oz...65.0
  cheesecake pie, without topping, 4 oz.............48.0
  cherry, 7 oz. 101.0
  chocolate–peanut butter, 6 oz. 64.0
  chocolate silk, 6 oz. 60.0
  Key lime, 6 oz. 79.0
  Oreo cookies & creme, 6 oz. 73.0
shake, chocolate or vanilla, 12 oz. 76.0
shake, malted milk, chocolate or vanilla, 12 oz............82.0

Denny's *(cont.)*

sherbet, rainbow, 4 oz.	25.0
sundae:	
Butterfinger hot fudge, 9 oz.	106.0
double scoop, 6 oz.	29.0
single scoop, 3 oz.	14.0
toppings, 2 oz., except as noted:	
blueberry or strawberry	17.0
cherry	14.0
chocolate	27.0
fudge	30.0
nut, 1 tsp., .3 oz.	1.0
whipped cream	2.0
yogurt, low-fat, chocolate/chocolate chip	19.0

Dessert filling, see "Pastry filling" and "Pie filling"

Dessert mix (see also "Cake, snack, mix" and "Cheesecake, mix"):

chocolate, double layer *(Jell-O No Bake)*, ⅛ dessert	34.0
chocolate silk, see "Pie mix"	
cookies and cream *(Jell-O No Bake)*, ⅙ dessert	51.0
lemon, double layer *(Jell-O No Bake)*, ⅛ dessert	36.0
peanut butter cup *(Jell-O No Bake)*, ⅛ dessert	41.0

Dill dip mix, garden *(Knorr)*, ½ tsp.	0
Dill seed:	
1 tbsp.	3.6
1 tsp.	1.2
Dill weed:	
fresh, 5 sprigs	.1
fresh, 1 cup	.6
dried, 1 tbsp.	1.7
dried, 1 tsp.	.6
Dock, fresh, raw, chopped, 1 cup	4.3
Dolphin fish, without added ingredients	0

Domino's Pizza:

classic hand tossed, 12" medium, 2 of 8 slices:

anchovy	54.7
bacon	54.8
banana peppers	55.6
beef	54.8
cheddar	54.9
cheese	54.7
cheese, extra	55.5

green peppers...55.6
ham...55.1
mushroom, fresh..55.9
olive, green...54.9
olive, ripe..55.6
onion...55.9
pepperoni..55.0
pineapple tidbits...57.9
sausage, Italian..56.9
classic hand tossed, 14" large, 2 of 8 slices:
anchovy...75.0
bacon...75.1
banana peppers..76.2
beef...75.0
cheddar...75.2
cheese...75.0
cheese, extra...76.0
green peppers..76.1
ham...75.5
mushroom, fresh..76.6
olive, green...75.2
olive, ripe..76.2
onion...76.5
pepperoni..75.3
pineapple tidbits...79.9
sausage, Italian..78.1
crunchy thin crust, 12" medium, ¼ pie:
anchovy...31.0
bacon...31.1
banana peppers..31.9
beef...31.1
cheddar...31.2
cheese...31.0
cheese, extra...31.8
green peppers..31.9
ham...31.5
mushroom, fresh..32.2
olive, green...31.2
olive, ripe..31.9
onion...32.2
pepperoni..31.3

Domino's Pizza, crunchy thin crust (cont.)

pineapple tidbits	34.3
sausage, Italian	33.3
crunchy thin crust, 14" large, ¼ pie:	
anchovy	43.5
bacon	43.7
banana peppers	44.7
beef	43.6
cheddar	43.7
cheese	43.5
cheese, extra	44.6
green peppers	44.6
ham	44.0
mushroom, fresh	45.1
olive, green	43.8
olive, ripe	44.7
onion	45.1
pepperoni	43.8
pineapple tidbits	48.5
sausage, Italian	46.6
ultimate deep dish, 6" small, whole pie:	
anchovy	68.4
bacon	68.6
banana peppers	69.8
beef	68.5
cheddar	68.8
cheese	68.4
cheese, extra	70.1
green peppers	69.7
ham	69.1
mushroom, fresh	69.9
olive, green	68.7
olive, ripe	69.8
onion	70.2
pepperoni	68.8
pineapple tidbits	72.8
sausage, Italian	71.8
ultimate deep dish, 12" medium, ¼ pie:	
anchovy	56.2
bacon	56.3
banana peppers	57.4

beef	56.2
cheddar	56.4
cheese	56.2
cheese, extra	57.2
green peppers	57.3
ham	56.7
mushroom, fresh	57.8
olive, green	56.4
olive, ripe	57.4
onion	57.7
pepperoni	56.5
pineapple tidbits	61.1
sausage, Italian	59.3

Donut, 1 piece, except as noted:

plain *(Awrey's)*, 2 oz.	31.0
plain *(Awrey's)* 1.5 oz.	18.0
chocolate, cake, sugared or glazed, 3¾" diam., 2.1 oz.	34.4
chocolate-coated or -frosted:	
(Awrey's), 1.75 oz.	23.0
(Hostess)	20.0
(Hostess Donettes), 3 pieces	34.0
(Little Debbie Singles), 2.5 oz.	40.0
cake, 2" diam., 1 oz.	13.4
chocolate *(Awrey's)*, 1.75 oz.	25.0
custard Bismark *(Awrey's)*, 3.7 oz.	44.0
ring *(Awrey's)*, 2.75 oz.	33.0
sour cream *(Awrey's)*, 3.75 oz.	54.0
sour cream *(Awrey's)*, 3 oz.	47.0
cinnamon sugar sour cream *(Awrey's)*, 2.5 oz.	39.0
coconut-topped *(Awrey's)*, 1.75 oz.	25.0
creme-filled, 3 oz.	25.5
cruller, glazed, 3" diam., 1.4 oz.	24.4
crunch *(Awrey's)*, 2.5 oz.	35.0
crunch-topped *(Awrey's)*, 1.75 oz.	19.0
devil's food, glazed *(Awrey's)*, 2.75 oz.	41.0
glazed:	
cake, 3" diam., 1.6 oz.	22.9
raised *(Hostess)*, 1.33 oz.	19.0
ring *(Awrey's)*, 2.5 oz.	30.0
sour cream *(Awrey's)*, 3.75 oz.	55.0
sour cream *(Awrey's)*, 3 oz.	34.0

Donut, glazed *(cont.)*
    stick *(Awrey's* Twin Pack), 2.75 oz. 41.0
hole, glazed or honeyed, .5 oz. 5.8
jelly, 3 oz. 33.2
jelly Bismark, vanilla-iced *(Awrey's),* 3.5 oz. 43.0
powdered sugar:
    (Awrey's), 2.25 oz...44.0
    (Awrey's), 1.5 oz...21.0
    (Little Debbie Singles), 2.5 oz. 38.0
    jelly Bismark *(Awrey's),* 2.75 oz....................................30.0
sour cream, plain *(Awrey's),* 3.25 oz....................................41.0
sprinkle-top *(Awrey's),* 1.75 oz. 19.0
stick:
    (Little Debbie), 1.6 oz. 24.0
    (Little Debbie Singles), 2.75 oz. 42.0
    cake, 1.8 oz. 25.8
sugared, cake, 3" diam., 1.6 oz. 22.9
vanilla-iced *(Awrey's* Long John), 3.5 oz. 44.0
wheat, cake, sugared or glazed, 2" diam., 1 oz. 11.9
white-iced *(Awrey's),* 1.75 oz..24.0
Dressing, see "Salad dressing" and specific listings
Dreyer's/Edy's Ice Cream Parlor, ½ cup, except as noted:
Classic ice cream:
    almond praline...21.0
    apple pie...19.0
    Bananafana..16.0
    black cherry vanilla..17.0
    black walnut..15.0
    blueberry cheesecake, New York....................................17.0
    bubble gum 20.0
    butter pecan..17.0
    Butterfinger Blast..19.0
    cappuccino crunch...21.0
    caramel decadence, double 16.0
    chocolate 15.0
    chocolate brownie chunk, fat-free 25.0
    chocolate chips!...18.0
    chocolate chocolate chip 17.0
    cinnamon swirl...18.0
    coconut pineapple 17.0
    coffee, kona 15.0

cookie dough	20.0
cookies and cream	18.0
espresso chip	17.0
fudge brownie, double	19.0
Girl Scouts thin mint cookie	18.0
green tea	16.0
macadamia nut	15.0
malt ball and fudge with *Whoppers*	21.0
mint chocolate chips!	18.0
mocha almond fudge	18.0
peanut butter cup	18.0
peppermint	17.0
pistachio nut	15.0
pumpkin	17.0
rocky road	17.0
root beer float	15.0
spumoni	17.0
strawberry	17.0
strawberry cheesecake chunk	18.0
vanilla	14.0
vanilla, French	16.0
vanilla, Tahitian	14.0
vanilla bean	15.0
vanilla-flavored, fat-free/no-sugar	19.0
waffle cone crunch	21.0
Grand soft ice cream:	
apple, deep dish	23.0
banana chocolate chunk	22.0
butter pecan	22.0
Butterfinger Blast	24.0
chocolate, fat free/no sugar	25.0
chocolate, double Dutch	19.0
chocolate chip cookie dough	23.0
Girl Scouts thin mint cookie	24.0
malt ball	25.0
mint chocolate chip	23.0
peppermint	23.0
rocky road	22.0
vanilla	21.0
vanilla, fat-free/no-sugar	26.0
vanilla with *Snickers*	23.0

Dreyer's/Edy's (cont.)

frozen yogurt:

chocolate, fat-free	18.0
Heath toffee crunch	19.0
peach	17.0
strawberry, fat-free	17.0
vanilla, fat-free	18.0

frozen yogurt, Grand soft:

cherry chocolate chip, low-fat	27.0
cookies and cream, low-fat	29.0
peaches and cream, fat-free	26.0
strawberry, fat-free	26.0
strawberry cheesecake, low-fat	25.0

sherbet, orange	29.0
sherbet, rainbow	27.0
sorbet, lemon	36.0
sorbet, raspberry	33.0

smoothie, 1 serving:

mango groove	94.0
strawberry fields	91.0
tropical oasis	90.0

Drum, freshwater, without added ingredients	0
Duck, domesticated or wild, without added ingredients, 4 oz.	0
Duck sauce, see "Sweet and sour sauce"	
Dumpling entree, frozen, Oriental style *(Lean Cuisine Everyday Favorites),* 9 oz.	51.0
Dumpling squash, see "Sweet dumpling squash"	

Dunkin' Donuts:

sandwich, *Omwich,* 1 piece:

bagel, bacon/cheddar or Spanish/cheese	79.0
bagel, three cheese	78.0
croissant, all varieties	33.0
English muffin, bacon/cheddar or three-cheese	33.0
English muffin, Spanish/cheese	34.0

sandwich, breakfast, ham/egg/cheese	31.0

bagel, 1 piece:

plain	73.0
blueberry	75.0
cinnamon raisin	74.0
egg	72.0
everything	74.0

garlic 76.0
onion 70.0
poppyseed 74.0
pumpernickel 75.0
salt 73.0
sesame 74.0
wheat 73.0
cream cheese, all varieties except salmon, 1 pkt. 3.0
cream cheese, salmon, 1 pkt. 2.0
cookie, 1 piece:
  chocolate chocolate chunk 26.0
  chocolate chunk 28.0
  chocolate chunk with nuts 27.0
  chocolate white chocolate chunk 28.0
  oatmeal raisin pecan 29.0
  peanut butter chocolate chunk with nuts 24.0
  peanut butter with nuts 24.0
croissant, 1 piece:
  plain 26.0
  almond 34.0
  chocolate 37.0
donuts, 1 piece:
  apple crumb 34.0
  apple fritter 41.0
  apple and spice 29.0
  Bavarian kreme 30.0
  black raspberry 32.0
  blueberry cake 35.0
  blueberry crumb 36.0
  Boston kreme 36.0
  bow tie 34.0
  butternut cake 36.0
  chocolate cake, double 37.0
  chocolate cake, glazed 33.0
  chocolate coconut cake 31.0
  chocolate-frosted 29.0
  chocolate-frosted cake 38.0
  chocolate-frosted coffee roll 36.0
  chocolate-iced, Bismark 50.0
  chocolate-kreme-filled 35.0
  cinnamon bun 85.0

Dunkin' Donuts, donuts (cont.)

cinnamon cake	31.0
coconut cake	33.0
coconut cake, toasted	35.0
coffee roll	33.0
cruller, chocolate, glazed	35.0
cruller, glazed	37.0
cruller, plain	25.0
cruller, sugar	27.0
Dunkin' Donut	25.0
éclair	39.0
glazed	25.0
glazed cake	33.0
glazed fritter	31.0
jelly-filled	32.0
jelly stick	44.0
lemon	28.0
maple-frosted	30.0
maple-frosted coffee roll	36.0
old-fashioned cake	26.0
powdered cake	32.0
powdered cruller	30.0
strawberry	32.0
strawberry-frosted	30.0
sugar-raised	22.0
sugared cake	27.0
vanilla-frosted	30.0
vanilla-frosted coffee roll	36.0
vanilla-kreme-filled	36.0
whole-wheat glazed	32.0

Munchkins, cake:

plain, 4 pieces	22.0
butternut, 3 pieces	25.0
chocolate, glazed, 3 pieces	26.0
cinnamon, 4 pieces	30.0
coconut, 3 pieces	23.0
coconut, toasted, 3 pieces	24.0
glazed, 3 pieces	27.0
powdered, 4 pieces	29.0
sugared, 4 pieces	28.0

Munchkins, yeast:

    glazed, 5 pieces 27.0

    jelly-filled, 5 pieces 30.0

    lemon-filled, 4 pieces 23.0

    sugar-raised, 7 pieces 26.0

muffin, 1 piece:

    apple cinnamon 74.0

    apple and spice 57.0

    apple and spice, low-fat 54.0

    banana, low-fat 57.0

    banana-nut 52.0

    blueberry, 6 oz. 76.0

    blueberry, 4 oz. 49.0

    blueberry, low-fat 55.0

    blueberry, reduced-fat 77.0

    bran 60.0

    bran, low-fat 57.0

    cherry 53.0

    cherry, low-fat 56.0

    chocolate, low-fat 53.0

    chocolate chip, 6 oz. 88.0

    chocolate chip, 4 oz. 58.0

    chocolate hazelnut chunk 87.0

    corn, 6 oz. 78.0

    corn, 4 oz. 57.0

    corn, low-fat 52.0

    corn, reduced-fat 79.0

    cranberry-orange 76.0

    cranberry-orange, low-fat 55.0

    cranberry-orange-nut 52.0

    honey bran raisin 84.0

    lemon poppyseed 56.0

    oat bran 55.0

beverages:

    coffee *Coolatta,* with cream, 16 oz. 51.0

    coffee *Coolatta,* with milk, whole, 2%, or skim, 16 oz. 52.0

    Dunkaccino, 20 oz. 71.0

    Dunkaccino, 18.75 oz. 67.0

    Dunkaccino, 14 oz. 51.0

    Dunkaccino, 10 oz. 34.0

    hot cocoa, 20 oz. 79.0

Dunkin' Donuts, beverages (cont.)
   hot cocoa, 18.75 oz...75.0
   hot cocoa, 14 oz...57.0
   hot cocoa, 10 oz...38.0
   orange-mango fruit *Coolatta*, 16 oz....................71.0
   pink lemonade fruit *Coolatta*, 16 oz..................88.0
   raspberry-lemonade *Coolatta*, 16 oz.................68.0
   strawberry fruit *Coolatta*, 16 oz..........................70.0
   vanilla *Coolatta*, 16 oz. 94.0
Durian:
raw or frozen, 1.3 lb..164.7
chopped or diced, 1 cup 65.8

E

FOOD AND MEASURE **CARBOHYDRATE GRAMS**

Edamame *(Frieda's)*, ½ cup, 2.6 oz...9.0
Edy's Ice Cream Parlor, see *"Dreyer's/Edy's Ice Cream Parlor"*
Eel, without added ingredients 0
Egg, chicken:
raw, whole:
    1 extra large 7
    1 large 6
    1 cup 3.0
    frozen, 1 oz. 3
raw, white only:
    1 large 3
    1 cup 2.5
    dried, 1 oz. 2.2
    frozen, 1 oz. 3
raw, yolk only[1]:
    1 large 3
    1 cup 4.3
    frozen, 8 oz...2.6
cooked:
    fried, 1 large egg 6
    hard-boiled, chopped, 1 cup...1.5
    hard-boiled, chopped, 1 tbsp. 1
    omelet, 1 large egg 6
    poached, 1 large.. .6
    scrambled, 1 cup...4.8
Egg, dried:
scrambled, freeze-dried *(AlpineAire)*, 2 eggs 2.0
scrambling/omelet mix *(AlpineAire)*, 2 eggs 3.0
whole, 1 tbsp. 2
whole, sifted, 1 cup..4.2
yolk, 1 tbsp. 1
Egg, duck, raw, whole, 1 egg..1.0

[1] *Includes a small portion of white.*

Egg, goose, raw, whole, 1 egg 1.9
Egg, quail, raw, whole, 1 egg...<0.1
Egg, turkey, raw, whole, 1 egg.. .9
Egg dish, dried:
scrambled *(AlpineAire Bandito Scramble)*, 1½ cups 19.0
ranch omelet, with beef *(AlpineAire)*, 1 cup..........................17.0
"Egg" salad, see "Tofu salad"
Egg sandwich, see "Breakfast sandwich"
Egg substitute, ¼ cup:
(Egg Beaters) 1.0
(Morningstar Farms Better'n Eggs)...0
(Morningstar Farms Scramblers)..2.0
(Tofutti Egg Watchers) 1.0
Eggnog, dairy pack:
(Crowley), ½ cup 23.0
(Crowley Light), ½ cup 22.0
(Crowley Nonfat), ½ cup...25.0
1 cup..34.4
1 fl. oz..4.3
Eggnog, canned *(Borden's* Premium), ½ cup 17.0
Eggnog mix, powder:
2 rounded tsp...27.6
prepared with milk, 8 fl. oz. 38.9
Eggplant, fresh:
raw, peeled, 1 lb. (yield from 1¼-lb. eggplant) 27.8
raw, 1" cubes, 1 cup..5.0
raw, Chinese or Japanese *(Frieda's)*, ⅔ cup, 3 oz. 5.0
boiled, drained, 1" cubes, 1 cup..6.6
Eggplant, in jar:
appetizer *(Progresso* Caponata), 2 tbsp......................................2.0
marinated *(Casa Visco)*, 1 oz. 1.0
roasted *(Peloponnese* Meze), 2 tbsp..2.0
sauteed *(Life in Provence)*, ½ cup 12.0
strips, in sunflower oil *(Rienzi)*, 1 oz. 0
Eggplant dip, 2 tbsp.:
(Peloponnese Babaganoush) 2.0
(Victoria) 2.0
caviar *(Cedarlane)* 3.0
roasted, and red pepper *(Cedarlane)*..2.0
Eggplant dip mix *(Casbah* Babaganoush), 2 oz., ½ cup* 25.0

Eggplant entree, frozen:
Parmesan *(Cedarlane)*, 5-oz. pkg. 16.0
Parmesan *(Mrs. Paul's)*, ½ cup 18.0
parmigiana, with linguine *(Michelina's)*, 8-oz. pkg. 42.0
Eggplant relish, Indian *(Patak's* Brinjal), 1 tbsp. 5.0
Eggroll, frozen:
(Empire Kosher), 3.1-oz. roll 28.0
chicken:
    (Chun King Restaurant Style), 3-oz. roll 22.0
    (La Choy Restaurant Style), 3-oz. roll 25.0
    (Michelina's Yu Sing), 6 rolls, 3 oz. 23.0
    mini *(Chun King/La Choy)*, 6 rolls 25.0
    sweet and sour *(La Choy* Restaurant Style), 3-oz. roll 29.0
    sweet and sour *(Michelina's Yu Sing)*, 6 rolls, 3 oz. 26.0
mini *(Empire* Kosher), 6 rolls, 4.9 oz. 43.0
pork *(La Choy* Restaurant Style), 3-oz. roll 24.0
pork, sweet and sour *(Michelina's Yu Sing)*, 6 rolls, 3 oz. 25.0
pork and shrimp:
    (Michelina's Yu Sing), 6 rolls, 3 oz. 23.0
    bite-size *(La Choy)*, 12 rolls 25.0
    mini *(Chun King/La Choy)*, 6 rolls 27.0
shrimp:
    (Chun King Restaurant Style), 3-oz. roll 24.0
    (La Choy Restaurant Style), 3-oz. roll 25.0
    (Michelina's Yu Sing), 6 rolls, 3 oz. 24.0
    mini *(Chun King/La Choy)*, 6 rolls 28.0
vegetable, with lobster, mini *(La Choy)*, 6 rolls 27.0
Eggroll, refrigerated, 1 roll with sauce pkt.:
shrimp *(Chung's)* 23.0
vegetable *(Chung's)* 24.0
Eggroll entree, frozen, vegetable *(Lean Cuisine Everyday
    Favorites)*, 9 oz. 57.0
Eggroll wrapper:
(Frieda's), 2 pieces, 1.65 oz. 28.0
(Nasoya), 2 pieces, 1.6 oz. 24.0
7"-square piece, 1.1 oz. 18.5
Elderberry, fresh, raw, 1 cup 26.7
Elderberry nectar *(R.W. Knudsen)*, 8 fl. oz. 28.0
Empanadilla, frozen, 2 pieces:
cheese *(Goya)* 44.0
pizza *(Goya)* 56.0

Enchilada (see also "Enchilada entree"), frozen:
black bean and vegetable *(Amy's)*, 4.75 oz. 20.0
black bean and vegetable *(Amy's* Family Size), 4.38 oz. 17.0
cheese *(Amy's)*, 4.75 oz. 13.0
cheese *(Amy's* Family Size), 5 oz. 13.0
chicken *(Stouffer's)*, 4.75 oz. 22.0
vegetable, garden *(Cedarlane)*, 4.5 oz. 24.0
Enchilada dinner, frozen:
beef *(Patio)*, 12 oz. 52.0
beef, chili, and beans *(Patio* Extra Large), 15.5 oz. 73.0
beef and cheese, chili, and beans *(Patio* Extra Large),
     15.5 oz. 80.0
black bean *(Amy's)*, 10 oz. 41.0
cheese *(Amy's)*, 9 oz. 38.0
cheese *(Patio)*, 12 oz. 54.0
chicken *(Patio)*, 12 oz. 60.0
chicken suprema *(Healthy Choice* Meal), 11.3 oz. 46.0
Enchilada entree, frozen, 1 pkg., except as noted:
beef:
     (Banquet), 11 oz. 54.0
     (Patio), 2 pieces with sauce 29.0
     bake *(Ortega* Family Fiesta), 9¼ oz., ¼ pkg. 54.0
beef and tamale, chili gravy with *(Morton)*, 10 oz. 40.0
beef and tamale combo *(Banquet)*, 11 oz. 56.0
cheese *(Banquet)*, 11 oz. 56.0
cheese *(Patio)*, 2 pieces with sauce 30.0
chicken *(Banquet)*, 11 oz. 54.0
chicken Suiza *(Healthy Choice* Entree), 10 oz. 43.0
combo, Mexican style *(Banquet)*, 11 oz. 55.0
pie, three-layer *(Cedarlane)*, ½ of 11-oz. pkg. 27.0
Suiza *(Lean Cuisine Everyday Favorites)*, 9 oz. 48.0
Enchilada sauce, ¼ cup:
(Gebhardt)...4.0
(La Victoria) 2.0
(Rosarita) 3.0
green *(La Victoria)* 3.0
green chili *(El Torito* Fire-Roasted)................................4.0
tomatillo *(El Torito)* 4.0
tomato *(El Torito* Fire-Roasted)......................................7.0
Enchilada seasoning mix *(Lawry's* Spices & Seasonings),
     2 tsp. 4.0

Endive, fresh, raw:

1 head, 1.1 lbs. 17.2

chopped, ½ cup... .8

Endive, Belgian, see "Chicory, witloof"

Entree sauce, see specific listings

Epazote, fresh, raw:

1 sprig 1

1 tbsp...<.1

Eppaw, fresh, raw, 1 cup 31.7

Escarole, see "Endive"

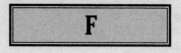

F

FOOD AND MEASURE   **CARBOHYDRATE GRAMS**

Fajita dinner kit:
(Chi-Chi's), 2 shells and seasonings 54.0
chicken *(Taco Bell Home Originals)*, 2 fajitas* 45.0
Fajita entree, see specific listings
Fajita pie, potato top *(Mrs. Patterson's Aussie Pie)*,
  5.5-oz. piece 33.0
Fajita seasoning mix:
(Chi-Chi's), ¼ pkg. 7.0
(El Torito), ¼ pkg. 7.0
(Lawry's Spices & Seasonings), 2 tsp. 3.0
chicken:
  (Lawry's Seasonings), 1 tsp. 2.0
  (Ortega), 1½ tsp. 3.0
  (Taco Bell Home Originals), about 1 tbsp. 5.0
Falafel mix, dry:
(Casbah), 1.5 oz. 20.0
(Fantastic Foods), ½ cup 42.0
(Near East), ¼ cup 18.0
Farina, see "Cereal, cooking/hot"
Fava beans, see "Broad beans, mature," and "Habas"
Feijoa, fresh, raw:
(Frieda's), 5 oz. 15.0
trimmed, 1 fruit, 1.75 oz. 5.3
pureed, 1 cup 25.8
Fennel, bulb, raw:
(Frieda's), ¾ cup, 3 oz. 6.0
1 bulb, 8.3 oz. 17.1
sliced, 1 cup 6.3
Fennel seeds:
1 tbsp. 3.0
1 tsp. 1.0
Fenugreek seeds:
1 tbsp. 6.5
1 tsp. 2.2

Fettuccine, plain:
dry, see "Pasta"
refrigerated:
    (Contadina Buitoni), 1¼ cups 45.0
    regular or flavored *(Di Giorno)*, 2.5 oz. 38.0
    spinach *(Contadina Buitoni)*, 1¼ cups 43.0
Fettuccine dish, mix:
Alfredo:
    (Knorr Classic), ¾ cup 43.0
    (Knorr TasteBreaks), 1 cont. 41.0
    (Pasta Roni), about 1 cup* 49.0
    (Pasta Roni Reduced Fat), about 1 cup* 50.0
creamy basil sauce *(Knorr* TasteBreaks), 1 cont. 40.0
Fettuccine entree, dried *(AlpineAire* Leonardo da Fettuccini),
    1¼ cups 44.0
Fettuccine entree, frozen, 1 pkg., except as noted:
Alfredo:
    (Banquet), 9.5 oz. 40.0
    (Freezer Queen Homestyle), 9 oz. 42.0
    (Healthy Choice Entree), 8 oz. 37.0
    (Lean Cuisine Everyday Favorites), 9.25 oz. 42.0
    (Marie Callender's Meals Supreme), 13 oz. 35.0
    (Michelina's), 9 oz. 45.0
    (Stouffer's), 11.5 oz. 64.0
    with broccoli and chicken *(Michelina's)*, 8.5 oz. 37.0
    and garlic bread *(Marie Callender's* Meals), 14 oz. ...82.0
with broccoli and chicken *(Marie Callender's* Meals), 13 oz. ...53.0
carbonara *(Michelina's)*, 8 oz. 40.0
with creamy pesto and vegetables *(Michelina's)*, 8.5 oz. ...37.0
primavera:
    (Lean Cuisine Everyday Favorites), 10 oz. 38.0
    (Michelina's), 8 oz. 36.0
    (Stouffer's), 10 oz. 45.0
    with chicken *(Michelina's)*, 8 oz. 37.0
    with tortellini *(Marie Callender's* Meals), 14 oz. 57.0
Fiddlehead fern, fresh, raw, 4 oz. 6.3
Fig, fresh:
1 large, 2.3 oz. 12.3
1 medium, 1.8 oz. 9.6
Fig, canned:
in water, 1 fig with liquid 3.8

Fig, canned *(cont.)*
in water, 1 cup 34.7
in light syrup, 1 fig with liquid 5.0
in light syrup, 1 cup 45.2
in heavy syrup:
   (Oregon Kadota), ½ cup..30.0
   1 fig with liquid...6.4
   1 cup 59.3
in extra heavy syrup, 1 cup 72.7
Fig, dried:
1 fig, ⅔ oz. 12.4
1 cup 130.0
California, all varieties, ¼ cup, 1.4 oz. 26.0
calimyrna *(Blue Ribbon Orchard Choice/Sun•Maid),* 1½ oz.,
   about 2 pieces..28.0
calimyrna or mission *(Sonoma* Organic), 3 figs, 1.4 oz..............26.0
mission *(Blue Ribbon Orchard Choice/Sun•Maid),* 1½ oz.,
   about 4 pieces..28.0
stewed, 1 cup..71.4
Filberts, shelled:
blanched, 1 oz..4.8
chopped, 1 cup 19.2
ground, 1 cup 12.6
dry-roasted, 1 oz..5.0
Fillo pastry, frozen, .7-oz. sheet...............................10.0
Finnan haddie, see "Haddock"
Finocchio, see "Fennel"
Fireweed leaves, fresh, raw:
1 plant...4.2
chopped, 1 cup 4.4
Fish, see specific listings
Fish batter mix, see "Fish seasoning and coating mix"
Fish cake, see "Fish dish" and specific fish listings
Fish dinner, frozen, 1 pkg.:
herb-baked *(Healthy Choice* Meal), 10.9 oz. 54.0
lemon pepper *(Healthy Choice* Meal), 10.7 oz. 50.0
Fish dish, frozen (see also "Fish entree"):
cakes *(Mrs. Paul's),* 2 cakes 24.0
with cheese and salsa *(Oven Poppers),* ½ pkg., 4.5 oz. 3.0
croquettes *(Dr. Praeger's),* 2.2-oz. piece....................12.0

fillet, battered:
    (Mrs. Paul's), 1 piece 14.0
    (Mrs. Paul's Hearty Size), 1 piece............................19.0
    (Van de Kamp's), 1 piece...13.0
fillet, breaded:
    (Dr. Praeger's), 2.1-oz. piece..................................11.0
    (Mrs. Paul's), 2 pieces...19.0
    (Mrs. Paul's Healthy Selects), 1 piece 19.0
    (Van de Kamp's), 2 pieces..17.0
    (Van de Kamp's Crisp & Healthy), 2 pieces...........25.0
    (Van de Kamp's Hearty Size), 1 piece....................10.0
garlic herb *(Mrs. Paul's* Healthy Selects), 1 piece 19.0
garlic and herb *(Van de Kamp's* Crisp & Healthy),
    2 pieces 25.0
lemon pepper *(Mrs. Paul's* Healthy Selects), 1 piece 19.0
lemon pepper *(Van de Kamp's* Crisp & Healthy), 2 pieces....25.0
sandwich *(Dr. Praeger's)*, 4-oz. piece.................................19.0
fillet, grilled, 1 piece:
    Cajun, garlic butter, or lemon pepper *(Mrs. Paul's)*....................0
    garlic butter, lemon butter, or lemon pepper *(Van de
      Kamp's)* 0
portion:
    battered *(Van de Kamp's)*, 1 piece...........................13.0
    breaded *(Van de Kamp's)*, 3 pieces 23.0
    breaded, heated, 2-oz. piece.....................................13.5
with shrimp, crab, and vegetables *(Oven Poppers)*, ½ pkg.,
    4.5 oz. 13.0
with spinach and cheese *(Oven Poppers)*, ½ pkg., 4.5 oz. 8.0
sticks, breaded:
    (Dr. Praeger's Fillet), 3 pieces, 2.9 oz. 14.0
    (Dr. Praeger's Minced), ⅔-oz. piece.........................3.0
    (Mrs. Paul's), 6 pieces...21.0
    (Mrs. Paul's Healthy Selects), 6 pieces 26.0
    (Mrs. Paul's Hearty Size), 5 pieces........................25.0
    (Van de Kamp's), 6 pieces.......................................22.0
    (Van de Kamp's Club), 6 sticks................................19.0
    (Van de Kamp's Crisp & Healthy), 6 pieces...........24.0
    (Van de Kamp's Mini), 13 pieces.............................19.0
    (Van de Kamp's Snack/Value), 6 pieces 20.0
    heated, 1-oz. piece 6.7
strips, breaded *(Mrs. Paul's/Van de Kamp's)*, 4 pieces...............25.0

Fish dish *(cont.)*
tenders, battered *(Mrs. Paul's)*, 4 pieces 26.0
tenders, battered *(Van de Kamp's)*, 4 pieces......................24.0
Fish entree, frozen, 1 pkg.:
baked *(Lean Cuisine Cafe Classics)*, 9 oz. 40.0
breaded, with macaroni and cheese *(Marie Callender's Meals)*,
    12 oz. 53.0
fillet, with macaroni and cheese *(Stouffer's* Homestyle),
    9 oz. 37.0
sticks *(Banquet)*, 6.6 oz. 33.0
sticks, with whipped potatoes and corn *(Freezer Queen* Meal),
    6.5 oz. 47.0
Fish roe, see "Caviar" and "Roe"
Fish sauce:
1 fl. oz. 1.0
1 tbsp... .7
Fish seasoning and coating mix:
(Shake 'n Bake Original Recipe), ⅛ pkt. 14.0
and chips *(Don's Chuck Wagon)*, ¼ cup.....................21.0
Fish sticks, see "Fish entree"
Flan, see "Pudding" and "Pudding and pie filling mix"
Flatbread, see "Cracker"
Flatfish, without added ingredients 0
Flavor enhancer *(Accent)*, ⅛ tsp. 0
Flax powder *(Arrowhead Mills* Nutri), 2 tbsp. 6.0
Flax seeds:
(Arrowhead Mills), 3 tbsp. 11.0
1 cup...53.1
1 tbsp..4.1
Flounder, fresh, without added ingredients 0
Flounder entree, frozen:
au gratin *(Oven Poppers)*, ½ pkg., 5 oz. 5.0
crab-stuffed *(Oven Poppers)*, ½ pkg., 5 oz. 15.0
fillet, breaded *(Mrs. Paul's)*, 1 piece.........................11.0
fillet, breaded *(Van de Kamp's* Premium), 1 piece 18.0
with spinach and cheese *(Oven Poppers)*, ½ pkg., 4.5 oz. 8.0
stuffed with broccoli and cheese *(Oven Poppers)*, ½ pkg., 5 oz. ...4.0
stuffed with garlic, shrimp, and almonds *(Oven Poppers)*,
    ½ pkg., 5 oz. 15.0
Flour, see "Wheat flour" and specific listings
Focaccia, sprouted five-grain *(Shiloh Farms)*, 4-oz. roll 52.0

Focaccia, stuffed, frozen:
Italian, cheese and peppers *(Cedarlane)*, ½ of 11-oz. pkg..........52.0
Mediterranian, spinach and cheese *(Cedarlane)*, ½ of
    11-oz. pkg. 51.0
Roma, tomato and basil *(Cedarlane)*, ½ of 11-oz. pkg. 46.0
Fondue, ready-to-serve:
(Swiss Knight), ¼ cup 2.0
(Swissrose), ¼ cup 0
Frankfurter (see also "Knockwurst"):
(Hormel Fat Free Hot Dogs), 1 link 5.0
(Light & Lean), 1 link..4.0
(Louis Rich Original 50% less Fat), 1.6-oz. link.........................2.0
(Oscar Mayer Wieners), 1.6-oz. link...1.0
(Russer Light Deli), 2-oz. link...3.0
beef:
    (Ball Park), 2-oz. link..3.0
    (Ball Park Fat Free), 1.75-oz. link...7.0
    (Ball Park Kosher), 1.5-oz. link...2.0
    (Ball Park Lite), 1.75-oz. link..3.0
    (Ball Park Singles), 1.6-oz. link..2.0
    (Boar's Head Natural Casing), 2-oz. link.................................1.0
    (Boar's Head Skinless/Lite), 1.6-oz. link..................................0
    (Healthy Choice), 1.75-oz. link..7.0
    (Hebrew National), 1.7-oz. link..1.0
    (Hebrew National Dinner), 4-oz. link 1.0
    (Hebrew National Family/Party Pack), 3-oz. link.....................1.0
    (Hebrew National 97% Fat Free), 1.7-oz. link.........................3.0
    (Hebrew National Reduced Fat), 1.7-oz. link 0
    (Hormel Fat Free), 1 link..5.0
    (Hormel Fat Free Hot Dogs), 1 link..5.0
    (Hormel Natural Casing), 1 link..0
    (Nathan's Famous), 2-oz. link..1.0
    (Russer Natural Casing), 2.6-oz. link.......................................1.0
    (Wranglers), 2-oz. link..1.0
    2-oz. link..1.0
    1.6-oz. link 8
beef and pork:
    (Ball Park Fat Free), 1.75-oz. link 6.0
    (Ball Park Lite), 1.75-oz. link..3.0
    (Ball Park Singles), 1.6-oz. link..3.0
    1.6-oz. link..1.1

Frankfurter *(cont.)*

cheese:

   (Ball Park Singles), 1.6-oz. link 2.0

   (Wranglers), 2-oz. link................................1.0

   smokie, 1.5-oz. link 6

chicken *(Empire* Kosher), 2-oz. link................................1.0

Chicken, 1.6-oz. link................................3.1

cocktail:

   (Johnsonville Little Wieners), 6 links, 2 oz. 2.0

   beef *(Hebrew National),* 5 links, 2 oz. 1.0

   beef, wrapped *(Hebrew National* Franks in a Blanket),

     5 pieces, 2.9 oz................................8.0

pork and beef *(Boar's Head* Natural Casing), 2-oz. link...................0

smoked:

   (Johnsonville Wieners), 1.7-oz. link 1.0

   (Oscar Mayer Big & Juicy Hot Dogs), 2.7-oz. link................1.0

   (Wranglers), 2-oz. link................................1.0

turkey *(Empire* Kosher), 2-oz. link ....<1.0

turkey, 1.6-oz. link 7

turkey, pork, beef *(Healthy Choice* Low Fat), 1.75-oz. link...........6.0

"Frankfurter," vegetarian:

canned:

   (Loma Linda Big Franks), 1.8-oz. link 2.0

   (Loma Linda Big Franks Low Fat), 1.8-oz. link.......................3.0

   (Loma Linda Little Links), 2 links, 1.6 oz. 2.0

   (Loma Linda Linketts), 1.2-oz. link................................1.0

   (Worthington Super Links), 1.7-oz. link 2.0

   (Worthington Veja-Links), 1.1-oz. link................................1.0

frozen:

   (Morningstar Farms America's Original Veggie Dog),

     2-oz. link................................6.0

   (Natural Touch Veggie Dog), 2-oz. link................................6.0

   (Worthington Leanies), 1.4-oz. link................................2.0

   corn dog *(Loma Linda),* 2.5-oz. piece 22.0

   corn dog *(Morningstar Farms Meat-Free),* 2.5-oz. piece.......22.0

   corn dog *(Natural Touch* Veggie), 2.5-oz. piece 22.0

   corn dog, mini *(Morningstar Farms Meat-Free),* 4 pieces,

     2.7 oz................................21.0

Frankfurter sandwich:

(Ball Park Fun Franks), 2 pkg.................................32.0

corn dog:
    (Ball Park), 2.6-oz. piece 21.0
    (Hormel Quick Meal), 3.5-oz. piece 32.9
    (Michelina's Corn Dawgs), 5.5-oz. pkg.................37.0
    mini *(Hormel Quick Meal)*, 10 pieces, 5.6 oz. 47.0
    mini *(Kid's Kitchen)*, 5 pieces, 2.8 oz. 23.0
French beans:
mature, raw, 1 cup 118.0
mature, boiled, 1 cup 42.5
French cut beans, see "Green bean"
French toast, frozen:
(Aunt Jemima Homestyle), 2 slices 35.0
2.1-oz. piece 18.9
cinnamon *(Aunt Jemima)*, 2 slices..........................35.0
cinnamon sticks *(Aunt Jemima)*, 4 pieces 52.0
Frosting, ready-to-spread, 2 tbsp.:
banana creme *(Pillsbury Creamy Supreme)*................23.0
butter cream *(Creamy Deluxe)* 24.0
cherry *(Creamy Deluxe)* 24.0
chocolate:
    (Betty Crocker Soft Whipped)..............................14.0
    (Creamy Deluxe)...22.0
    (Pillsbury Creamy Supreme) 21.0
    (Sweet Rewards) 24.0
    dark *(Creamy Deluxe)*..21.0
    milk *(Betty Crocker* Soft Whipped).......................14.0
    milk *(Creamy Deluxe)* 22.0
    milk *(Sweet Rewards)* 25.0
    milk or fudge *(Pillsbury Creamy Supreme)* 21.0
    white *(Creamy Deluxe)*...24.0
coconut pecan *(Creamy Deluxe)* 17.0
cookies and creme *(Pillsbury Creamy Supreme)*........23.0
cream cheese *(Betty Crocker* Soft Whipped) 15.0
cream cheese *(Creamy Deluxe)*...............................24.0
lemon:
    (Betty Crocker Soft Whipped)..............................15.0
    (Creamy Deluxe)...24.0
    creme *(Pillsbury Creamy Supreme)* 24.0
rainbow chip *(Creamy Deluxe)*.................................24.0
sour cream, chocolate *(Creamy Deluxe)* 22.0
sour cream, white *(Creamy Deluxe)*.........................24.0

Frosting *(cont.)*
strawberry *(Betty Crocker Soft Whipped)* 15.0
strawberry cream cheese *(Creamy Deluxe)* 24.0
strawberry creme *(Pillsbury Creamy Supreme)* 24.0
vanilla:
    (Betty Crocker Soft Whipped)...15.0
    (Creamy Deluxe)...24.0
    (Pillsbury Creamy Supreme) 23.0
    (Pillsbury Creamy Supreme Funfetti) 25.0
    (Sweet Rewards)..27.0
    French *(Creamy Deluxe)* 24.0
    French *(Pillsbury Creamy Supreme)* 26.0
    white, fluffy *(Betty Crocker Soft Whipped)* 15.0
Frosting mix:
(Estee), ⅕ pkg. 20.0
chocolate, 1.5 oz. 30.1
coconut-pecan *(Betty Crocker)*, 3 tbsp. 21.0
fluffy, .9 oz. 16.3
fudge *("Jiffy")*, ¼ cup* 28.0
vanilla, 1.5 oz. 30.4
white *("Jiffy")*, ¼ cup* 27.0
white, fluffy *(Betty Crocker)*, 3 tbsp. 24.0
Fructose:
(Estee), 1 pkt. 3.0
(Estee), 1 tsp. 4.0
(Featherweight), 1 tsp. 4.0
Fruit, see specific listings
Fruit, candied, see specific listings
Fruit, mixed, candied *(S&W Glace Cake Mix)*, 2 tbsp. 25.0
Fruit, mixed, canned (see also "Fruit cocktail"):
(Dole FruitBowls), 4-oz. bowl 22.0
in water, 1 cup 19.3
in juice:
    (Del Monte Chunky Fruit Naturals), ½ cup..........................15.0
    (Del Monte Fruit Naturals Snack Cup), 4-oz. cup 13.0
    1 cup 32.5
    chunky *(Libby's Lite)*, ½ cup..14.0
    chunky *(S&W)*, ½ cup...19.0
    tropical, with pineapple/passion fruit juices *(Del Monte)*,
      ½ cup 16.0

in extra light syrup:
    (Del Monte Chunky Lite), ½ cup 15.0
    (Del Monte Lite Snack Cup), 4-oz. cup..................13.0
in light syrup:
    (Del Monte Fruit-to-Go), 4-oz. cup 18.0
    (Del Monte Orchard Select California), ½ cup.......19.0
    1 cup 38.2
    cherry-flavored *(Del Monte Fruit Pleasures)*, ½ cup 22.0
    cherry-flavored *(Del Monte Fruitrageous)*, 4-oz. cup 22.0
    tropical *(Dole* Fruit Salad), ½ cup 20.0
    tropical, with passion fruit juices *(Del Monte)*, ½ cup 21.0
in heavy syrup:
    (Del Monte Chunky), ½ cup 24.0
    (Del Monte Snack Cup), 4-oz. cup 20.0
    1 cup 48.7
    tropical, 1 cup 57.5
in extra heavy syrup, 1 cup 59.0
tropical *(Dole FruitBowls)*, 4-oz. bowl.......................16.0
Fruit, mixed, dried:
(Sonoma Organic), 7 pieces, 1.4 oz......................30.0
diced *(Sonoma* Organic), ⅓ cup, 1.4 oz. 31.0
Fruit, mixed, frozen, sweetened *(Birds Eye)*, ½ cup 23.0
Fruit bar, frozen (see also "Ice bar"), 1 bar:
banana, creamy, chocolate-dipped *(Dreyer's/Edy's)*....................23.0
banana cream *(Frozfruit)*...20.0
berry, orange, or punch *(Hi-C)*,................................16.0
berry, wild *(Edy's)* 21.0
cantaloupe *(Frozfruit)*...15.0
cherry *(Frozfruit)*...16.0
cherry, grape, or orange *(Minute Maid)* 14.0
coconut *(Frozfruit)* 18.0
grape *(Welch's)* 19.0
lemon *(Frozfruit)*..19.0
lemonade or lime *(Dreyer's/Edy's)* 20.0
lime *(Frozfruit)*...22.0
mango *(Frozfruit)*...26.0
peach *(Edy's)*...22.0
peach *(Smoothie.Yum* Give Peach a Chance) 21.0
piña colada *(Frozfruit)*..22.0
pineapple *(Frozfruit)*..20.0

Fruit bar *(cont.)*
strawberry:
    (Dreyer's/Edy's) 21.0
    (Frozfruit) 23.0
    cream *(Frozfruit)* 22.0
    creamy, chocolate-dipped *(Dreyer's/Edy's)* 21.0
strawberry-banana *(Smoothie.Yum Yumtonic)* 34.0
tangerine *(Edy's)* 20.0
tropical *(Frozfruit)* 21.0
tropical blends *(Welch's* Variety Pack) 11.0
watermelon *(Frozfruit)* 17.0
Fruit cocktail, canned:
(Del Monte Very Cherry), ½ cup 22.0
in water, 1 cup 20.7
in juice:
    (Del Monte Fruit Naturals), ½ cup..............................15.0
    (Libby's Lite), ½ cup 15.0
    (S&W Natural Style), ½ cup...20.0
    1 cup 28.1
in extra light syrup *(Del Monte* Lite), ½ cup.....................15.0
in extra light syrup, 1 cup 14.3
in light syrup, 1 cup 36.1
in heavy syrup:
    (Del Monte), ½ cup 24.0
    (S&W), ½ cup 23.0
    1 cup 46.9
in extra heavy syrup, 1 cup 59.5
in extra heavy syrup, ½ cup..29.8
Fruit glacé, see "Fruit, mixed, candied," and specific listings
Fruit glaze, see "Strawberry pie glaze"
Fruit ice, see "Ice"
Fruit juice, see specific fruit listings
Fruit juice bar, see "Fruit bar"
Fruit juice blend, 8 fl. oz., except as noted:
(After the Fall Maui Grove)...23.0
(After the Fall Sangria de la Noche) 30.0
(R.W. Knudsen Natural Breakfast)...................................27.0
(R.W. Knudsen Simply Nutritious) 31.0
(R.W. Knudsen Simply Nutritious Vita Juice)...................29.0
punch *(Minute Maid* Calcium)..36.0
punch *(Mott's)* 30.0

tropical *(Juicy Juice)*..32.0
tropical *(Juicy Juice)*, 8.45-fl.-oz. box.......................34.0
Fruit juice drink, sparkling, see "Soft drink"
Fruit juice drink blend, 8 fl. oz., except as noted:
(Capri Sun Surfer Cooler), 1 pouch 27.0
(Dole Fruit Fiesta)...34.0
(Kool-Aid Bursts Great Bluedini), 1 bottle.................24.0
(Rocket Juice Ginkgo Think), 16 fl. oz. 38.0
(Snapple Bali Blast)..28.0
citrus:
    (WhipperSnapple Power Citrus Smoothie), 10 fl. oz. 30.0
    cooler *(Turkey Hill* Calypso).................................30.0
    punch *(Tropicana)*...36.0
    punch *(Tropicana Twister)*, 10 fl. oz. 45.0
punch:
    (AriZona) 28.0
    (Crystal Light) 0
    (Dole), 10 fl. oz...39.0
    (Hawaiian Punch Fruit Juicy Red) 29.0
    (Snapple Hydro) 22.0
    (Tropicana) 32.0
    (Turkey Hill Flamenco)...................................30.0
    tropical *(Kool-Aid Bursts)*, 1 bottle......................24.0
    tropical *(Kool-Aid Splash)* 31.0
    tropical *(R.W. Knudsen)* 29.0
tropical fruit smoothie *(Rocket Juice Orange Blast)*, 16 fl. oz.....71.0
frozen*, punch 28.9
mix*:
    punch *(Crystal Light)*....................................0
    punch, tropical *(Kool-Aid)* 25.0
    punch, tropical *(Kool-Aid* Sugar Sweetened)...............16.0
Fruit leather, see "Fruit snack"
Fruit pectin:
(Sure•Jell), ¼ tsp. 1.0
unsweetened, 1¾-oz. pkg. 45.2
Fruit protector *(Sure•Jell Ever-Fresh)*, ¼ tsp......<1.0
Fruit salad, canned, see "Fruit, mixed, canned"
Fruit snack, all fruits:
(Fruit by the Foot), .75-oz. roll............................17.0
(Fruit Roll-Ups), .5-oz. roll...............................12.0

Fruit snack *(cont.)*
leather:
    bar, .8-oz. bar 18.1
    pieces, 1-oz. pkg. 21.2
    roll, large, ¾ oz. 17.7
    roll, small, .5 oz. 11.8
Fruit spread (see also "Jam and preserves"), 1 tbsp.:
all varieties:
    (Dickenson's) 13.0
    (Estee Fructose) 4.0
    (Kraft Reduced Calorie) 5.0
    (Polaner) 10.0
    (Smucker's) 10.0
apricot, blackberry, raspberry, or strawberry *(Kraft)* 13.0
grape *(Featherweight)* 4.0
peach, pineapple, or orange marmalade *(Kraft)* 14.0
Fruit-nut mix, see "Trail mix"
Fudge topping, see "Chocolate topping"
Fusilli pasta dish, mix:
with creamy pesto sauce *(Knorr)*, ⅔ cup 46.0
and red beans *(Marrakesh Express* Pasta & Sauce), ⅓ cup,
    1 cup* 41.0

G

Gai lan, see "Broccoli, Chinese"
Galanga *(Frieda's),* ⅔ cup, 3 oz. 13.0
Garbanzo beans:
dry:
    (Arrowhead Mills), ¼ cup...29.0
    (Frieda's), ⅓ cup, 3 oz. 23.0
    1 cup 121.3
boiled, 1 cup 45.0
Garbanzo beans, canned, ½ cup:
(Allens/East Texas Fair) 19.0
(Eden Organic) 19.0
(Goya Chick Peas)..20.0
(Hain Chick Peas)...20.0
(Joan of Arc) 18.0
(Progresso Chickpeas)..20.0
(Seneca)...19.0
(Shari Ann's Organic) 18.0
(Westbrae Natural) 18.0
Garlic, fresh:
raw *(Frieda's* Elephant), 1 tbsp...1.0
raw, 1 tsp. 9
Garlic, chopped or crushed, in jar *(Christopher Ranch),* 1 tsp....1.0
Garlic, pickled, in jar *(Christopher Ranch),* 3 pieces 0
Garlic, roasted, in jar, lightly seasoned *(Christopher Ranch),*
    2–3 cloves...2.0
Garlic paste, in jar *(Italia in Tavola),* 1 tbsp. 3.0
Garlic pepper:
(Lawry's), ¼ tsp. 0
1 tsp. 1.8
Garlic powder:
1 tbsp..6.1
1 tsp. 2.0
with parsley *(Lawry's),* ¼ tsp. 1.0
Garlic relish, Indian, in jar *(Patak's),* 1 tbsp. 3.0

Garlic salt:
(Lawry's), ¼ tsp. 0
1 tsp. 5
Garlic spread:
(Lawry's), 1 tbsp. 2.0
concentrate *(Lawry's),* 2 tsp. 1.0
Garlic sprouts *(Jonathan's),* 1 cup 14.0
Gefiltefish, sweet, 1.5-oz. pc. 3.1
Gelatin, dry, unsweetened, 1 envelope or 1 tbsp. 0
Gelatin dessert, ready-to-eat:
all flavors:
    (Jell-O Snacks), 3.5-oz. cont. 17.0
    (Jell-O Snacks Sugar Free), 3.25-oz. cont. 0
    (Kozy Shack), 4-oz. cont. 23.0
    (Kraft Handi-Snacks), 3.5-oz. cont. 20.0
orange or strawberry *(Kozy Shack Sugar Free),* 4-oz. cont. 2.0
Gelatin dessert mix, ½ cup*:
all flavors:
    (Jell-O) 19.0
    (Jell-O Sugar Free) 0
    (Royal) 17.0
    except cherry *(Royal Sugar Free)* 1.0
cherry *(Hain),* ¼ pkg. 20.0
cherry *(Royal Sugar Free)* 2.0
strawberry *(Jell-O 1-2-3)* 26.0
Gelatin drink mix, orange flavor, .6-oz. pkt.* 10.5
Gelato, see "Ice cream"
Gemelli pasta dish, mix, and white beans *(Marrakesh*
    Express Pasta & Sauce), ⅓ cup, 1 cup* 43.0
Giardiniera, see "Vegetables, mixed, pickled"
Ginger, root, fresh:
(Frieda's), 1 tbsp. 1.0
1 tsp. 1
sliced, 1" diam., ¼ cup 3.6
Ginger, crushed, in jar *(Budarim),* 1 tsp. ....<1.0
Ginger, crystallized:
(Frieda's), 9 pieces, 1.1 oz. 26.0
(Sonoma), 1.5-oz. pouch 34.0
Ginger, ground:
1 tbsp. 3.8
1 tsp. 1.3

Ginger, pickled:
(*Budarim* Sushi), 1 oz. 5.0
(*Eden*), 1 tbsp. 3.0
Japanese, 1 oz. 2.1
Ginger, Thai or Siamese, see "Galanga"
Ginger beverage:
(*Rocket Juice Ginger Ginseng*), 16 fl. oz. 39.0
nectar, Hawaiian (*Santa Cruz Organic*), 8 fl. oz. 27.0
Gingerbread, see "Bread, mix, sweet"
Ginkgo nut, shelled:
raw, 1 oz. 10.7
dried, 1 oz. 20.5
Ginkgo nut, canned, 1 cup...................................34.3
Gizzard:
chicken, raw, 1.3-oz. gizzard 2
chicken, simmered, chopped or diced, 1 cup 2
turkey, raw, 4-oz. gizzard 7
turkey, simmered, chopped, or diced, 1 cup................... .9
Glaze, ham, see "Ham glaze"
Glaze, pie, see "Strawberry pie glaze"
Glaze mix, see "Seasoning and coating mix"
Gluten, see "Wheat flour"
Goa beans, see "Winged beans"
Goat, without added ingredients...............................0
Goatfish, without added ingredients..........................0
Gobo root, see "Burdock root"
Godfather's Pizza:
original crust, cheese:
    jumbo, 1/10 pie...53.0
    large, 1/10 pie..36.0
    medium, 1/8 pie..34.0
    mini, 1/4 pie...19.0
original crust, combo:
    jumbo, 1/10 pie...56.0
    large, 1/10 pie..38.0
    medium, 1/8 pie..36.0
    mini, 1/4 pie...21.0
golden crust:
    cheese, large, 1/10 pie...28.0
    cheese, medium, 1/8 pie...26.0

206 *Corinne T. Netzer*

Godfather's Pizza, golden crust *(cont.)*
combo, large, ¹⁄₁₀ pie 31.0
combo, medium, ⅛ pie 28.0
Golden nugget squash *(Frieda's)*, ¾ cup, 3 oz. 7.0
Goose, without added ingredients, 4 oz. 0
Goose fat 0
Goose liver, see "Liver" and "Paté"
Gooseberries, fresh, raw, 1 cup 15.3
Gooseberries, canned:
in light syrup *(Oregon)*, ½ cup 22.0
in light syrup, 1 cup 47.3
Gourd:
dishcloth:
raw, 6.3-oz. gourd 7.8
raw, 1" pieces, 1 cup 4.1
boiled, drained, 1" pieces, 1 cup 25.5
boiled, drained, 1" slices, ½ cup 12.8
white-flower:
raw, 1.7-lb. gourd 26.1
raw, 1" pieces, ½ cup 2.0
boiled, drained, 1" cubes, 1 cup 5.4
Gourd strips, see "Kanpyo"
Grains, see specific listings
Granadilla, see "Passion fruit"
Granola, see "Cereal"
Granola and cereal bar, 1 bar, except as noted:
all fruit varieties:
(Barbara's Nature's Choice Cereal Fat Free), 1.3 oz. 27.0
(Hain Breakfast Bar), 1.4 oz. 29.0
(Health Valley Fruit Bars), 1.5 oz. 35.0
(Health Valley Granola Bars), 1.5 oz. 35.0
(Health Valley Granola Bars Moist and Chewy), 1 oz. 22.0
(Health Valley Bakes), 1 oz. 19.0
(Health Valley Breakfast Bakes), 1.3 oz. 26.0
(Health Valley Tarts), 1.4 oz. 28.0
(Kellogg's Nutri-Grain), 1.3 oz. 27.0
(Kellogg's Nutri-Grain Fruit-full Squares), 1.7 oz. 35.0
(Nabisco Fruit 'n Grain), 1.3 oz. 25.0
(Sunbelt Cereal Bar), 1.3 oz. 28.0
(Sweet Rewards Fat Free), 1.3 oz. 29.0
all varieties *(Nature Valley Crunchy Granola)*, 2 bars, 1.5 oz. 29.0

almond *(Sunbelt* Chewy Granola), 1 oz...17.0
apple, blueberry, or strawberry cobbler *(Health Valley* Cereal
    Bar), 1.3 oz..27.0
apple cinnamon:
    (Quaker Fruit & Oatmeal), 1.3 oz...................................26.0
    (Quaker Granola Low Fat), 1 oz.......................................21.0
    (Sunbelt Chewy Granola Low Fat), 1.2 oz. 28.0
    brown sugar *(Kellogg's Nutri-Grain Twists),* 1.3 oz...............27.0
banana-nut *(Sunbelt* Granola), 1.9 oz. 37.0
banana-strawberry *(Kellogg's Nutri-Grain Twists),* 1.3 oz...........26.0
Bavarian or vanilla creme *(Health Valley* Cereal Bar), 1.3 oz.......28.0
berry *(Quaker* Fruit & Oatmeal Very Berry), 1.3 oz. 27.0
berry *(Sunbelt* Cereal Basic), 1.9 oz.................................40.0
blueberry *(Quaker* Fruit & Oatmeal), 1.3 oz. 26.0
blueberry or strawberry *(Nabisco* Fruit 'n Grain), 1.3 oz. 25.0
carob chip *(Barbara's Nature's Choice* Granola), .75 oz. 16.0
cherry or berry *(Barbara's Nature's Choice* Cereal Low Fat),
    1.3 oz..28.0
(Chex), 1.4 oz..26.0
chocolate *(Health Valley Tars),* 1.4 oz. 28.0
chocolate chip:
    (Health Valley Granola Bars), 1.5 oz. 35.0
    (Quaker Chewy Granola), .6 oz.......................................13.0
    (Quaker Chewy Granola Low Fat Chocolate Chunk), 1 oz. 22.0
    (Sunbelt Chewy Granola), 1.2 oz....................................23.0
    (Sunbelt Chew Granola Singles), 1.8 oz. 33.0
    fudge-dipped *(Sunbelt),* 1.5 oz.......................................27.0
    fudge-dipped *(Sunbelt* Singles), 2 oz. 36.0
    or fudge *(Kudos* Enrobed), 1 oz.....................................20.0
cinnamon and raisin *(Barbara's Nature's Choice* Granola),
    .75 oz. 16.0
cinnamon and raisin *(Sunbelt* Granola Low Fat), 1.9 oz. 42.0
(Cinnamon Toast Crunch), 1.6 oz. 31.0
cocoa *(Kellogg's Rice Krispies Treats* Squares), .8 oz. 16.0
cookies and cream *(Quaker* Chewy Granola), 1 oz.......................22.0
fruit *(Sunbelt* Jammers), 1 oz..23.0
fruit and nut *(Sunbelt* Granola), 1.9 oz. 40.0
fudge, double *(Sweet Rewards* Fat Free Supreme), 1.1 oz. 25.0
(Honey Nut Cheerios), 1.4 oz...26.0
(Kellogg's Rice Krispies Treats Squares Original), .8 oz...............18.0
(Kudos with M&M's), .8 oz. 17.0

Granola and cereal bar *(cont.)*

(Kudos with Snickers), .8 oz. 16.9
macaroon, fudge-dipped *(Sunbelt)*, 1.4 oz.......................24.0
macaroon, fudge-dipped *(Sunbelt* Singles), 2 oz. 33.0
marshmallow *(Golden Grahams Treats)*, .8 oz. 17.0
marshmallow, regular or chocolate chip *(Health Valley)*.............24.0
oatmeal raisin *(Quaker* Chew Granola Low Fat)*, 1 oz. 22.0
oatmeal raisin *(Sunbelt* Chewy Granola Low Fat)*, 1.2 oz............27.0
oats and honey:
    (Barbara's Nature's Choice Granola)*, .75 oz. 15.0
    (Sunbelt Chewy Granola)*, 1.2 oz.....................................19.0
    (Sunbelt Chewy Granola Singles)*, 1.7 oz. 32.0
peanut *(Health Valley* Granola Bars Moist and Chewy)*, 1 oz. 19.0
peanut butter:
    (Barbara's Nature's Choice Granola)*, .75 oz. 14.0
    (Kudos), 1 oz...19.0
    chocolate *(Golden Grahams Treats)*, .8 oz...........................15.0
    chocolate *(Kellogg's Rice Krispies Treats* Squares)*, .8 oz. 16.0
    chocolate chip *(Quaker* Chewy Granola)*, 1 oz.......................19.0
rice bar:
    caramel, double chocolate, or peanut butter crunch
      (Hain Mini Munchie Snack Bar)*, 1 oz. 20.0
    chocolate, chocolate chip, or peanut butter *(Estee)* 15.0
    vanilla *(Estee)*..14.0
S'mores:
    (Quaker Chewy Granola Low Fat)*, 1 oz. 22.0
    (Sunbelt Granola Treats)*, 1.1 oz....................................21.0
    chocolate chunk *(Golden Grahams Treats)*, .8 oz. 17.0
    chocolate chunk *(Golden Grahams Treats* King Size)*,
      1.6 oz..34.0
strawberry *(Quaker* Fruit & Oatmeal)*, 1.3 oz. 26.0
strawberry and blueberry *(Kellogg's Nutri-Grain Twists)*,
    1.3 oz. 27.0
strawberry and creme *(Kellogg's Nutri-Grain Twists)*, 1.3 oz......26.0
Grapes, fresh, raw:
American type (slipskin)*, 1 grape 4
American type (slipskin)*, 1 cup 15.8
red or green, European type (adherent skin):
    (Dole), 1½ cups 24.0
    with seeds, 1 cup 27.4
    seedless, 1 cup 28.4

Grapes, canned, seedless:
in water, 1 cup 25.2
in light syrup *(Oregon* Thompson), ½ cup 23.0
in heavy syrup, 1 cup...50.3
Grape drink, 8 fl. oz., except as noted:
(After the Fall Hearty)...37.0
(Kool-Aid Bursts), 1 bottle 25.0
(Mott's) 31.0
(R.W. Knudsen Aseptic) 35.0
(Snapple Hydro)...23.0
punch *(Hawaiian Punch Grape Geyser)*...................30.0
white *(Snapple* Diet)..2.0
white *(Welch's)* 35.0
Grape drink blend, 8 fl. oz., except as noted:
berry *(Kool-Aid Splash)* 31.0
berry *(Rocket Juice "Zinful" Anti Oxidant),* 16 fl. oz. 48.0
mix*, berry *(Kool-Aid Grape Berry Splash* Sugar Sweetened)....17.0
Grape drink mix* *(Kool-Aid* Sugar Sweetened), 8 fl. oz............16.0
Grape juice, 8 fl. oz.:
(R.W. Knudsen) 37.0
(Welch's) 42.0
Concord *(R.W. Knudsen)* 40.0
white *(Juicy Juice)* 38.0
white *(Santa Cruz Organic)* 28.0
frozen*, sweetened 31.9
Grape juice blend:
(Mott's), 11.5 fl. oz..43.0
(Mott's), 8 fl. oz..31.0
Grape leaves, fresh:
raw, 1 leaf 5
raw, 1 cup 2.4
Grape leaves, in jar:
(Krinos), 1 leaf 0
1 leaf 5
Grape leaves, stuffed *(Cedarlane),* 1 piece 8.0
Grapefruit, fresh, raw:
(Dole), ½ medium...14.0
(Ocean Spray), ½ medium, 5.5 oz............................16.0
pink or red:
  ½ large, 4½" diam..13.4
  ½ medium, 3¾" diam..9.4

Grapefruit, pink or red *(cont.)*

large sections with juice, 1 cup 18.6
medium sections with juice, 1 cup 17.7
California or Arizona, ½ medium, 3¾" diam. 11.9
California or Arizona, medium sections with juice, 1 cup......22.8
Florida, ½ medium, 3¾" diam. 9.2
Florida, medium sections with juice, 1 cup 17.3
white:
  ½ large, 4½" diam. 13.4
  ½ medium, 3¾" diam. 9.9
  large sections with juice, 1 cup 18.6
  medium sections with juice, 1 cup 19.3
  California, ½ medium, 3¾" diam. 10.7
  California, medium sections with juice, 1 cup.....................20.9
  Florida, ½ medium, 3¾" diam. 9.7
  Florida, sections with juice, 1 cup 18.8

Grapefruit, canned or chilled:

in water, 1 cup 22.3
in juice, 1 cup...22.9
in light syrup, 1 cup...39.2

Grapefruit juice, 8 fl. oz., except as noted:

fresh, raw, pink or white 22.7
canned, dairy-pack, or bottled:
  (Goya), 6 fl. oz..13.0
  (Mott's)..27.0
  (Ocean Spray)..24.0
  (R.W. Knudsen) 23.0
  (R.W. Knudsen Organic) 23.0
  (R.W. Knudsen Rio Red) 35.0
  (Season's Best)..22.0
  (Tropicana Pure Premium Golden) 22.0
  (Tropicana Pure Premium Ruby Red Calcium).....................22.0
  unsweetened 22.1
  sweetened 27.8
  pink *(Ocean Spray)*..28.0
frozen*, unsweetened 24.0

Grapefruit juice drink:

pink *(Tropicana Twister),* 10 fl. oz..34.0
ruby red:
  (Ocean Spray), 8 fl. oz...33.0

(Snapple Diet), 8 fl. oz. 2.0
(Tropicana Twister), 10 fl. oz. 42.0
Grapefruit juice drink blend, 8 fl. oz.:
ginkgo extract *(R.W. Knudsen Simply Nutritious Ginkgo*
    Alert) 31.0
mango, ruby red *(Ocean Spray)*..33.0
ruby red *(Minute Maid* with Calcium) 27.0
strawberry, ruby red *(Ocean Spray)*....................................34.0
tangerine, ruby red *(Ocean Spray)*......................................32.0
Gravy, see specific listings
Great northern beans:
dry, 1 cup 114.1
boiled, 1 cup 37.3
Great northern beans, canned, ½ cup:
(Allens)..19.0
(Joan of Arc)..18.0
(Westbrae Natural)..16.0
with sausage *(Trappey's)*...18.0
Green beans, fresh:
raw, 10 beans, 4" long 3.9
raw, 1 cup 7.8
boiled, drained, 1 cup 9.9
Green beans, canned, ½ cup, except as noted:
(Allens Shell Outs)...6.0
(Green Giant Kitchen Sliced)...4.0
(Walnut Acres Organic Farms)..4.0
all styles *(Seneca)*...5.0
drained, 10 beans 2.8
drained, 1 cup 6.1
all varieties, except Italian *(Del Monte)* 4.0
whole *(Green Giant)*...5.0
cut *(Allens* No Salt) 3.0
cut *(Allens/Sunshine/GaBelle/Alma/Crest Top)*.....................6.0
cut or French style:
    (Green Giant)..4.0
    (Greene's Farm)..4.0
    (Hain) 4.0
French style *(Allens)* 4.0
Italian style *(Allens/Sunshine)*...7.0
Italian style *(Del Monte)* 6.0
and potatoes *(Allens/Sunshine)* 7.0

Green beans, canned *(cont.)*

seasoned, all styles 4.0

yellow or wax, see "Wax beans, canned"

Green beans, frozen:

all styles:

    10-oz. pkg. 21.5

    1 cup 9.4

    boiled, drained, 1 cup...8.7

whole:

    (Birds Eye), 21 beans 5.0

    (Freshlike), 1 cup...4.0

    (Seabrook Farms), ¾ cup..4.0

cut:

    (Freshlike), ⅔ cup...4.0

    (Freshlike Stir-fry), 1 cup..5.0

    (Green Giant), ¾ cup...5.0

cut or French cut *(Birds Eye)*, ½ cup...............................6.0

French cut *(Freshlike)*, 1 cup..4.0

Italian cut *(Birds Eye)*, ½ cup 8.0

Green beans, pickled, in jar, hot and spicy *(Hogue Farms)*,

    ¼ cup 3.0

Green bean combination, frozen:

and almonds *(Green Giant)*, ⅔ cup 4.0

and carrots *(Birds Eye/Freshlike* Baby Blend), 1 cup 5.0

casserole *(Green Giant)*, ⅔ cup 9.0

mushroom casserole *(Stouffer's)*, ½ cup 12.0

with spaetzle *(Birds Eye* Bavarian Style), 1 cup 15.0

whole, stir-fry *(Birds Eye* Farm Fresh), 1¾ cups 19.0

Green peas, see "Peas, green"

Green pepper, see "Pepper, sweet"

Greens, see specific listings

Greens, Chinese *(Frieda's* Yu Choy Sum), 1 cup, 3 oz................3.0

Greens, mixed, canned *(Allens/Sunshine)*, ½ cup.....................8.0

Grenadine syrup *(Rose's)*, 2 tbsp...22.0

Grilling sauce (see also "Marinade" and specific listings):

(San-J SJ Grilling), 2 tbsp. 8.0

chipotle *(Chi-Chi's)*, 2 tbsp..15.0

ginger, sweet, sesame *(House of Tsang* Hibachi), 1 tbsp.............9.0

pepper, see "Pepper sauce"

salsa *(Chi-Chi's)*, 2 tbsp. 12.0

teriyaki *(House of Tsang)*, 1 tbsp. 10.0

Tex-Mex *(Chi-Chi's)*, 2 tbsp...8.0
Grits, see "Corn grits"
Ground-cherry, fresh, raw, trimmed, 1 cup 15.7
Grouper, without added ingredients 0
Guacamole, refrigerated *(Calavo)*, 2 tbsp. 3.0
Guacamole seasoning mix:
(Bearitos), ½ tsp...1.0
(El Torito), 1/12 pkg..1.0
(Lawry's Spices & Seasonings), ½ tsp. 1.0
Guanabana nectar *(Goya)*, 6 fl. oz. 27.0
Guava, fresh, raw:
(Frieda's), 3-oz. fruit..10.0
common, trimmed, 3.2-oz. fruit.....................................10.7
common, 1 cup..19.6
strawberry, trimmed, .2-oz. fruit.....................................1.0
strawberry, 1 cup..42.4
Guava drink blend:
berry *(Fruit Works)*, 12 fl. oz..46.0
strawberry *(R.W. Knudsen)*, 8 fl. oz..............................27.0
Guava juice blend *(After the Fall Guava Maya)*, 8 fl. oz. 26.0
Guava nectar:
(Goya), 6 fl. oz. 27.0
(Libby's), 11.5-fl.-oz. can...52.0
Guava sauce, cooked, 1 cup.......................................22.6
Guavadilla, see "Passion fruit"
Guinea hen, without added ingredients, 4 oz.................0
Gyro mix, dry *(Casbah)*, .65 oz. 12.0

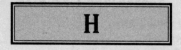

H

FOOD AND MEASURE   **CARBOHYDRATE GRAMS**

Habañero chili, see "Pepper, chili"
Habas *(Frieda's),* ½ cup, 3 oz..17.0
Haddock, fresh or smoked, without added ingredients 0
Haddock entree, frozen:
fillet:
    battered *(Van de Kamp's),* 2 pieces.............................17.0
    breaded *(Mrs. Paul's* Premium), 1 piece 17.0
    breaded *(Van de Kamp's* Premium), 1 piece 18.0
with shrimp, crab and vegetables *(Oven Poppers),*
    ½ pkg., 5 oz...12.0
Hake, see "Whiting"
Halibut, Atlantic or Pacific, without added ingredients..................0
Halibut entree, frozen, fillet, battered *(Van de Kamp's),*
    3 pieces 19.0
Halvah, 2 oz.:
chocolate, marble, or vanilla *(Joyva)* 18.0
chocolate-covered *(Joyva)*..20.0
Ham, fresh, without added ingredients....................................0
Ham, cured:
whole leg, unheated, 4 oz. or 1 cup ....<.1
whole leg, roasted, 4 oz. or 1 cup chopped or diced 0
boneless:
    (11% fat), unheated, 1 oz...9
    (11% fat), unheated, diced, 1 cup.................................4.2
    (11% fat), roasted, 3 oz. or 1 cup chopped or diced 0
    extra lean (5% fat), unheated, 1 oz. 3
    extra lean (5% fat), unheated, diced, 1 cup..................1.3
    extra lean (5% fat), roasted, 3 oz..............................1.3
    extra lean (5% fat), roasted, chopped or diced, 1 cup 2.1
Ham, refrigerated or canned, 3 oz., except as noted:
(Boar's Head Sweet Slice) 1.0
(Black Label) 0
(Black Label Refrigerated)...7
(Hormel), 2 oz..0

(Hormel Cure 81/Curemaster)..0

(Spiral Cure 81) 1.0

13% fat, unheated...0

13% fat, roasted 4

extra lean, 4% fat, roasted 6

extra lean, 4% fat, roasted, 1 cup 7

all varieties *(Jones Dairy Farm)* 0

all varieties, except maple *(Jones Dairy Farm Country Carved)*.......0

maple *(Jones Dairy Farm Country Carved)* 1.0

steak *(Jones Dairy Farm Lean Choice)*............................1.0

Ham entree, frozen, smoked steak, with macaroni and cheese
   (Marie Callender's Meals), 14-oz. pkg. 63.0

Ham glaze:

(Crosse & Blackwell), 1 tbsp...8.0

(Reese), 1 tbsp..5.0

brown sugar and spice *(Boar's Head),* 2 tbsp...............30.0

Ham lunch meat, (see also "Prosciutto" and "Turkey ham"),
   2 oz., except as noted:

(Black Bear Lower Sodium) 1.0

(Boar's Head Deluxe)..2.0

(Boar's Head Deluxe Lower Sodium) ....<1.0

(Carl Buddig Lean), 9 slices, 2 oz. 1.0

(Hansel 'n Gretel Healthy Deli Cinnamon Apple Grove)...............4.0

(Hansel 'n Gretel Healthy Deli Deluxe) 1.0

(Hansel 'n Gretel Healthy Deli Less Sodium) 2.0

(Hansel 'n Gretel Healthy Deli Olde Tyme Taverne 99%
   Fat Free) 1.0

(Hansel 'n Gretel Healthy Deli Shattuck) 2.0

(Healthy Choice 10 oz.), 1-oz. slice...............................1.0

(Light & Lean 97), 1-oz. slice..0

(Light & Lean 97), 3 slices, 3 oz. 2.0

(Oscar Mayer Lower Sodium), 3 slices, 2.2 oz. 2.0

baked:

   (Russer) 4.0

   (Sara Lee Homestyle) 2.0

   cooked *(Healthy Choice),* 1-oz. slice 1.0

   or cooked *(Healthy Choice Deli Traditions),* 6 slices, 1.9 oz....1.0

Black Forest *(Boar's Head)*..2.0

Black Forest *(Russer)*..0

boiled *(Sara Lee* Deli), 2 slices, 1.6 oz...........................1.0

Ham lunch meat *(cont.)*
brown sugar:
    (Sara Lee)...5.0
    (Sara Lee Deli), 2 slices, 1.6 oz...4.0
    baked *(Carl Buddig* Premium Lean Slices), 2.5-oz. pkg. 3.0
    cured *(Healthy Choice Hearty Deli Flavor)*, 3 slices, 2 oz. 3.0
cappicola *(Boar's Head* Cappy) 3.0
cappicola *(Hansel 'n Gretel Healthy Deli* Cappi) 2.0
chopped:
    (Black Label)...2.0
    ¾-oz. slice 0
    canned, ¾-oz. slice 1
cooked:
    (Healthy Choice)..1.0
    (Healthy Choice), 1-oz. slice..2.0
    (Hormel)..2.0
    (Russer/Russer Fat Free/Light)..2.0
    (Sara Lee Old Fashioned) 1.0
glazed *(Hansel 'n Gretel Healthy Deli* Pear Shape)......................2.0
honey:
    (Carl Buddig Lean), 2.5-oz. pkg...3.0
    (Carl Buddig Lean), 9 slices, 2 oz...2.0
    (Hansel 'n Gretel Healthy Deli Honey Valley) 2.0
    (Healthy Choice)..2.0
    (Healthy Choice), 1-oz. slice..1.0
    (Healthy Choice Savory Selections), 6 slices, 1.9 oz...............2.0
    (Oscar Mayer), 3 slices, 2.2 oz..2.0
    baked *(Carl Buddig* Premium Lean Slices), 2.5-oz. pkg. 3.0
    baked *(Healthy Choice* Hearty Deli Flavor), 3 slices, 2 oz........3.0
    cured *(Russer/Russer* Fat Free)...2.0
    cured *(Sara Lee)*..2.0
    cured *(Sara Lee* Deli), 2 slices, 1.6 oz..................................1.0
    maple *(Healthy Choice)* 3.0
    maple *(Healthy Choice Savory Selections)*, 6 slices, 1.9 oz. ...3.0
    and maple-cured *(Russer)*...3.0
    oven-roasted *(Sara Lee* Bavarian Brand) 2.0
honey mustard *(Healthy Choice Savory Selections)*, 6 slices,
    1.9 oz..3.0
hot *(Hansel 'n Gretel Healthy Deli* Rodeo)...................................1.0
hot *(Russer)*...3.0
jalapeño *(Hansel 'n Gretel Healthy Deli)*......................................3.0

maple:
- (Boar's Head Maple Glazed Honey Coat) 3.0
- (Hansel 'n Gretel Healthy Deli Flame Seared/Vermont) 3.0
- (Russer Canadian Brand) 4.0
- glazed (Black Bear)..2.0
- honey (Sara Lee) 4.0

minced, ¾-oz. slice.. .4

pepper (Boar's Head) 2.0

pepper (Hansel 'n Gretel Healthy Deli Tutta Bella)..................3.0

rosemary and sun-dried tomato (Boar's Head)............................2.0

smoked:
- (Carl Buddig Premium Lean Slices), 2.5-oz. pkg..................1.0
- (Healthy Choice) 2.0
- (Healthy Choice), 1-oz. slice......................................1.0
- (Healthy Choice Deli Traditions), 6 slices, 1.9 oz. 2.0
- (Oscar Mayer), 3 slices, 2.2 oz.....................................0
- (Russer Old Fashioned) 0
- (Sara Lee Smokehouse) 1.0
- Black Forest (Hansel 'n Gretel Healthy Deli 99% Fat Free) 1.0
- double (Hansel 'n Gretel Healthy Deli 99% Fat Free)............1.0
- Virginia (Boar's Head)..2.0
- Virginia (Hansel 'n Gretel Healthy Deli) 2.0
- Virginia (Russer/Russer Fat Free)................................3.0
- spiced (Boar's Head) 1.0
- spiced (Russer)..5.0

Virginia:
- (Black Bear)..2.0
- (Hansel 'n Gretel Healthy Deli) 2.0
- (Hansel 'n Gretel Healthy Deli Less Sodium)....................3.0
- (Healthy Choice) 1.0
- baked (Hansel 'n Gretel Healthy Deli) 3.0
- baked (Sara Lee Deli), 3 slices, 1.8 oz. 2.0
- fruited (Hansel 'n Gretel Healthy Deli) 2.0
- pineapple-topped (Boar's Head) 3.0

Ham patty:
(Hormel), 2-oz. patty..1.0
unheated, 1 patty, 2.3 oz...1.1
grilled, 1 patty, 2.1 oz. (2.3 oz. unheated)..........................1.0
grilled, 14.6 oz. (yield from 1 lb. unheated) 7.0

Ham spread:
deviled (Hormel Cure 81), 4 tbsp....................................2.0

Ham spread *(cont.)*
deviled *(Underwood)*, 4 tbsp..3.0
salad, 1 tbsp. 1.6
Ham-cheese croissant, Swiss *(Sara Lee)*, 3.7-oz. piece............27.0
Ham-cheese loaf:
(Oscar Mayer), 1-oz. slice..<1.0
(Russer), 2 oz. 5.0
1-oz. slice..4
Ham-cheese patty *(Hormel)*, 2-oz. patty 0
Ham-cheese sandwich/pocket, 1 piece:
(Deli Stuffs), 4.5 oz. 41.0
(Healthy Choice Hearty Handfuls), 6.1 oz. 48.0
(Hot Pockets), 4.5 oz. 40.0
(Toaster Breaks Melts), 2.2 oz. 22.0
cheddar *(Croissant Pockets)*, 4.5 oz. 40.0
cheddar *(Lean Pockets)*, 4.5 oz...42.0
"Ham-cheese" style sandwich, vegetarian *(Morningstar
    Farms* Stuffed Sandwich), 4.5-oz. piece................................45.0
Hamburger, see "Beef, sandwich/pocket" and specific restaurant
    listings
"Hamburger," vegetarian, see "Burger, vegetarian"
Hamburger entree, mix, 1 cup*, except as noted:
bacon cheeseburger *(Hamburger Helper)*.....................................35.0
barbecue beef *(Hamburger Helper)*..37.0
beef pasta *(Hamburger Helper)*...26.0
beef Romanoff *(Hamburger Helper)*...29.0
beef stew *(Hamburger Helper)*...26.0
beef taco *(Hamburger Helper)*..31.0
beef teriyaki *(Hamburger Helper)*...34.0
cheddar and bacon *(Hamburger Helper)*.......................................27.0
cheddar and broccoli *(Hamburger Helper)*.....................................33.0
cheddar cheese melt *(Hamburger Helper)* 31.0
cheddar spirals *(Hamburger Helper* Reduced Sodium)...............27.0
cheese, three *(Hamburger Helper)*...32.0
cheese pizza, double *(Hamburger Helper)* 35.0
cheeseburger macaroni *(Hamburger Helper)*.................................33.0
cheesy hash browns *(Hamburger Helper)*.......................................39.0
cheesy Italian *(Hamburger Helper)* 28.0
cheesy shells *(Hamburger Helper)*..30.0
chili macaroni *(Hamburger Helper)*...30.0
fettuccine Alfredo *(Hamburger Helper)* 26.0

Italian, zesty *(Hamburger Helper)* 32.0
Italian herb *(Hamburger Helper* Reduced Sodium) 29.0
Italian Parmesan *(Hamburger Helper)*..............................31.0
lasagna *(Hamburger Helper)*..............................29.0
lasagna, four-cheese *(Hamburger Helper)* 31.0
meat loaf *(Hamburger Helper)*, ⅙ loaf* 11.0
Mexican, zesty *(Hamburger Helper)*..............................31.0
mushroom and wild rice *(Hamburger Helper)* 30.0
nacho cheese *(Hamburger Helper)* 30.0
pepperoni pizza *(Hamburger Helper)* 20.0
Philly cheesesteak *(Hamburger Helper)* 25.0
pizza pasta with cheese topping *(Hamburger Helper)*................31.0
potatoes au gratin *(Hamburger Helper)* 25.0
potatoes Stroganoff *(Hamburger Helper)*..............................24.0
ravioli with white cheese topping *(Hamburger Helper)*...............34.0
rice Oriental *(Hamburger Helper)*..............................32.0
Salisbury *(Hamburger Helper)* 26.0
Southwestern beef *(Hamburger Helper* Reduced Sodium) 32.0
spaghetti *(Hamburger Helper)*..............................27.0
Stroganoff *(Hamburger Helper)* 30.0
Hard sauce, brandied *(Crosse & Blackwell)*, 2 tbsp...................26.0
Hardee's, 1 serving:
breakfast biscuit:
    apple cinnamon 'n' raisin 42.0
    bacon, egg, cheese..............................45.0
    Biscuit 'N' Gravy..............................56.0
    chicken 62.0
    ham 45.0
    ham, country..............................44.0
    jelly..............................57.0
    Made from Scratch biscuit..............................44.0
    Omelet..............................45.0
    sausage 44.0
    sausage and egg..............................45.0
    steak..............................56.0
other breakfast items:
    Frisco sandwich, ham..............................42.0
    Hash Rounds, regular..............................24.0
burgers:
    All-Star, Famous Star, or Super Star 41.0
    Frisco or *Monster Burger*..............................37.0

Hardee's, burgers (cont.)
    hamburger 29.0
sandwiches:
    bacon Swiss crispy chicken 45.0
    chicken, grilled 28.0
    chicken fillet 44.0
    Fisherman's Fillet 45.0
    hot dog, with condiments 25.0
    hot ham 'n' cheese 34.0
    Monster Roast Beef 26.0
    roast beef, regular, or *Big Roast Beef* 26.0
chicken, 1 piece:
    breast 29.0
    leg 15.0
    thigh 30.0
    wing 23.0
sides:
    coleslaw, 4 oz. 13.0
    Crispy Curls, large 62.0
    Crispy Curls, medium 41.0
    Crispy Curls, monster 70.0
    fries, large 59.0
    fries, monster 67.0
    fries, regular 45.0
    gravy, 1.5 oz. 3.0
    mashed potatoes, small, 4 oz. 14.0
desserts/shakes:
    apple turnover 38.0
    peach cobbler, 6 oz. 60.0
    shake, chocolate 67.0
    shake, vanilla 65.0
Hazelnuts, see "Filberts"
Head cheese:
(Boar's Head), 2 oz. ....<1.0
1-oz. slice 1
Heart:
beef, raw, 1 oz. 7
beef, simmered, 9.1 oz. (yield from 1 lb. raw) 1.1
chicken, raw, .2 oz. 0
chicken, simmered, chopped or diced, 1 cup 1
lamb, raw, 4 oz. 2.2

lamb, braised, 6.7 oz. (yield from 1 lb. raw) 3.7
pork, raw, 8 oz. 3.0
pork, braised, 1 heart, 4.6 oz. 5
turkey, raw, 1 oz. 2
turkey, simmered, chopped or diced, 1 cup 3.0
veal, raw, 4 oz. 1
veal, braised, 7 oz. (yield from 1 lb. raw) 3
Hearts of palm, see "Palm"
Herbs, see specific listings
Herbs, mixed (*Lawry's* Pinch of Herbs), ¼ tsp. 0
Herring, fresh, kippered, or smoked, without added ingredients 0
Herring, canned, see "Sardine"
Herring, pickled, ¼ cup, except as noted:
1 cup 13.5
in dill sauce (*Elf/Vita*) 7.0
roll mops (*Elf*) 8.0
slices (*Vita* Lunch), 2 oz. 5.0
in sour cream:
   (*Elf*) 5.0
   (*Nathan's Famous*) 11.0
   (*Vita*) 8.0
in wine sauce:
   (*Elf*) 8.0
   (*Elf* Old Fashioned) 5.0
   (*Skansen* Tidbits), 5 pieces, 1.9 oz. 7.0
   (*Vita* Party Snacks), 2 oz., about ¼ cup 8.0
   (*Vita* Party Snacks Tastee Bits), 2 oz. 10.0
Herring salad, chopped (*Blue Ridge Farms*), ⅓ cup, 3 oz. 17.0
Hickory nuts, dried, shelled, 1 cup 21.9
Hiziki, see "Seaweed"
Hoisin sauce:
(*House of Tsang*), 1 tsp. 4.0
1 tbsp. 7.1
Hollandaise sauce, in jar, 2 tbsp.:
(*Melba*) 1.0
(*Reese*) 1.0
Hollandaise sauce mix, dry:
(*Concord Foods*), 1½ tbsp. 4.0
(*Knorr* Classic Sauces), 1 tsp. 2.0

Hollandaise sauce mix *(cont.)*
with butter fat, 1.2-oz. pkt..10.8
with vegetable oil, .9-oz. pkt. 15.5
Hominy, canned:
golden:
   (Allens/Uncle William), ½ cup........................27.0
   (Allens/Uncle William Pepi), ½ cup..............25.0
   1 cup 22.8
white:
   (Allens/Uncle William), ½ cup........................22.0
   (Goya), ¼ cup..39.0
   1 cup 23.5
Hominy grits, see "Corn grits"
Honey:
(Goya), 1 tbsp. 17.0
(Sioux), 1 tbsp. 17.0
1 tbsp..17.3
Honey bun, see "Bun, sweet"
Honey butter *(Downey's),* 1 tbsp. 11.0
Honey mustard, see "Mustard blend"
Honey spread, all flavors *(Bigelow),* 1 tbsp. 17.0
Honeydew melon, fresh, raw:
(Dole), ¹⁄₁₀ melon..12.0
¹⁄₁₀ melon, 7" X 2" slice, 8 oz.................................11.8
balls, 1 cup 16.2
cubed, 1 cup, approx. 20 pieces.............................15.6
Horseradish, fresh:
(Frieda's), 1 tbsp. 1.0
leafy tips, raw, chopped, 1 cup 1.7
leafy tips, boiled, drained, chopped, 1 cup 4.7
Horseradish, prepared:
(Boar's Head), 1 tsp. 0
1 tbsp...1.7
1 tsp. 6
all styles *(Gold's),* 1 tsp. 0
regular or cream style *(Kraft),* 1 tsp.........................0
Horseradish mustard, see "Mustard blend"
Horseradish sauce *(Kraft),* 1 tsp.....................<1.0
Horseradish-tree:
leafy tips, boiled, drained, chopped, 1 cup 4.7

pods:

raw, 15⅓"-long pod	.9
raw, sliced, 1 cup	8.5
boiled, drained, sliced, 1 cup	9.7

Hot dog, see "Frankfurter"

Hot dog sauce, see "Chili sauce"

Hot fudge sauce, see "Chocolate topping"

Hot sauce (see also specific listings), 1 tsp., except as noted:

(Frank's RedHot)	0
(Grace Original Jamaican)	0
(Helen's Tropical Exotics)	1.0
(Lottie's Traditional Barbados Recipe)	1.0
(Tabasco)	0
(Taco Bell Home Originals The Restaurant Hot Sauce)	0
(Trappey's Bull Louisiana/Indi-Pep West Indian Style/Cayenne Buffalo/Mexi-Pep)	<1.0
(Trappey's Cayenne)	0
chili (Sun Luck)	<1.0
chili pepper garlic (A Taste of Thai)	2.0
habañero (D. L. Jardine's Blazin' Saddles XXX)	0
habañero (Shotgun Willie's XXXX), 2 tbsp.	2.0

jalapeño:

(Búfalo)	0
(D. L. Jardine's Texapeppa)	0
(Trappey's Red Devil)	0

Hubbard squash, fresh:

raw (Frieda's), ¾ cup, 3 oz.	7.0
raw, cubed, 1 cup	10.1
baked, cubed, 1 cup	22.2
boiled, mashed, 1 cup	15.2

Hummus:

1 cup	35.7
1 tbsp.	2.0
all varieties (Cedar's), 2 tbsp.	5.0
basil and sun-dried tomato or roasted red pepper (Cedarlane), 2 tbsp.	6.0
garlic, roasted (Cedarlane), 2 tbsp.	5.0

Hummus dip mix:

(Casbah), 1 oz., ¼ cup*	14.0
(Fantastic Foods), 2 tbsp.	9.0

Hungarian pepper, see "Paprika"
Hunter gravy mix *(Knorr* Gravy Classics), 1 tbsp., ¼ cup* 4.0
Hyacinth beans:
immature, raw, 1 cup 7.4
immature, boiled, drained, 1 cup 8.0
mature, raw, 1 cup 127.6
mature, boiled, 1 cup 40.2

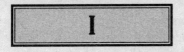

FOOD AND MEASURE   **CARBOHYDRATE GRAMS**

Ice (see also "Sorbet"):
cherry:
    (Icee), 3-fl.-oz. tube...18.0
    (Luigi's Real Italian), 6 fl. oz...............................27.0
    (Mama Tish's), 4 fl. oz..22.0
chocolate *(Mama Tish's* No Sugar), 4 fl. oz. 25.0
chocolate fudge *(Luigi's* Real Italian), 6 fl. oz. 25.0
grape *(Luigi's* Real Italian), 6 fl. oz. 27.0
lemon:
    (Luigi's Real Italian), 6 fl. oz...............................26.0
    (Mama Tish's), 4 fl. oz..21.0
    (Mama Tish's No Sugar), 4 fl. oz.......................19.0
lemonade *(Minute Maid)*, 1 tube..............................25.0
orange *(Chill Orange Overload)*, ¾ of 6-oz. cup 24.0
orange *(Icee)*, 3-fl.-oz. tube 13.0
raspberry:
    (Mama Tish's), 4 fl. oz..24.0
    blue *(Icee)*, 3-fl.-oz. tube....................................18.0
    with lemon *(Chill Blue Raspberry Blast)*, ¾ of 6-oz. cup 26.0
strawberry:
    (Chill Verry Strawberry), ¾ of 6-oz. cup 23.0
    (Icee), 3-fl.-oz. tube...14.0
    (Luigi's Real Italian), 6 fl. oz...............................27.0
    (Mama Tish's), 4 fl. oz..20.0
    (Mama Tish's No Sugar), 4 fl. oz.......................18.0
watermelon *(Chill Watermelon Wipeout)*, ¾ of 6-oz. cup 18.0
Ice bar (see also "Fruit bar"), 1 bar:
(Popsicle Firecracker 12 Pack), 1.6 fl. oz.............10.0
(Popsicle Micro Pops 6 Pack), 2.2 fl. oz...............10.0
all flavors:
    (Mr. Freeze) 11.0
    (Popsicle La Fruita Loca 12 Pack), 3.5 fl. oz......22.0
    (Popsicle Great White* 12 Pack), 1.75 fl. oz...........11.0
    (Popsicle Lick-A-Color 10 Pack), 2 fl. oz.............13.0

Ice, all flavors *(cont.)*

    (Popsicle Nickelodeon Green Slime 12 Pack), 1.75 fl. oz......17.0
    (Popsicle Pokémon 6 Pack), 3 fl. oz....................................19.0
    (Popsicle Rainbow), 1.75 fl. oz. 11.0
    (Popsicle Scribblers 24 Pack), 1.2 fl. oz. 16.0
    (Welch's Double Dare Double Sours/Mega Sours),
       1.75 fl. oz..10.0
orange/cherry/grape *(Popsicle* 12 Pack), 1.75 fl. oz. 11.0
orange/cherry/grape *(Popsicle* Sugar Free 12 Pack),
    1.75 fl. oz. 3.0
orange/raspberry/strawberry *(Popsicle* All Natural 12 Pack),
    1.75 fl. oz. 12.0
root beer/banana/lemon lime *(Popsicle* 12 Pack), 1.75 fl. oz......11.0

Ice cream, ½ cup:

almond, toasted *(Dreyer's* Grand) 15.0
almond praline *(Dreyer's* Grand) 21.0
apple pie à la mode *(Dreyer's/Edy's* Homemade)........................19.0
banana:
    nut *(Blue Bell* Half Gallon) 18.0
    nut *(Blue Bell* Pint) 17.0
    peanut butter *(Dreamery Banana Boogie)* 27.0
    pudding *(Blue Bell)*...24.0
    split *(Blue Bell)*..22.0
    split *(Blue Bell* Light)..20.0
    split *(Blue Bell* Low Fat/No Sugar) 15.0
(Ben & Jerry's Blondies are a Swirl's Best Friend Low Fat) 41.0
(Ben & Jerry's Bovinity Divinity) 30.0
(Ben & Jerry's Cherry Garcia) 26.0
(Ben & Jerry's Chubby Hubby) 33.0
(Ben & Jerry's Chunky Monkey) 32.0
(Ben & Jerry's Dilbert's World Totally Nuts)................................27.0
(Ben & Jerry's Everything but the . . . 2-Twisted) 30.0
(Ben & Jerry's From Russia With Buzz 2-Twisted) 26.0
(Ben & Jerry's Half Baked 2-Twisted) 36.0
(Ben & Jerry's Jerry Jubilee 2-Twisted) 29.0
(Ben & Jerry's Monkey Wrench 2-Twisted).................................28.0
(Ben & Jerry's Nutty Waffle Cone) 32.0
(Ben & Jerry's Phish Food)..41.0
(Ben & Jerry's Pulp Addiction 2-Twisted) 25.0
(Ben & Jerry's Urban Jumble 2-Twisted) 28.0
(Ben & Jerry's Wavy Gravy)...32.0

berry pie *(Dreamery Blue Ribbon Berry Pie)*................................31.0
black raspberry *(Dreamery Avalanche)* 27.0
black raspberry *(Turkey Hill Premium)* 18.0
black walnut *(Blue Bell)*...16.0
blackberry pie *(Dreyer's/Edy's Grand Light)* 17.0
blackberry swirl *(Edy's Grand)* 17.0
blueberry cobbler *(Dreyer's/Edy's Fat Free/No Sugar)*.........22.0
blueberry hill *(Healthy Choice Old Fashioned)* 23.0
brownies à la mode *(Dreyer's/Edy's Homemade)*.................18.0
butter almond *(Breyers All Natural)* 14.0
butter pecan:
    (Breyers All Natural) 14.0
    (Breyers Homemade) 16.0
    (Dreyer's/Edy's Grand)...15.0
    (Dreyer's/Edy's Grand Light)..16.0
    (Dreyer's/Edy's No Sugar) 14.0
    (Dreyer's/Edy's Homemade Old Fashioned)....................14.0
    (Eskimo Pie Reduced Fat) 16.0
    (Häagen-Dazs)..20.0
    (Turkey Hill Gourmet) 17.0
    (Turkey Hill Premium) 16.0
    crunch *(Healthy Choice)*...22.0
buttered pecan:
    (Blue Bell)...17.0
    (Blue Bell Light)...22.0
    (Blue Bell Low Fat/No Sugar) 16.0
butterscotch *(Healthy Choice Blondie Old Fashioned)* 26.0
cappuccino:
    (Häagen-Dazs Gelato)...39.0
    (Häagen-Dazs Cappuccino Commotion).............................25.0
    chocolate chunk *(Healthy Choice)* 22.0
    mocha crunch *(Healthy Choice)* 22.0
    mocha fudge *(Healthy Choice)* 23.0
caramel:
    (Ben & Jerry's Triple Caramel Chunk) 32.0
    (Edy's Grand Light Crazy for Caramel) 19.0
    brownie vanilla *(Turkey Hill Fat Free)*.............................25.0
    cashew crunch *(Turkey Hill Premium)*..............................18.0
    crème *(Dreamery)* 32.0
    crème, pecan *(Häagen-Dazs)*...29.0
    fudge *(Turkey Hill Decadence Fat Free/No Sugar)* 23.0

Ice cream, caramel *(cont.)*

    pecan fudge *(Blue Bell)* 21.0
    peanut brittle *(Dreyer's/Edy's Homemade)* 22.0
    praline crunch *(Breyers All Natural)* 22.0
    praline crunch *(Dreyer's/Edy's Fat Free)* 25.0
    sundae crunch *(Blue Bell)* 24.0
    toffee bar *(Dreamery Heaven)* 32.0
cashew praline *(Dreamery Cashew Praline Parfait)* 30.0
cherries, chocolate-covered *(Blue Bell)*...............................24.0
cherry, black *(Turkey Hill Premium)*....................................18.0
cherry vanilla:
    (Blue Bell)...19.0
    (Breyers All Natural) 17.0
    (Häagen-Dazs)...23.0
    (Healthy Choice Old Fashioned) 22.0
    black cherry *(Dreyer's/Edy's Grand)* 17.0
    fudge *(Turkey Hill Fat Free/No Sugar)* 20.0
chocolate:
    (Breyers All Natural) 18.0
    (Breyers Rainbow)..16.0
    (Dreyer's/Edy's Grand) 16.0
    (Häagen-Dazs)...22.0
    (Häagen-Dazs Gelato) 37.0
    (Starbucks Double Shot) 28.0
    dark, Belgian *(Godiva)* 26.0
    Dutch *(Blue Bell)* 18.0
    Dutch *(Turkey Hill Fat Free/No Sugar)* 20.0
    Dutch *(Turkey Hill Premium)* 19.0
    Dutch, double *(Blue Bell Light)* 23.0
    French *(Breyers All Natural Light)* 22.0
    milk *(Blue Bell)*..22.0
    triple *(Blue Bell Half Gallon)* 21.0
    triple *(Blue Bell Pint)* 20.0
    triple *(Dreyer's/Edy's Grand Thunder)* 18.0
    triple *(Dreyer's/Edy's No Sugar)* 15.0
chocolate, with caramel and brownies *(Starbucks*
    Brownies au Caramel) 31.0
chocolate, white, macadamia toffee *(Godiva)* 21.0
chocolate, white, raspberry *(Godiva)* 31.0
chocolate-almond, white *(Blue Bell)*...................................17.0
chocolate-almond-marshmallow *(Blue Bell)* 23.0

chocolate chip:
- *(Blue Bell)* 18.0
- *(Breyers* All Natural) 17.0
- *(Dreyer's/Edy's* Grand Chocolate Chips!) 18.0
- *(Dreyer's/Edy's Homemade* Cookie Jar) 18.0
- cherry *(Edy's* Grand) 18.0
- chocolate *(Häagen-Dazs)* 26.0

chocolate chip cookie dough:
- *(Ben & Jerry's)* 34.0
- *(Blue Bell)* 23.0
- *(Breyers* All Natural) 20.0
- *(Turkey Hill* Premium) 21.0

chocolate chunk:
- cherry *(Healthy Choice)* 19.0
- chocolate *(Healthy Choice)* 21.0
- double *(Dreyer's/Edy's Homemade)* 19.0
- peanut butter *(Edy's* Fat Free) 26.0
- triple *(Healthy Choice)* 18.0

chocolate cream pie *(Dreyer's/Edy's Homemade)* 19.0

chocolate fudge:
- *(Dreyer's/Edy's* Fat Free) 25.0
- *(Dreyer's/Edy's* Fat Free/No Sugar) 22.0
- brownie *(Ben & Jerry's)* 32.0
- brownie *(Häagen-Dazs* Low Fat) 34.0
- chocolate *(Häagen-Dazs)* 27.0
- double *(Breyers* Homemade) 22.0
- mousse *(Dreyer's/Edy's* Grand Light) 17.0
- mousse *(Healthy Choice)* 21.0
- mousse or sundae *(Edy's* Grand) 19.0

chocolate-hazelnut truffle *(Godiva)* 31.0

chocolate-marshmallow:
- *(Eskimo Pie* Reduced Fat) 23.0
- *(Turkey Hill* Premium) 24.0
- swirl *(Dreamery Galactic Chocolate Swirl)* 37.0

chocolate–peanut butter chunk *(Dreamery)* 29.0

chocolate-raspberry *(Dreyer's/Edy's Chocolate Raspberry Escape* Grand Light) 19.0

chocolate-raspberry soufflé *(Godiva)* 31.0

chocolate–Swiss almond *(Häagen-Dazs)* 25.0

chocolate truffle *(Dreamery* Explosion) 30.0

cinnamon *(Häagen-Dazs)* 21.0

Ice cream *(cont.)*

coconut:

    (Häagen-Dazs Gelato)..38.0

    cream pie *(Ben & Jerry's* Low Fat)..........................29.0

    cream pie *(Healthy Choice)* 23.0

    nutty *(Blue Bell)*..16.0

coffee (see also "cappuccino," above):

    (Blue Bell)..18.0

    (Breyers All Natural) 14.0

    (Dreamery Cuppa Joe) 24.0

    (Dreyer's/Edy's Grand)...16.0

    (Häagen-Dazs)..21.0

    (Starbucks Italian Roast)..26.0

    (Starbucks Java Chip) 29.0

    (Starbucks Latte Low Fat) 30.0

    (Turkey Hill Premium Colombian) 16.0

    almond fudge *(Starbucks)*.......................................28.0

    with cinnamon and coffee cake *(Starbucks Coffee Cake*
        Streusel) 34.0

    crunch *(Ben & Jerry's Heath Bar)* 32.0

    espresso chip *(Edy's* Grand).................................17.0

    espresso fudge chip *(Dreyer's/Edy's* Grand Light) ...18.0

    fudge *(Edy's* Fat Free/No Sugar).............................22.0

    fudge *(Häagen-Dazs* Low Fat) 32.0

    hazelnut *(Ben & Jerry's Coffee Hazelnut Swirl* Special
        Batch) 26.0

    mocha *(Ben & Jerry's* Mocha Latte Low Fat) 28.0

    mocha *(Starbucks Mocha Frappuccino* Low Fat) 32.0

    mocha-almond fudge *(Blue Bell)*.............................21.0

    mocha-almond fudge *(Dreyer's* Grand) 17.0

    mocha chip *(Häagen-Dazs)* 25.0

    mousse crunch *(Dreyer's/Edy's* Grand Light) 17.0

    toffee *(Starbucks* Java Toffee) 30.0

cookie:

    (Dreamery Grandma's Cookie Jar) 32.0

    (Dreyer's Girl Scouts Samoas Grand)......................21.0

    (Dreyer's Girl Scouts Tagalongs Grand Light) 17.0

    (Edy's Girl Scouts Samoas Limited Edition) 21.0

    (Edy's Girl Scouts Tagalongs Limited Edition).........17.0

    chunk *(Dreyer's/Edy's* Fat Free) 24.0

    thin mint *(Dreyer's Girl Scouts* Grand) 18.0

thin mint *(Edy's Girl Scouts* Limited Edition) 18.0
cookie crème de menthe *(Healthy Choice)*...............................21.0
cookie dough:
    (Dreyer's/Edy's Grand)...21.0
    (Dreyer's/Edy's Grand Light)..19.0
    chip *(Häagen-Dazs)*..29.0
    chocolate *(Dreyer's Scooby-Doo Dough* Grand Light) 19.0
cookies and cream:
    (Blue Bell)..21.0
    (Blue Bell Light)...20.0
    (Blue Bell Low Fat/No Sugar) 18.0
    (Breyers Cookies In Cream All Natural) 18.0
    (Dreyer's/Edy's Grand)...19.0
    (Dreyer's/Edy's Grand Light)...17.0
    (Häagen-Dazs)...23.0
    (Healthy Choice)..24.0
    (Turkey Hill Fat Free) 23.0
    (Turkey Hill Gourmet)...21.0
    (Turkey Hill Premium)...19.0
    mint *(Turkey Hill* Premium)...19.0
cookies and fudge *(Häagen-Dazs* Low Fat) 33.0
(Dreamery Sticky Bun)...30.0
(Dreamery Hot Chilly Chili) 27.0
(Dreamery Nuts About Malt)..29.0
(Dreyer's Grand Gold Miner's Dream) 19.0
(Dreyer's Checkered Flag Sundae Grand) 18.0
(Dreyer's Infinity Divinity Grand Light).......................................19.0
(Dreyer's Orbit City Swirl/Scooby Snack Grand) 19.0
(Dreyer's/Edy's Chips 'N Swirls No Sugar)...............................16.0
(Dreyer's/Edy's French Silk Grand Light)..................................19.0
(Dreyer's/Edy's Halloween Bash Limited Edition) 18.0
(Dreyer's/Edy's M&M's Grand) 22.0
(Dreyer's/Edy's Milky Way Grand) 21.0
(Dreyer's/Edy's Snickers Grand)...24.0
(Dreyer's/Edy's 3 Musketeers Grand) 22.0
(Dreyer's/Edy's Twix Grand) 23.0
dulce de leche:
    (Blue Bell)..22.0
    (Breyers All Natural) 21.0
    (Dreyer's/Edy's Grand) 20.0
    (Häagen-Dazs)...28.0

Ice cream, dulce de leche *(cont.)*

(Starbucks)	31.0
(Edy's Baseball Sundae Limited Edition)	21.0
(Edy's Checkered Flag Sundae Limited Edition)	18.0
(Edy's Chunky Toy Funilla Limited Edition)	19.0
(Edy's Infinity Divinity Grand Light Limited Edition)	19.0
eggnog *(Turkey Hill* Premium)	17.0
eggnog and cream *(Dreyer's/Edy's* Homemade)	17.0
espresso, see "coffee," above	
fruit *(Breyers* Rainbow)	16.0

fudge brownie:

(Breyers Homemade)	22.0
(Healthy Choice)	22.0
à la mode *(Healthy Choice)*	22.0
double *(Dreyer's/Edy's* Grand)	19.0
double *(Edy's* No Sugar)	16.0
nut *(Blue Bell)*	21.0
fudge cake, turtle *(Healthy Choice)*	25.0
fudge chunk, super *(Ben & Jerry's* New York)	28.0
fudge ripple *(Eskimo Pie* Reduced Fat)	19.0
fudge ripple *(Turkey Hill* Premium)	20.0
fudge sundae, hot *(Blue Bell)*	20.0
gingerbread *(Dreyer's/Edy's Gingerbread Man* Grand Light)	19.0
hazelnut *(Häagen-Dazs* Gelato)	33.0
ice cream sandwich *(Dreyer's/Edy's* Grand)	19.0
Irish cream *(Häagen-Dazs* Bailey's)	23.0
macadamia brittle *(Häagen-Dazs)*	25.0
mango *(Häagen-Dazs)*	28.0
mint *(Ben & Jerry's Entangled Mints* 2-Twisted)	30.0
mint *(Dreamery* Cool)	34.0
mint chip *(Häagen-Dazs)*	26.0
mint chocolate *(Dreyer's Jeff's Mint Chocolate Sundae* Grand)	19.0

mint chocolate chip:

(Blue Bell Half Gallon)	18.0
(Blue Bell Pint)	17.0
(Breyers All Natural)	17.0
(Breyers All Natural Light)	21.0
(Dreyer's/Edy's Grand Light Mint Chocolate Chips!)	17.0
(Dreyer's/Edy's Grand Mint Chocolate Chips!)	18.0
(Healthy Choice)	21.0

    (Turkey Hill Gourmet) 19.0
    (Turkey Hill Premium) 17.0
mint chocolate cookie *(Ben & Jerry's)* 28.0
mint fudge *(Turkey Hill* Midnight Mint Fat Free) 24.0
mocha, see "coffee," above
Neapolitan:
    (Blue Bell Half Gallon) 17.0
    (Blue Bell Pint) 16.0
    (Breyers Homemade) 17.0
    (Dreyer's Grand) 16.0
    (Eskimo Pie Reduced Fat) 18.0
    (Turkey Hill Fat Free) 21.0
    (Turkey Hill Gourmet) 19.0
    (Turkey Hill Premium) 18.0
orange and cream *(Ben & Jerry's)* 23.0
peach:
    (Breyers All Natural) 17.0
    (Dreamery Harvest) 26.0
    (Dreyer's Homemade Grovestand) 15.0
peaches and homemade vanilla *(Blue Bell)* 23.0
peaches and homemade vanilla *(Blue Bell* Light) 24.0
peanut butter:
    (Dreyer's Blitz Grand) 16.0
    (Edy's NFL Blitz Limited Edition) 16.0
    cookie *(Dreyer's/Edy's* All About PB No Sugar) 15.0
    cup *(Ben & Jerry's)* 32.0
    cup *(Dreyer's/Edy's* Grand Light Peanut Butter Cups!) 17.0
    cup *(Healthy Choice)* 19.0
    cup, chocolate *(Turkey Hill* Premium) 18.0
    ripple *(Turkey Hill* Premium) 16.0
peanut-toffee crunch *(Dreyer's Cracker Jack* Grand) 20.0
pecan *(Ben & Jerry's Southern Pecan Pie)* 26.0
pecan-caramel truffle *(Godiva)* 32.0
pecan pralines and cream *(Blue Bell* Half Gallon) 23.0
pecan pralines and cream *(Blue Bell* Pint) 22.0
peppermint:
    (Blue Bell) 20.0
    (Dreyer's Grand) 17.0
    (Edy's/Edy's Grand Light Limited Edition) 17.0
pineapple-coconut *(Häagen-Dazs)* 25.0
pineapple and homemade vanilla *(Blue Bell)* 21.0

Ice cream *(cont.)*

pistachio *(Ben & Jerry's Pistachio Pistachio)* 20.0
pistachio *(Häagen-Dazs)* 22.0
pistachio-almond *(Blue Bell)* 17.0
praline:
   and caramel *(Breyers All Natural Light)* 24.0
   and caramel *(Healthy Choice)* 25.0
   caramel cluster *(Healthy Choice)* 25.0
   and cream *(Häagen-Dazs)* 27.0
pumpkin *(Dreyer's Grand/Edy's Limited Edition)* 17.0
raspberry:
   (Häagen-Dazs Gelato) 40.0
   marble chunk *(Dreyer's/Edy's Fat Free)* 25.0
   truffle, wild *(Healthy Choice)* 22.0
   vanilla swirl *(Dreyer's/Edy's Fat Free/No Sugar)* 19.0
rocky road:
   (Blue Bell Low Fat/No Sugar) 15.0
   (Blue Bell/Blue Bell Light) 18.0
   (Breyers All Natural) 24.0
   (Breyers All Natural Light) 22.0
   (Dreyer's/Edy's Grand/Grand Light) 17.0
   (Healthy Choice) 28.0
   (Turkey Hill Premium) 23.0
rum raisin *(Häagen-Dazs)* 22.0
rum raisin *(Turkey Hill Premium)* 19.0
S'mores:
   (Ben & Jerry's Low Fat) 35.0
   (Dreyer's S'mores & More Grand Light) 22.0
   (Edy's S'mores & More Grand Light) 20.0
strawberries and homemade vanilla:
   (Blue Bell Half Gallon) 23.0
   (Blue Bell Light) 24.0
   (Blue Bell Pint) 22.0
strawberry:
   (Blue Bell Half Gallon) 20.0
   (Blue Bell Pint) 19.0
   (Breyers All Natural) 15.0
   (Breyers All Natural Light) 19.0
   (Edy's No Sugar) 13.0
   (Häagen-Dazs) 23.0
   (Healthy Choice Old Fashioned) 20.0

cheesecake *(Blue Bell)*..............................22.0
cheesecake, New York *(Dreamery)*..............27.0
and cream *(Dreyer's/Edy's Homemade)* 15.0
and cream *(Turkey Hill* Premium)................19.0
real *(Dreyer's/Edy's* Grand)......................16.0
tin roof *(Blue Bell* Half Gallon) 22.0
tin roof *(Blue Bell* Pint) 21.0
(Turkey Hill Gourmet Tin Roof Sundae) 20.0
(Turkey Hill Premium Tin Roof Sundae).........19.0
vanilla:
    (Ben & Jerry's World's Best)...................22.0
    (Blue Bell Country) 16.0
    (Blue Bell Country Low Fat/No Sugar)..........15.0
    (Blue Bell Homemade Half Gallon) 21.0
    (Blue Bell Homemade Light)...................22.0
    (Blue Bell Homemade One Gallon) 20.0
    (Blue Bell Homemade Pint) 19.0
    (Breyers All Natural) 15.0
    (Breyers All Natural Light)....................19.0
    (Breyers Calcium Rich Natural) 14.0
    (Breyers Fat Free)............................19.0
    (Breyers Homemade) 16.0
    (Breyers Light) 18.0
    (Breyers No Sugar Added) 11.0
    (Dreamery)..................................25.0
    (Dreyer's Grand) 20.0
    (Dreyer's/Edy's Fat Free)....................22.0
    (Dreyer's/Edy's Fat Free/No Sugar)...........19.0
    (Dreyer's/Edy's Grand Light).................15.0
    (Dreyer's/Edy's No Sugar) 13.0
    (Dreyer's/Edy's Homemade All Natural)........14.0
    (Edy's Grand)...............................15.0
    (Eskimo Pie Reduced Fat) 17.0
    (Häagen-Dazs)..............................21.0
    (Häagen-Dazs Low Fat) 29.0
    (Healthy Choice).............................18.0
    (Turkey Hill Premium) 16.0
    bean *(Blue Bell)*..............................20.0
    bean *(Blue Bell* Fat Free/No Sugar)...........17.0
    bean *(Dreyer's/Edy's* Grand) 15.0
    bean *(Healthy Choice)* 19.0

Ice cream, vanilla *(cont.)*
    bean *(Turkey Hill Fat Free)* 21.0
    bean *(Turkey Hill Fat Free/No Sugar)* 20.0
    bean *(Turkey Hill Gourmet)* 18.0
    bean *(Turkey Hill Premium)* 16.0
    custard *(Edy's Homemade)* 13.0
    French *(Blue Bell)* 18.0
    French *(Breyers All Natural)* 15.0
    French *(Breyers All Natural Light)* 18.0
    French *(Dreyer's Grand)* 17.0
    French *(Edy's Grand)* 16.0
    French *(Turkey Hill Premium)* 16.0
vanilla-almond *(Starbucks Bliss)* 27.0
vanilla-caramel *(Edy's Fat Free/No Sugar)* 21.0
vanilla-caramel *(Häagen-Dazs Low Fat)* 32.0
vanilla-caramel fudge *(Ben & Jerry's)* 33.0
vanilla-caramel fudge *(Edy's Grand)* 18.0
vanilla cashew crunch *(Starbucks)* 30.0
vanilla and chocolate:
    (Breyers Take Two All Natural) 16.0
    (Edy's Grand) 16.0
    (Turkey Hill Gourmet) 19.0
    (Turkey Hill Premium) 17.0
    swirl *(Dreyer's/Edy's Fat Free/No Sugar)* 20.0
vanilla, chocolate, and strawberry:
    (Breyers All Natural) 16.0
    (Breyers All Natural Light) 19.0
    (Breyers No Sugar Added) 11.0
    (Edy's Grand) 16.0
vanilla fudge:
    swirl *(Dreyer's Grand Chunky Toy Funilla)* 19.0
    twirl *(Breyers All Natural)* 18.0
    twirl *(Breyers No Sugar Added)* 14.0
vanilla and orange sherbet, see "Sherbet"
vanilla and orange sorbet, see "Sorbet"
vanilla–Swiss almond *(Häagen-Dazs)* 23.0
vanilla–toffee bar *(Ben & Jerry's Heath)* 30.0
"Ice cream," nondairy, ½ cup:
(Tofutti Premium Supreme) 18.0
all flavors, soft-serve *(Tofutti/Tofutti Lite)* 20.0
Better Pecan (Tofutti Premium) 22.0

carob or carob-almond *(Rice Dream)* 24.0
cappuccino *(Rice Dream)*...23.0
cappuccino-almond fudge *(Rice Dream* Supreme) 24.0
cherry-chocolate chunk *(Rice Dream* Supreme) 27.0
cherry-vanilla *(Rice Dream)* 24.0
chocolate *(Rice Dream)*...24.0
chocolate-almond chunk *(Rice Dream* Supreme) 25.0
chocolate chip *(Rice Dream)*...26.0
chocolate cookie crunch *(Tofutti* Premium) 26.0
chocolate fudge *(Tofutti* Low Fat) 25.0
chocolate fudge brownie *(Rice Dream* Supreme) 28.0
chocolate fudge sundae or vanilla *(Tofutti* Fat/Sugar Free) 20.0
chocolate supreme *(Tofutti* Premium)..18.0
cocoa marble fudge *(Rice Dream)* 25.0
coffee-marshmallow swirl *(Tofutti* Low Fat)...............................24.0
espresso bean, double *(Rice Dream* Supreme)............................24.0
honey-vanilla chamomile *(Tofutti)*..20.0
mint carob chip *(Rice Dream)*...26.0
mint chocolate cookie *(Rice Dream* Supreme)............................26.0
Neapolitan *(Rice Dream)*...24.0
orange-vanilla swirl *(Rice Dream)*..23.0
peach-mango *(Tofutti* Low Fat) 23.0
peanut butter cup *(Rice Dream* Supreme) 25.0
praline *(Rice Dream* Supreme Pralines N' Dream) 24.0
strawberry *(Rice Dream)*...24.0
strawberry-banana *(Tofutti* Low Fat) 23.0
vanilla:
    (Rice Dream) 23.0
    (Tofutti Premium) 20.0
    with almonds *(Rice Dream* Swiss Almond) 25.0
    with almonds *(Tofutti Vanilla Almond Bark* Premium)...........21.0
vanilla fudge *(Tofutti* Low Fat)..24.0
vanilla fudge *(Tofutti* Premium)..25.0
vanilla fudge sundae *(Tofutti)*...20.0
vanilla-strawberry sundae *(Tofutti)* 19.0
wildberry *(Tofutti* Premium Supreme)...24.0
Ice cream bar, 1 bar:
(Ben & Jerry's Phish Stick)...32.0
(Good Humor Variety 30 Pack), 2.75 fl. oz. 19.0
berry *(Ben & Jerry's Berry Wild Whirl)*..28.0
candy bar swirl *(Klondike)* 29.0

Ice cream bar *(cont.)*
cappuccino *(Klondike)* 26.0
caramel or strawberry, soft *(Breyers* Magnum) 35.0
caramel crunch *(Klondike)* 30.0
chocolate:
   (Klondike Variety 12 Pack) 21.0
   chocolate-coated *(Klondike)* 25.0
   dark-chocolate-coated *(Häagen-Dazs)* 28.0
   milk-chocolate-and-almond-coated *(Häagen-Dazs)* 23.0
   eclair *(Good Humor),* 3 fl. oz. 21.0
chocolate peanut butter swirl, milk-chocolate-coated
   (Häagen-Dazs) 21.0
coconut-pineapple, white-chocolate-coated *(Häagen-Dazs)* 25.0
coffee:
   (Starbucks Frappuccino) 20.0
   almond crunch *(Häagen-Dazs)* 27.0
   caramel *(Starbucks Frappuccino)* 22.0
   mocha *(Starbucks Frappuccino)* 21.0
cookie dough *(Ben & Jerry's)* 45.0
cookies and cream:
   (Good Humor) 24.0
   (Oreo) 18.0
   crunch *(Häagen-Dazs)* 30.0
dulce de leche, caramel-coated *(Häagen-Dazs)* 28.0
mint, dark-chocolate-coated *(Häagen-Dazs)* 27.0
mocha java *(Weight Watchers Smart Ones)* 15.0
Neapolitan *(Klondike)* 25.0
nut *(Ben & Jerry's Totally Nuts)* 24.0
peanut butter *(Good Humor Reese's Peanut Butter Cup)* 24.0
passion fruit *(Ben & Jerry's Passionfruit Smooch)* 26.0
S'mores *(Ben & Jerry's)* 34.0
strawberry, white-chocolate-coated *(Häagen-Dazs)* 20.0
strawberry shortcake *(Good Humor),* 3 fl. oz. 21.0
strawberry shortcake *(Good Humor* Variety 30 Pack),
   2.75 fl. oz. 20.0
strawberry swirl *(Klondike)* 28.0
toffee crunch, English *(Weight Watchers Smart Ones),* 12.0
vanilla:
   (Ben & Jerry's) 29.0
   (Klondike Original) 25.0
   (Klondike Reduced Fat/No Sugar) 19.0

(Klondike Variety 12 Pack) 21.0
almond-coated *(Klondike)* 26.0
almond-coated, toasted *(Good Humor)*, 3 fl. oz. 22.0
chocolate-and-crisps-coated *(Klondike* Krispy Krunch) 28.0
chocolate-and-sprinkle-coated *(Popsicle* Sprinklers),
   2.1 fl. oz. 18.0
dark-chocolate-coated *(Eskimo Pie)*, 2.5 fl. oz. 14.0
dark-chocolate-coated *(Eskimo Pie* No Sugar), 2.5 fl. oz. 13.0
dark-chocolate-coated *(Klondike)* 25.0
dark- or milk-chocolate-coated *(Good Humor)*, 3 fl. oz. 16.0
milk-chocolate-coated *(Eskimo Pie* Original), 2.5 fl. oz. 12.0
milk-chocolate-coated *(Häagen-Dazs)* 24.0
milk-chocolate-and-almond-coated *(Häagen-Dazs)*...............26.0
milk-chocolate-and-crisps-coated *(Eskimo Pie* No Sugar),
   2.5 fl. oz. 13.0
toffee-coated *(Klondike* Heath) 27.0
vanilla and sherbet, see "Sherbet bar"
vanilla and sorbet, see "Sorbet bar"
vanilla-toffee *(Ben & Jerry's* Heath Bar) 32.0
"Ice cream" bar, nondairy, 1 bar:
chocolate, chocolate-coated *(The Rice Dream Bar)* 32.0
chocolate, chocolate-and-nut-coated *(The Nutty Rice*
   Dream Bar)..............................23.0
chocolate fudge *(Tofutti* Fudge Treats) 6.0
chocolate fudge *(Tofutti* Teddy Fudge) 19.0
fruit, mixed, chocolate-coated *(Tofutti* Frutti)..............................15.0
peanut butter *(Tofutti* Monkey Bars) 22.0
strawberry, carob-coated *(The Rice Dream Bar)*..............................31.0
strawberry or vanilla fudge, crumb-coated *(Tofutti)*..................20.0
vanilla, carob-coated *(The Rice Dream Bar)*..............................33.0
vanilla, chocolate-and-nut-coated *(The Nutty Rice*
   Dream Bar)..............................23.0
Ice cream cake, ½ cup:
cappuccino *(Viennetta)* 19.0
chocolate, triple *(Viennetta)* 16.0
vanilla *(Viennetta)* 19.0
vanilla *(Viennetta* Snack Size) 21.0
Ice cream cone, filled, 1 piece:
(Good Humor Variety 30 Pack), 4 fl. oz. 31.0
caramel or fudge *(Klondike* Big Bear), 5 fl. oz. 40.0
cookies and cream *(Oreo)*..............................27.0

Ice cream cone *(cont.)*
rocky road *(Turkey Hill* Sundae)................................35.0
vanilla *(Klondike Big Bear),* 5 fl. oz. 35.0
vanilla, chocolate-and-nut-topped *(Eskimo Pie* No Sugar),
    4.2 fl. oz. 24.0
vanilla fudge chip *(Turkey Hill* Sundae)..................34.0
"Ice cream" cone, nondairy, filled, 1 piece:
chocolate *(Rice Dream)*......................................37.0
vanilla *(Rice Dream)*..36.0
Ice cream cone and cup, unfilled, 1 piece:
cone:
    chocolate *(Oreo)*..10.0
    chocolatey *(Keebler)*..................................10.0
    fudge-dipped *(Keebler)*................................6.0
    sugar *(Comet)* 12.0
    sugar *(Keebler)*..10.0
    waffle, cone or bowl *(Keebler)*...................10.0
cup *(Comet)* 4.0
cup *(Keebler)* 4.0
"Ice cream" dessert roll, nondairy *(Tofutti* Rock Roll),
    1 slice 22.0
Ice cream mix, ½ cup:
chocolate *(Junket)* 26.0
vanilla *(Junket)*..27.0
Ice cream pie or patty, see "Ice cream sandwich"
Ice cream sandwich, 1 piece:
(Klondike Choco Taco) 30.0
chocolate chip cookie *(Klondike Big Bear),* 4 fl. oz. 41.0
chocolate chip mint *(Turkey Hill)* 28.0
cookies and cream *(Oreo Big Stuff)*....................33.0
Neapolitan *(Klondike Big Bear)* 30.0
peanut butter swirl *(Turkey Hill)*..........................27.0
raspberries and cream *(Turkey Hill)*....................27.0
vanilla:
    (Eskimo Pie), 3.8 fl. oz. 27.0
    (Good Humor), 3 fl. oz. 26.0
    (Klondike Big Bear)....................................31.0
    (Weight Watchers Smart Ones) 28.0
    (SnackWells's Low Fat), 2.3 fl. oz. 18.0
    (Turkey Hill) 26.0
    fudge center *(Eskimo Pie Arctic Madness)*............26.0

"Ice cream" sandwich, nondairy, 1 piece:
chocolate *(Rice Dream Pie)*..39.0
chocolate, wafer *(Tofutti Cuties)* 16.0
chocolate chip, cookie *(Tofutti Too-Too's)*.................................30.0
mint *(Rice Dream Pie)*...39.0
mocha *(Rice Dream Pie)* 40.0
peanut butter, wafer *(Tofutti Cuties)*..20.0
vanilla:
    (Rice Dream Pie) 40.0
    cookie *(Tofutti Too-Too's)* 28.0
    dark-chocolate-coated *(Tofutti Cutie Pie)* 18.0
vanilla or wildberry, wafer *(Tofutti Cuties)* 17.0
Ice cream and sherbet, see "Sherbet"
Ice cream and sorbet, see "Sorbet"
Icing, see "Frosting"
Italian cut beans, see "Green beans"
Italian sausage, see "Sausage"
Italian seasoning, 1 tsp... .6

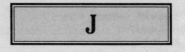

FOOD AND MEASURE   **CARBOHYDRATE GRAMS**

Jack in the Box, 1 serving:
breakfast items:
    bacon..0
    biscuit..24.0
    biscuit, sausage..25.0
    biscuit, sausage, egg, and cheese...............................27.0
    Breakfast Jack...28.0
    Country Crock Spread...0
    croissant, sausage or supreme 37.0
    French toast sticks 53.0
    grape jelly...10.0
    hash browns..14.0
    sandwich, ultimate..39.0
    syrup 30.0
burgers:
    cheeseburger, bacon bacon..39.0
    cheeseburger, double 31.0
    cheeseburger, ultimate, with or without bacon..............37.0
    hamburger...30.0
    hamburger with cheese 31.0
    Jumbo Jack..43.0
    Jumbo Jack with cheese 44.0
    Sourdough Jack 36.0
chicken and more:
    cheese, American or Swiss style, 1 slice.......................1.0
    chicken breast, 5 pieces 24.0
    chicken sandwiches:
        chicken 38.0
        chicken fajita pita..34.0
        chicken fillet, grilled..39.0
        chicken supreme...66.0
        Jack's Spicy Chicken...52.0
    dipping sauces, 1 oz.:
        barbecue..11.0

buttermilk house...3.0
Frank's RedHot Buffalo 2.0
sweet and sour 11.0
fish and chips 86.0
taco 12.0
taco, monster 19.0
tartar sauce or salsa......................................2.0

salad and teriyaki bowl:
chicken teriyaki bowl.....................................128.0
garden chicken salad......................................8.0
side salad 3.0
croutons..8.0
soy sauce 1.0

salad dressings:
blue cheese...11.0
buttermilk house..6.0
Italian, low-calorie 2.0
Thousand Island 10.0

sides:
fries, curly, chili cheese 60.0
fries, curly, seasoned...................................45.0
fries, jumbo 58.0
fries, regular 46.0
fries, super scoop..82.0
ketchup...2.0
onion rings 50.0
potato wedges, bacon-cheddar 55.0

snacks:
egg rolls, 1 piece..13.0
egg rolls, 3 pieces 40.0
jalapeños, stuffed, 3 pieces.......................20.0
jalapeños, stuffed, 7 pieces.......................46.0
sour cream 1.0

shakes, regular:
cappuccino 80.0
chocolate 85.0
Oreo cookie 91.0
strawberry 85.0
vanilla 73.0

desserts:
apple turnover, hot 41.0

Jack in the Box, desserts (cont.)
   cheesecake 32.0
   double fudge cake 50.0
Jackfruit, fresh:
(Frieda's), ⅓ cup, 1.4 oz. 30.0
raw, sliced, 1 cup 39.6
Jackfruit, canned, in syrup, drained, 1 cup 42.6
Jackfruit, dried *(Frieda's),* ½ cup, 3 oz. 20.0
Jalapeño, see "Pepper, jalapeño"
Jalapeño dip *(Kraft),* 2 tbsp. 3.0
Jalapeño jelly, see "Jelly, hot"
Jalapeño sauce, see "Hot sauce"
Jalfrezi sauce, see "Curry sauce"
Jam and preserves (see also "Fruit spread" and "Jelly"),
   1 tbsp., except as noted:
all fruits:
   (Knott's Berry Farm), 1 tsp. 4.0
   (Smucker's) 13.0
   (Smucker's Low Sugar) 6.0
   (Smucker's Light Sugar Free) 5.0
amaretto, peach and pecan *(D.L. Jardine's),* 2 tbsp. 19.0
apricot 12.9
apricot, .5-oz. pkt. 9.0
grape *(Kraft)* 14.0
marmalade, orange *(Crosse & Blackwell)* 16.0
strawberry or red plum *(Kraft)* 13.0
Jamaican jerk dipping sauce *(Helen's Tropical Exotics),*
   2 tbsp. 10.0
Jamaican jerk marinade *(Helen's Tropical Exotics),* 1 tbsp. 1.0
Jamaican jerk seasoning *(Helen's Tropical Exotics),* 1 tbsp. 7.0
Japanese burdock, see "Burdock root"
Java-plum, fresh, raw:
3 pieces, .3 oz. 1.4
1 cup 21.0
Jelly, fruit, 1 tbsp:
all fruits *(Smucker's)* 13.0
all fruits, except apple and grape *(Kraft)* 13.0
apple *(Musselman's)* 13.0
apple, mint-flavored *(Crosse & Blackwell)* 14.0
apple or grape *(Kraft)* 14.0
guava *(Goya)* 12.0

guava or red currant *(Crosse & Blackwell)* 14.0
Jelly, hot, 2 tbsp., except as noted:
habañero *(D.L. Jardine's)* 19.0
jalapeño *(D.L. Jardine's* Hotter) 20.0
jalapeño cherry *(D.L. Jardine's* Hotter) 21.0
pepper *(Reese),* 1 tbsp 13.0
Jerusalem artichoke:
(Frieda's Sunchoke), ½ cup, 3 oz. 14.0
raw, sliced, 1 cup 26.2
Jicama, see "Yam bean tuber"
Jujube:
raw, with seeds, 1 lb. 85.3
raw, seeded, 1 oz. 5.7
dried, 1 oz. 20.1
Jute, potherb:
raw, 1 cup 1.6
boiled, drained, 1 cup 6.4

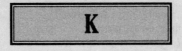

K

FOOD AND MEASURE	CARBOHYDRATE GRAMS

Kabocha squash *(Frieda's)*, ¾ cup, 3 oz. 7.0
Kale, fresh:
raw, chopped, 1 cup..6.7
boiled, drained, chopped, 1 cup..............................7.3
Kale, canned *(Allens/Sunshine)*, ½ cup 3.0
Kale, frozen:
unprepared, 10-oz. pkg. 13.9
unprepared, ⅓ of 10-oz. pkg. 4.6
boiled, drained, chopped, 1 cup..............................7.4
boiled, drained, chopped, ½ cup 3.7
Kale, Chinese, see "Broccoli, Chinese"
Kale, Scotch, fresh:
raw, chopped, 1 cup..5.6
boiled, drained, chopped, 1 cup..............................7.3
Kamranga, see "Carambola"
Kamut flakes, see "Cereal, ready-to-eat"
Kamut flour *(Arrowhead Mills)*, ¼ cup 25.0
Kanpyo:
2-oz. strip...4.1
½ cup..17.6
Kasha, see "Buckwheat groats"
Kelp, see "Seaweed"
Ketchup, 1 tbsp.:
(Del Monte)..4.0
(Estee)...5.0
(Heinz)...4.0
(Hunt's) 4.0
(Muir Glen Organic) 3.0
unsweetened *(Westbrae Natural)* 1.0
fruit-sweetened *(Westbrae Natural)* 4.0
spicy *(Muir Glen Organic)* 3.0
KFC, 1 serving:
chicken, *Original Recipe:*
    breast 16.0

    drumstick 4.0
    thigh 6.0
    wing, whole 5.0
chicken, *Extra Crispy:*
    breast 17.0
    drumstick 7.0
    thigh 14.0
    wing, whole 10.0
chicken, hot and spicy:
    breast 23.0
    drumstick 9.0
    thigh 13.0
    wing, whole 9.0
chicken, popcorn, large..36.0
chicken, popcorn, small 21.0
chicken pot pie, chunky 69.0
chicken sandwiches, with sauce:
    honey BBQ flavored...37.0
    Original Recipe 39.0
    Tender Roast 26.0
    Triple Crunch/Triple Crunch Zinger.....................39.0
chicken wings, honey BBQ, 6 pieces.........................33.0
chicken wings, *Hot Wings,* 6 pieces 18.0
Crispy Strips, Colonel's, 3 pieces..........................18.0
Crispy Strips, spicy, 3 pieces 23.0
salads and sides:
    BBQ baked beans 33.0
    biscuit, 2-oz. piece 20.0
    coleslaw..26.0
    corn on the cob 35.0
    macaroni and cheese...21.0
    mashed potatoes with gravy..................................17.0
    potato salad 23.0
    potato wedges 28.0
desserts:
    chocolate chip cake, double 41.0
    Colonel's pies, 1 slice:
        apple 44.0
        pecan 66.0
        strawberry creme..32.0

KFC, desserts (cont.)
Little Bucket parfaits:
chocolate cream 37.0
fudge brownie...44.0
lemon creme...62.0
strawberry shortcake 33.0
Kidney, braised:
beef, 6.9 oz. (yield from 1 lb. raw)......................................1.9
lamb, 9 oz. (yield from 1 lb. raw)..2.5
pork, 4 oz. 0
veal, 4 oz. 0
Kidney beans, mature:
all types:
dry, 1 cup 110.4
boiled, 1 cup..40.4
boiled, 1 tbsp..2.5
red:
dry *(Arrowhead Mills),* ¼ cup 29.0
dry, 1 cup 112.8
dry, 1 tbsp. 7.5
boiled, 1 cup..40.4
boiled, 1 tbsp..2.5
red, California, dry, 1 cup...110.0
red, California, boiled, 1 cup..40.0
red, royal, dry, 1 cup...107.3
red, royal, boiled, 1 cup...38.7
Kidney beans, canned, ½ cup:
red:
(Allens/Trappey's) 22.0
(Eden Organic) 18.0
(Goya Spanish Style) 18.0
(Joan of Arc) 20.0
(Progresso) 20.0
(Seneca) 20.0
(Westbrae Natural) 15.0
dark *(Hain)* 18.0
light *(Joan of Arc)* 20.0
with bacon, light *(Trappey's* New Orleans Style) 20.0
with chili gravy *(Trappey's)*...20.0
Creole style *(Trappey's)* 19.0
with jalapeños, light *(Trappey's)*......................................19.0

white:
  (Eden Organic) 17.0
  (Progresso Cannellini) 18.0
  (Shari Ann's Organic Cannellini) 18.0
Kidney beans, sprouted, raw, 1 cup 7.5
Kielbasa (see also "Polish sausage"):
(Boar's Head), 2 oz. 0
(Johnsonville), 3-oz. link, grilled 1.0
(Russer Loaf), 2 oz. 5.0
pork and beef, .9-oz. slice 6
turkey (Louis Rich Polska), 2 oz. 2.0
turkey, pork, and beef (Healthy Choice Polska), 2 oz. 6.0
Kimchee, in jars (Frieda's), ¼ cup, 2 oz. 2.0
Kiwi, fresh:
(Dole), 2 fruits 18.0
peeled, 1 large, 3.2 oz. 13.5
peeled, 1 medium, 2.7 oz. 11.3
regular, baby, or gold (Frieda's), 5 oz. 21.0
Kiwi drink blend, 8 fl. oz., except as noted:
lime (Kool-Aid Bursts Kickin' Kiwi-Lime), 1 bottle 24.0
strawberry:
  (Crystal Light) 0
  (Kool-Aid Splash) 29.0
  (R.W. Knudsen) 30.0
  (Snapple Diet) 5.0
mix*, lime (Kool-Aid Kickin' Kiwi-Lime Sugar Sweetened) 16.0
Kiwi juice blend (After the Fall Kiwi Bear), 8 fl. oz. 24.0
Knockwurst:
(Karl Ehmer), 4-oz. link 1.0
beef:
  (Ball Park), 4-oz. link 1.0
  (Boar's Head), 4-oz. link 1.0
  (Hebrew National), 3-oz. link 1.0
beef and pork (Ball Park), 4-oz. link 4.0
Kohlrabi, fresh:
raw:
  (Frieda's), ⅔ cup, 3 oz. 5.0
  .6-oz. slice 1.0
  1 cup 8.4
boiled, drained, sliced, 1 cup 12.0

Krispy Kreme Doughnuts, 1 piece:
blueberry, glazed 37.0
blueberry-filled, powdered 26.0
cake:
    chocolate-iced 28.0
    powdered..26.0
    traditional 22.0
chocolate-iced:
    plain..30.0
    creme-filled 32.0
    custard-filled 38.0
    with sprinkles 31.0
cinnamon apple–filled 29.0
cinnamon bun 26.0
creme-filled, glazed 32.0
cruller, chocolate-iced 26.0
cruller, glazed...22.0
devil's food, glazed..29.0
Krispy Kreme original glazed..17.0
lemon-filled, yeast..28.0
maple-iced 28.0
raspberry-filled..27.0
Kumquat, fresh:
(Frieda's), 5 oz. 23.0
untrimmed, 1 lb. 69.3
1 medium, .7-oz. fruit 3.1
seeded, 1 oz..4.7
Kumquat, pickled, in jar, sweet *(Haddon House)*, 1 piece 2.0
Kun choy, see "Celery, Chinese"
Kuri squash, red *(Frieda's)*, ¾ cup, 3 oz. 7.0

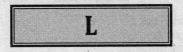

FOOD AND MEASURE CARBOHYDRATE GRAMS

Lamb, without added ingredients 0
Lamb's-quarter, fresh, boiled, drained, chopped, 1 cup..............9.0
Lard, pork 0
Lasagna, canned or packaged:
(Dinty Moore American Classics), 1 bowl...................28.0
with meat sauce *(Hormel* Microcup Meals), 1 cup 31.0
Lasagna, frozen, 1 pkg., except as noted:
(Healthy Choice Roma Entree), 13.5 oz. 59.0
(Stouffer's Bake), 11.5 oz...51.0
Alfredo *(Michelina's),* 9 oz. 38.0
cheese:
    (Amy's), 10.25 oz. 37.0
    (Lean Cuisine Everyday Favorites), 11.5 oz....................38.0
    casserole *(Lean Cuisine Everyday Favorites),* 10 oz. 40.0
    extra *(Marie Callender's* Meals), 15 oz. 61.0
    five *(Lean Cuisine* Family Style Favorites), 1/12 of 96-oz.
      pkg., 8 oz..27.0
    five *(Stouffer's),* 10.75 oz..40.0
    four *(Michelina's),* 8 oz..43.0
cheese with chicken scallopini *(Lean Cuisine Cafe Classics),*
    10 oz. 27.0
chicken:
    (Lean Cuisine Family Style Favorites), 1/12 of 96-oz. pkg.,
      8 oz..26.0
    (Lean Cuisine Everyday Favorites), 10 oz. 34.0
    (Stouffer's), 1 cup 29.0
with meat sauce:
    (Banquet), 9.5 oz..38.0
    (Banquet Family Size), 1 cup.....................................33.0
    (Freezer Queen Deluxe Family Entree), 1 cup 39.0
    (Freezer Queen Homestyle), 10 oz................................42.0
    (Lean Cuisine Everyday Favorites), 10½ oz............35.0
    (Marie Callender's Family), 1 cup 35.0
    (Marie Callender's Meals), 15 oz. 59.0

Lasagna, frozen *(cont.)*

   (Michelina's), 9 oz. 39.0
   (Stouffer's), 10.5 oz. 39.0
   (Stouffer's 96 oz.), 1 cup 29.0
   (Stouffer's 2¼ oz.), 1 cup 28.0
   layered *(Michelina's),* 8 oz. 29.0
   layered *(Michelina's),* 10 oz. 47.0
pollo *(Michelina's),* 8 oz. 33.0
Pomodoro, layered *(Michelina's),* 8 oz. 29.0
primavera *(Michelina's),* 8 oz. 34.0
tomato sauce and Italian sausage *(Stouffer's),* 10⅞ oz. 43.0
vegetable:
   (Amy's), 9.5 oz. 39.0
   (Amy's Family Size), 7 oz. 26.0
   (Cedarlane Low Fat Garden), 10 oz. 48.0
   (Lean Cuisine Everyday Favorites), 10½ oz. 35.0
   (Stouffer's), 10½ oz. 34.0
   (Stouffer's 96 oz.), 1 cup 36.0
   tofu *(Amy's),* 9.5 oz. 41.0
with vegetables *(Michelina's),* 8.5 oz. 35.0
with vegetables, layered *(Michelina's),* 8 oz. 30.0
with white sauce, layered *(Michelina's),* 10 oz. 51.0
Lasagna mix*, frozen, skillet *(Green Giant Create a Meal!),*
   1¼ cups 31.0
Leek, fresh, lower leaf and bulb portion:
raw *(Frieda's),* ⅓ cup, 3 oz. 12.0
raw, 1 cup, 3.1 oz. 12.6
boiled, drained, 1 leek, 4.4 oz. 9.4
boiled, drained, chopped, or diced, ¼ cup 2.0
Leek, freeze-dried, lower leaf and bulb portion:
¼ cup 6
1 tbsp. 1
Lemon, fresh, raw:
(Dole), 1 fruit 4.0
with peel, seeded, 3.8 oz. 11.6
peeled, 2⅛" diam. 5.4
peeled sections, 1 cup 19.8
Lemon curd, 1 tbsp.:
(Crosse & Blackwell) 13.0
(Dickenson's) 15.0

Lemon drink blend, ginger enchinacea *(R.W. Knudsen Simply Nutritious),* 8 fl. oz. 25.0
Lemon filling, see "Pie filling"
Lemon herb sauce mix *(Knorr* Classic Sauces), 1 tbsp. 4.0
Lemon juice:
fresh, 8 fl. oz. 21.8
fresh, 2 tbsp. 2.6
canned or bottled:
   (Santa Cruz Organic), 1 tsp. 0
   8 fl. oz. 15.8
   1 tbsp. 1.0
   from concentrate *(ReaLemon),* 1 tsp. 0
frozen, unsweetened, single strength, 2 tbsp. 2.0
Lemon peel, fresh, raw:
1 tbsp. 1.0
1 tsp. 3
Lemon pepper:
(Lawry's), ¼ tap. 0
1 tsp. 1.5
Lemonade, 8 fl. oz., except as noted:
(After the Fall) 23.0
(Crystal Light) 0
(R.W. Knudsen Aseptic) 27.0
(R.W. Knudsen Natural) 29.0
(Santa Cruz Organic) 24.0
(Snapple) 30.0
(Turkey Hill) 29.0
(Turkey Hill Diet) 5.0
pink:
   (AriZona) 28.0
   (Fruit Works), 12 fl. oz. 46.0
   (Snapple) 26.0
   (Snapple Diet) 2.0
frozen*, pink 25.9
frozen*, white 26.0
Lemonade fruit blend, see specific fruit listings
Lemonade mix, 8 fl. oz.*:
(Kool-Aid Sugar Sweetened) 17.0
1-oz. powder or 8 fl. oz.* 26.9
regular or pink:
   (Country Time Sugar Free) 0

Lemonade mix, regular or pink *(cont.)*
   (Crystal Light) 0
   (Kool-Aid) 25.0
Lemon-lime drink, 8 fl. oz.:
(Snapple Hydro) 24.0
mix* *(Crystal Light)* 0
mix* *(Kool-Aid)* 25.0
Lemongrass, fresh:
1 cup 16.9
1 tbsp. 1.2
Lemongrass hearts, in jars *(A Taste of Thai)*, 1 piece 1.0
Lentils, mature:
dry:
   (Goya), ¼ cup 19.0
   1 cup 109.6
   1 tbsp. 6.9
   green or red *(Arrowhead Mills)*, ¼ cup 27.0
   pink, 1 cup 113.6
boiled, 1 cup 39.9
boiled, 1 tbsp. 2.5
Lentils, canned, ½ cup:
(Eden Organic) 13.0
(Westbrae Natural) 13.0
Lentils, sprouted, raw, 1 cup 17.0
Lentil chili, see "Chili, canned or packaged"
Lentil rice dish, mix, see "Rice dish, mix"
Lentil rice loaf, frozen *(Natural Touch)*, 1" slice 14.0
Lettuce (see also "Salad" and "Salad blends"), fresh:
bibb or Boston, 1 head, 5" diam. 3.8
bibb or Boston, chopped or shredded, 1 cup 1.3
iceberg:
   (Andy Boy), ⅙ medium head 3.0
   (Dole), ⅙ medium head, 3.2 oz. 3.0
   1 large head, 1⅔ lbs. 15.8
   chopped or shredded, 1 cup 1.1
   shredded *(Dole* Classic), 3 oz. 3.0
leaf, shredded *(Andy Boy)*, 1½ cups 4.0
leaf, shredded *(Dole)*, 1½ cups, 3 oz. 4.0
limestone *(Frieda's)*, ⅔ cup, 3 oz. 2.0
looseleaf, 1 leaf, approx. .4 oz. 4
looseleaf, shredded, ½ cup 1.0

Romaine or cos:
  (Andy Boy), 6 leaves 3.0
  (Dole), 6 leaves, 3 oz. 3.0
  1 inner leaf 2
  shredded, ½ cup 7
Lily root, see "Lotus root"
Lima beans:
immature or green:
  raw *(Frieda's)*, ⅓ cup, 3 oz. 20.0
  raw, 1 cup 31.4
  boiled, drained, 1 cup 40.2
mature:
  baby, dry *(Goya)*, ¼ cup 23.0
  baby, dry, 1 cup 126.9
  baby, boiled, 1 cup 42.4
  large, dry, 1 cup 112.8
  large, boiled, 1 cup 39.3
Lima beans, canned
immature:
  (Allens/East Texas Fair Green), ½ cup 23.0
  (Del Monte Green), ½ cup 15.0
  (Sunshine Green Butterbeans), ½ cup 23.0
  16-oz. can 60.5
  ½ cup 16.5
  with bacon *(Trappey's)* 22.0
mature:
  baby *(Allens* Butterbeans) 22.0
  baby *(Eden* Original) 17.0
  baby, with bacon *(Trappey's)* 21.0
  large *(Allens* Butterbeans) 20.0
  large, 1 cup 35.9
  large, with sausage *(Trappey's* Butterbeans) 21.0
Lima beans, frozen:
(Seabrook Farms Petite), ½ cup 22.0
baby:
  (Birds Eye), ½ cup 24.0
  (Freshlike), ½ cup 22.0
  (Green Giant), ½ cup 16.0
  (Green Giant Harvest Fresh), ½ cup 15.0
  (Seneca), ⅔ cup 23.0
  unprepared, 10-oz. pkg. 71.4

Lima bean, frozen, baby *(cont.)*

unprepared, ½ cup 20.6
boiled, drained, 10-oz. pkg. 60.5
boiled, drained, ½ cup 17.5
in butter sauce *(Green Giant)*, ⅔ cup...................18.0

Fordhook:

(Birds Eye), ½ cup 19.0
(Freshlike), ½ cup 17.0
(Seneca), ⅔ cup 17.0
unprepared, 10-oz. pkg. 56.3
unprepared, ½ cup 15.9
boiled, drained, 10-oz. pkg. 58.5
boiled, drained, ½ cup 16.0

mature, regular or speckled *(Birds Eye Southern Butterbeans)*,
½ cup 20.0

Lime, fresh, raw:

2"-diam. fruit, 2.4 oz. 7.1
Key *(Frieda's)*, 3-oz. fruit 9.0

Lime drink blend, 8 fl. oz.:

(After the Fall Key West Lime) 25.0
cactus *(R.W. Knudsen* Quencher) 29.0

Lime juice:

fresh, 8 fl. oz. 22.2
fresh, 2 tbsp. 2.8

canned or bottled:

(Santa Cruz Organic), 1 tsp. 0
unsweetened, 8 fl. oz. 16.5
unsweetened, 2 tbsp. 21.1
from concentrate *(ReaLime)*, 1 tsp. 0
sweetened *(Rose's)*, 1 tsp. 2.0

Lime relish, Indian, 1 tbsp.:

hot *(Patak's)*..5
mild *(Patak's)* 0

Limeade, frozen*, 8 fl. oz. 27.2

Ling, without added ingredients 0

Ling cod, without added ingredients 0

Linguine, plain:

dry, see "Pasta"
refrigerated *(Contadina Buitoni)*, 1¼ cups 45.0
refrigerated, regular or herb *(Di Giorno)*, 2.5 oz. 38.0

Linguine dish, mix:
with chicken and broccoli *(Pasta Roni)*, about 1 cup*...............49.0
creamy chicken Parmesan *(Pasta Roni)*, about 1 cup* 51.0
garlic and butter *(Lipton* Pasta & Sauce), ⅓ cup, 1 cup*..........40.0
Linguine entree, frozen, with clams and sauce
   (Michelina's), 8.5 oz. 52.0
Litchee, see "Lychee"
Little Caesar's:
pizza, 1 slice:
   12" round, cheese only 22.0
   12" round, pepperoni..21.0
   14" round, cheese only 23.0
   14" round, meatsa 24.0
   14" round, pepperoni, 3.1 oz. 23.0
   14" round, supreme, 4 oz. 25.0
   14" round, veggie, 3.9 oz..25.0
   16" round, cheese only 30.0
   16" round, pepperoni..31.0
   18" round, cheese only or pepperoni...................................32.0
   12" or 14" square, deep dish, cheese only or pepperoni 19.0
   12" thin crust, cheese only or pepperoni.............................12.0
   14" thin crust, cheese only or pepperoni.............................13.0
pizza by the slice, cheese only or pepperoni, ⅙ of 14" pie 39.0
sandwiches, cold, 1 piece:
   deli ham and cheese or Italian...68.0
   deli veggie 71.0
salad, antipasto, 6.6 oz. 10.0
salad, tossed side..9.0
salad dressings:
   Italian...2.0
   Italian, fat-free 5.0
   ranch 1.0
other menu items:
   cinnamon Caesar stick 57.0
   crazy bread, 1 slice..14.0
   crazy sauce, 4 oz...9.0
   Baby Pan! Pan!, 4.6 oz...32.0
Liquor[1], all proofs, 1 fl. oz...0

[1] *Includes all pure distilled liquors: bourbon, brandy, gin, rum, scotch, tequila, vodka, etc.*

Liver:
beef:
    raw, 4 oz. 6.4
    braised, 11.85 oz. (yield from 1 lb. raw) 11.5
    pan-fried, 10.4 oz. (yield from 1 lb. raw) 23.2
chicken, raw, 1.1 oz. 1.1
chicken, simmered, chopped or diced, 1 cup 1.2
duck, raw, 1.6 oz. 1.6
goose, raw, 3.3 oz. 5.9
lamb:
    raw, 4 oz. 2.0
    braised, 11.9 oz. (yield from 1 lb. raw) 8.5
    pan-fried, 11.4 oz. (yield from 1 lb. raw) 12.2
pork, raw, 4 oz. 2.8
pork, braised, 12.5 oz. (yield from 1 lb. raw) 13.3
turkey, raw, 3.6 oz. 4.2
turkey, simmered, chopped, 1 cup 4.8
veal (calves'):
    raw, 4 oz. 0
    braised, 8.8 oz. (yield from 1 lb. raw) 6.1
    pan-fried, 9.6 oz. (yield from 1 lb. raw) 10.7
Liver cheese, 1.3-oz. slice 8
Liver paté, see "Paté"
Liverwurst (see also "Braunschweiger") *(Boar's Head*
    Strassburger), 2 oz. 1.0
Lo bok, see "Radish, Oriental"
Loaf seasoning mix *(Natural Touch),* 4 tbsp. 10.0
Lobster, northern, meat only:
raw, 1 lobster, 5.3 oz. 8
boiled or steamed, 4 oz. 1.5
boiled or steamed, 1 cup, 5.1 oz. 1.9
Lobster sauce, canned *(Progresso),* ½ cup 6.0
Loganberries, frozen, unthawed, 1 cup 19.1
Long beans, see "Yard-long beans"
Long John Silver's:
entrees:
    chicken plank, battered, 1 piece 9.0
    clams, breaded, 1 order 26.0
    fish:
        battered, 1 piece 16.0
        battered, junior, 1 piece 8.0

breaded, country style, 1 piece..17.0
lemon crumb, 2 pieces 10.0
lemon crumb, à la carte, 2 pieces with rice......................52.0
lemon crumb, add-a-piece, 1 piece with rice..................9.0
lemon crumb, meal, 1 meal..................................89.0
shrimp, battered, 1 piece..................................3.0
shrimp, popcorn, 1 serving..................................33.0
sandwiches, 1 sandwich:
    chicken, regular or with cheese 40.0
    fish, regular, ultimate or with cheese................................46.0
sides:
    broccoli-cheese soup, 1 bowl..................................13.0
    cheese sticks, 5 pieces 12.0
    coleslaw, 4 oz. 23.0
    corn cobbett, 1 piece..................................19.0
    fries, large, 5 oz...................................46.0
    fries, regular, 3 oz...................................28.0
    hush puppy, 1 piece 9.0
    rice, 4 oz...................................34.0
salads:, 1 serving:
    chef, ocean 15.0
    chicken, grilled 10.0
    garden 9.0
    side..................................3.0
salad dressings, 1 pkt.:
    French, fat-free 10.0
    Italian..................................2.0
    ranch 1.0
    ranch, fat-free..................................9.0
    Thousand Island 5.0
condiments, 1 pkt.:
    honey mustard sauce 5.0
    ketchup..................................2.0
    malt vinegar..................................0
    shrimp sauce..................................3.0
    sweet and sour sauce..................................5.0
    tartar sauce..................................2.0
desserts, 1 piece:
    apple pie, Dutch..................................44.0
    banana split sundae pie..................................34.0
    chocolate creme pie 29.0

Long John Silver's, desserts (cont.)
lemon pie, double..41.0
pecan pie...53.0
pineapple creme cheesecake pie 36.0
strawberries n'creme pie 32.0
Longan:
fresh, raw, trimmed, 1 longan, .1 oz...................................5
dried, 1 oz...20.9
Loquat:
(Frieda's), 5 oz...17.0
untrimmed, 1 lb. 34.1
1 large, .7 oz. 2.4
cubed, 1 cup...18.1
Lotus root, fresh:
raw:
   (Frieda's 1 cup, 3 oz. 15.0
   untrimmed, 1 lb. 61.8
   9½"-long root 19.8
   sliced, 2½" diam., 10 slices...14.0
boiled, drained, ½ cup 9.6
boiled, drained, sliced, 2½" diam., 10 slices...................14.3
Lotus seeds:
fresh, raw, 1 oz. 4.9
dried, 1 oz., 42 medium...18.3
dried, 1 cup 20.6
Lox, see "Salmon, smoked"
Lunch meat, loaf (see also specific listings):
all varieties *(Spam),* 2 oz. 0
barbecue, .8-oz. slice 1.5
berliner, .8-oz. slice 6
Dutch brand *(Russer),* 2 oz..6.0
honey, 1-oz. slice 1.5
Italian brand *(Russer),* 2 oz. 5.0
jalapeño, with Monterey jack cheese *(Russer),* 2 oz. 4.0
luxury, pork, 1-oz. slice..1.4
mother's, pork, ¾-oz. slice 1.6
old-fashioned *(Russer* Light), 2 oz....................................4.0
olive:
   (Boar's Head), 2 oz. ....<1.0
   (Russer), 2 oz...4.0
   pork, 1-oz. slice...2.6

pepper *(Russer)*, 2 oz. 6.0
pepper, pork, and beef, 1-oz. slice 1.3
pickle and pimento *(Russer/Russer Light)*, 2 oz. 4.0
pickle and pimento, pork, 1-oz. slice 1.7
picnic, 1-oz. slice 1.3
pork and beef, 2-oz. slice..1.3
sausage, honey roll, beef, .8-oz. slice............................. .5
sausage, luncheon, pork, and beef, .8-oz. slice 4
Lunch "meat," vegetarian *(Wham)*, 2 slices................1.0
Lupin, mature:
raw, 1 cup 72.7
boiled, 1 cup 16.4
Lychee:
fresh, raw:
   (Frieda's), 1 fruit...14.0
   shelled and seeded, 1 oz. 18.0
   shelled and seeded, 1 cup...31.4
dried, 1 oz. 79.0
Lyonnaise gravy mix *(Knorr* Gravy Classics), 2 tsp., ¼ cup* 4.0

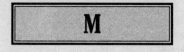

FOOD AND MEASURE   **CARBOHYDRATE GRAMS**

Macadamia nuts, shelled:
(Frieda's), 5 pieces, 1.1 oz. 4.0
raw, 1 oz., 10–12 kernels 3.9
raw, whole or halves, 1 cup 18.5
dry-roasted:
    unsalted, 1 oz. 3.8
    unsalted, whole or halves, 1 cup 17.9
    salted, 1 oz. 3.6
    salted, 1 cup 17.2
Macaroni, uncooked (see also "Pasta, dry, uncooked"), 2 oz.,
   except as noted:
(Creamette) 42.0
elbow *(Westbrae Natural)*, ½ cup 40.0
elbow or spiral 42.3
protein-fortified, small shells 37.2
vegetable (tri-color) 42.5
whole-wheat 42.5
Macaroni, cooked (see also "Pasta, dry, cooked"), 1 cup:
elbow 39.7
protein-fortified, small shells 35.5
spirals 38.0
vegetable (tri-color) 35.7
whole-wheat 37.2
Macaroni dish, see "Macaroni entree"
Macaroni entree, canned or packaged:
and beef:
    (Chef Boyardee Beefaroni), 1 cup....................................37.0
    (Kid's Kitchen Beefy Macaroni), 1 cup...............................23.0
    in tomato sauce *(Chef Boyardee Beefaroni)*, 1 cup 35.0
    in tomato sauce *(Chef Boyardee Beefaroni* Microwave),
       1 bowl..27.0
and cheese:
    (Chef Boyardee), ½ of 15-oz. can 35.0
    (Franco-American), 1 cup..29.0

(Hormel), 7.5-oz. can 30.0
(Hormel Microcup Meals), 1 cup...........................30.0
(Kid's Kitchen), 1 cup 30.0
and beef *(Kid's Kitchen* Cheezy Mac & Beef), 1 cup..............33.0
in cheese sauce *(Chef Boyardee)*, 1 cup 30.0
with *Cure 81* ham *(Dinty Moore American Classics)*,
   1 bowl..30.0
and franks *(Kid's Kitchen* Cheezy Mac & Franks), 1 cup 30.0
chili, see "Chili, canned or packaged"
Macaroni entree, dried, and cheese *(AlpineAire*
   Forever Young), 1 cup 54.0
Macaroni entree, frozen, 1 pkg., except as noted:
and beef:
   (Freezer Queen Homestyle), 9 oz........................32.0
   (Healthy Choice Entree), 8.5 oz. 34.0
   (Lean Cuisine Everyday Favorites), 10 oz..............43.0
   (Michelina's), 8 oz. 36.0
   (Michelina's Socceroni), 8 oz. 42.0
   (Stouffer's), 11½ oz. 37.0
and cheese:
   (Amy's), 9 oz. 47.0
   (Banquet), 12 oz. 57.0
   (Banquet Family Size), 1 cup.............................33.0
   (Boston Market Home Style Meals), 10 oz. 58.0
   (Freezer Queen Family Side Dish), 1 cup.............43.0
   (Freezer Queen Homestyle), 8 oz........................46.0
   (Healthy Choice Entree), 9 oz. 36.0
   (Howard Johnson's), 10 oz. 42.0
   (Lean Cuisine Everyday Favorites), 10 oz..............42.0
   (Marie Callender's Family), 1 cup 41.0
   (Marie Callender's Meals), 12 oz. 55.0
   (Morton), 1 cup 34.0
   (Stouffer's), 12 oz. 31.0
   (Stouffer's 76 oz.), 1 cup..................................37.0
   (Stouffer's 40 oz.), 1 cup..................................40.0
   (Stouffer's 20 oz.), 1 cup..................................32.0
   (Tofutti), 6 oz. 31.0
   with broccoli *(Stouffer's)*, 10½ oz......................43.0
   with ham *(Michelina's)*, 8 oz. 33.0
   pot pie *(Banquet)*, 6.5 oz. 34.0
   pot pie *(Morton)*, 6.5 oz. 34.0

Macaroni entree, frozen, and cheese *(cont.)*
    and sharp cheddar *(Michelina's)*, 10 oz.............................49.0
    soy *(Amy's* Cheeze), 9 oz...42.0
Macaroni entree, mix, and cheese:
(Bowl Appétit!), 1 bowl 54.0
(Creamette), 2.5 oz. 50.0
(Fantastic Foods Ready, Set Pasta! Cup), 2.1 oz. 41.0
(Kraft Deluxe Dinner Original), about 1 cup* 44.0
(Kraft Light Deluxe Dinner), about 1 cup* 48.0
(Kraft Original Dinner), 2.5 oz. 47.0
(Kraft Original Dinner), about 1 cup* 49.0
(Kraft Thick 'N Creamy Premium Dinner), about 1 cup* 50.0
(Land O Lakes), 2.5 oz. 49.0
(Land O Lakes Deluxe Plus), 3.5 oz., 1 cup* 46.0
Alfredo, cheesy *(Kraft* Premium Dinner), about 1 cup* 49.0
four-cheese *(Kraft* Deluxe Dinner), about 1 cup* 44.0
three-cheese *(Knorr* TasteBreaks), 1 cont. 41.0
three-cheese or mild white cheddar *(Kraft* Premium Dinner),
    about 1 cup* 49.0
Macaroni salad, refrigerated:
(Blue Ridge Farms), ½ cup 25.0
(Chef's Express), 4 oz. 21.0
Mace:
ground, 1 tbsp. 2.7
ground, 1 tsp. 9
Mackerel, fresh, canned, or smoked, meat only 0
Madras sauce, see "Curry sauce"
Mahimahi, fresh, without added ingredients.....................0
Mai tai drink mixer:
(Mr & Mrs T), 4.5 fl. oz...33.0
(Trader Vic's), 4 fl. oz..32.0
Malanga *(Frieda's)*, ⅔ cup, 3 oz. 23.0
Malt beverage, 8 fl. oz..31.9
Malt cooler, 12 fl. oz.:
(Bartles & Jaymes Original) 29.0
berry *(Bartles & Jaymes)* 33.0
black cherry *(Bartles & Jaymes)* 32.0
fuzzy navel, kiwi-strawberry, or hard lemonade
    (Bartles & Jaymes)...39.0
Margarita *(Bartles & Jaymes)* 46.0
peach *(Bartles & Jaymes)*...33.0

piña colada *(Bartles & Jaymes)* 48.0
strawberry daiquiri *(Bartles & Jaymes)* 36.0
tropical *(Bartles & Jaymes)*..37.0
Malt syrup, 1 tbsp.:
barley or wheat *(Eden* Organic)......................................14.0
rye *(Eden* Organic) 13.0
Malted milk powder:
natural:
    (Carnation Original), 3 tbsp. 15.0
    without added nutrients, 3 heaping tsp. or ¾-oz. pkt. 15.9
    without added nutrients, prepared with milk, 8 fl. oz. 27.3
    with added nutrients, 4–5 heaping tsp. or ¾-oz. pkt..............17.1
    with added nutrients, prepared with milk, 8 fl. oz. 28.4
chocolate flavor:
    (Carnation), 3 tbsp. 18.0
    without added nutrients, 3 heaping tsp. or ¾-oz. pkt. 18.4
    without added nutrients, prepared with milk, 8 fl. oz. 29.9
    with added nutrients, 3 heaping tsp. or ¾-oz. pkt..............17.7
    with added nutrients, prepared with milk, 8 fl. oz. 29.2
Mammy apple, fresh, untrimmed, 1 fruit, 1.9 lb. 105.8
Mandarin orange, see "Tangerine, canned"
Mandioca, see "Yuca root"
Mango, fresh:
(Frieda's Pango), 5-oz. fruit...24.0
untrimmed, 1 lb. 53.2
peeled, 1 fruit, 7.3 oz. 35.2
peeled and sliced *(Dole),* ½ cup 14.0
peeled and sliced, 1 cup 28.1
Mango, dried:
(Frieda's), 4 pieces, 1.4 oz. 32.0
(Sonoma), 6 pieces, 1.1 oz. 23.0
spiced *(Sonoma* Macho Mango), 6 pieces, 1.1 oz. 24.0
Mango, in jar, sliced:
in light syrup *(Ka•Me),* 4 pieces.......................................55.0
in syrup *(Haddon House),* ½ cup 22.0
Mango chutney, see "Chutney"
Mango drink, 8 fl. oz.:
(AriZona Mucho) 27.0
mix* *(Tang)* 25.0
Mango drink blend, 8 fl. oz.:
berry, mix* *(Kool-Aid Man-O-Mango-Berry)*...........................25.0

Mango drink blend *(cont.)*
berry, mix* *(Kool-Aid Man-O-Mango-Berry)* Sugar
    Sweetened)..16.0
peach *(R.W. Knudsen)* 30.0
Mango juice blend *(After the Fall Mango Montage)*, 8 fl. oz. 27.0
Mango nectar:
(Goya), 6 fl. oz. 27.0
(Libby's), 11.5-fl.-oz. can 51.0
(Libby's), 8 fl. oz. 36.0
Mango relish, Indian, 1 tbsp.:
hot *(Patak's)*..1.5
mild *(Patak's)*...1.0
Mangosteen, canned:
in syrup, 1 cup 38.7
in syrup, drained, 1 cup 35.1
Manicotti entree, frozen, 1 pkg.:
cheese *(Stouffer's)*, 9 oz. 34.0
cheese, three *(Healthy Choice* Entree), 11 oz..................40.0
cheese and spinach *(Lean Cuisine Hearty Portions Meal)*,
    15½ oz. 50.0
Mao du, see "Edamame"
Maple syrup (see also "Pancake syrup"), ¼ cup:
(Camp)..53.0
(Cary's/Maple Orchard's/MacDonald's) 52.0
(Maple Grove Farms) 53.0
Maple syrup granules, pure *(AlpineAire)*, ⅓ cup......................23.0
Margarine:
(Weight Watchers Lite), 1 tbsp. 2.0
regular, all varieties and blends, 1 tbsp..............................0
Margarine spread, all varieties and blends, 1 tbsp. 0
Margarita mixer, 4 fl. oz., except as noted:
bottled:
    (D.L. Jardine's Texarita), 1 fl. oz. 22.0
    (Holland House) 29.0
    (Mr & Mrs T)..29.0
    peach *(Daily's)*...48.0
    raspberry *(Daily's)*..46.0
    strawberry *(Mr & Mrs T)*, 3.5 fl. oz. 34.0
    strawberry *(Trader Vic's)*...40.0
frozen *(Bacardi)*, 2 fl. oz...25.0

Marinade (see also "Grilling sauce," "Stir-fry sauce," and specific listings) 1 tbsp.:
(House of Tsang Mandarin)..6.0
(Mary Rose Sari Sauce Marinade & Barbecue)............................1.0
Caribbean jerk, with papaya juice *(Lawry's)*................................6.0
citrus grill, with orange juice *(Lawry's)*....................................3.0
curry, see "Curry sauce, marinade"
Dijon and honey, with lemon juice *(Lawry's)* 3.0
fajitas meat *(D.L. Jardine's)* 1.0
ginger, Thai, with lime juice *(Lawry's)*.....................................2.0
Hawaiian, with tropical fruit juices *(Lawry's)* 4.0
herb and garlic, with lemon juice *(Lawry's)*................................2.0
hickory, with apple cider *(Lawry's)* 5.0
lemon pepper, with lemon juice *(Lawry's)*..................................2.0
London broil *(Lawry's* Weekday Gourmet)..................................2.0
Mediterranean, with lemon juice *(Lawry's)*.................................2.0
mesquite, with lime juice *(Lawry's)*..1.0
tequila lime, with lime juice *(Lawry's)*.....................................4.0
teriyaki:
   (Kikkoman Marinade & Sauce)..2.0
   (Kikkoman Marinade & Sauce Lite) 3.0
   (Mary Rose Sumi Sauce Barbecue and Marinade) 7.0
   (Soy Vey Veri Veri Teriyaki) 6.0
   garlic, roasted *(Kikkoman* Marinade & Sauce) 5.0
   with pineapple juice *(Lawry's)* 6.0
   steak *(Lawry's* Weekday Gourmet) 5.0
Marinade seasoning mix:
Cajun, spicy *(Adolph's For the Grill)*, 1 tbsp. 1.0
chicken tenderizing *(Adolph's Marinade in Minutes)*, ¾ tsp. 1.0
garlic, roasted *(Adolph's For the Grill)*, 1 tsp. 1.0
garlic flavor tenderizing *(Adolph's Marinade in Minutes)*,
   ¾ tsp...1.0
lemon herb, with cracked black pepper *(Adolph's For the Grill)*,
   ½ tsp..1.0
meat tenderizing *(Adolph's Marinade in Minutes)*, ¾ tsp. 1.0
meat tenderizing *(Adolph's Marinade in Minutes* Sodium Free)*,
   ¾ tsp...2.0
mesquite *(Adolph's For the Grill)*, ¾ tsp. 1.0
steak sauce tenderizing *(Adolph's Marinade in Minutes)*,
   ¾ tsp...1.0

Marjoram, dried:

1 tbsp..1.0

1 tsp... .4

Marmalade, see "Jam and preserves"

Marrow squash, raw, trimmed, 1 oz. 1.0

Marshmallow topping, 2 tbsp.:

(Marshmallow Fluff) 15.0

(Smucker's Spoonable) 29.0

(Solo Marshmallow Creme) 10.0

raspberry or strawberry *(Marshmallow Fluff)* 15.0

Marzipan, see "Almond paste"

Masa, see "Corn flour" and "Cornmeal"

Masala paste, see "Curry paste"

Masala sauce, see "Curry sauce"

Matzo, see "Cracker"

Matzo balls, in jar *(Mrs. Adler's),* 3 balls with liquid.................24.0

Mayonnaise, 1 tbsp.:

(Hain Canola/Safflower) 0

(Hain Eggless) 1.0

(Hain Lite Safflower) 2.0

(Hellmann's/Best Foods) 0

(Hellmann's/Best Foods Light) 1.0

(Henri's) 0

(Kraft)..0

(Kraft Light) 2.0

(Smart Balance Light) 2.0

(Weight Watchers Fat Free)...3.0

(Weight Watchers Light) 1.0

Mayonnaise dressing, 1 tbsp., except as noted:

(Kraft)..2.0

(Smart Beat)...3.0

(Weight Watchers) 3.0

1 cup...56.2

1 tbsp..3.5

all varieties *(Kraft Miracle Whip)*.................................2.0

imitation:

    milk cream...1.7

    soybean 2.4

    soybean, no cholesterol..2.2

low-fat *(Hellmann's/Best Foods),* 1 pkt. 3.0

soybean 4

whipped:
    (Hellmann's/Best Foods)......1.0
    fat-free *(Hellmann's/Best Foods)*......5.0
    fat-free *(Hellmann's/Best Foods)*, 1 pkt. 3.0
Mayonnaise mustard, see "Mustard blends"
McDonald's, 1 serving:
breakfast:
    bagel, ham and egg cheese......58.0
    bagel, Spanish omelet or steak and egg cheese......59.0
    biscuit, plain......34.0
    biscuit, bacon, egg, and cheese 36.0
    biscuit, sausage or sausage and egg......35.0
    breakfast burrito......21.0
    Egg McMuffin......27.0
    eggs, scrambled, 2......1.0
    English muffin, plain......25.0
    hash browns......14.0
    hotcakes, plain......58.0
    hotcakes, with syrup, margarine 104.0
    sausage 0
    Sausage McMuffin......26.0
    Sausage McMuffin, with egg......27.0
Danishes and muffins:
    apple bran muffin, low-fat......61.0
    apple Danish......47.0
    cheese Danish 45.0
    cinnamon roll 50.0
sandwiches:
    Big Mac......45.0
    Big Xtra!......51.0
    Big Xtra! with cheese 52.0
    cheeseburger......35.0
    Chicken McGrill......46.0
    Chicken McGrill, without mayo......45.0
    Crispy Chicken......54.0
    Filet-O-Fish......45.0
    hamburger......35.0
    Quarter Pounder......37.0
    Quarter pounder with cheese 38.0
Chicken McNuggets:
    4 pieces......13.0

McDonald's, Chicken McNuggets (cont.)
6 pieces	20.0
9 pieces	29.0

McNuggets sauce pkt.:
barbeque	10.0
honey	12.0
honey mustard	3.0
hot mustard	7.0
mayonnaise, light	<1.0
sweet and sour	11.0

french fries:
large	68.0
medium	57.0
super size	77.0
small	26.0

salads, without dressing:
chef salad	5.0
garden salad	4.0
grilled chicken Caesar salad	3.0
croutons, 1 pkg.	9.0

salad dressing, 1 pkg.:
Caesar	5.0
honey mustard	13.0
ranch	2.0
red French, reduced-calorie	18.0
Thousand Island	11.0
vinaigrette, herb	7.0

desserts and shakes:
baked apple pie	34.0
chocolate chip cookie	22.0
fruit 'n yogurt parfait	76.0
fruit 'n yogurt parfait, without granola	53.0
McDonaldland Cookies, 1 pkg.	32.0
McFlurry, Butterfinger or *M&M's*	90.0
McFlurry, Nestlé Crunch	89.0
McFlurry, Oreo	82.0
shake, chocolate or strawberry, small	60.0
shake, vanilla, small	59.0
sundae, hot caramel	61.0
sundae, hot fudge	52.0
sundae, strawberry	50.0

sundae nuts..2.0
vanilla cone, reduced-fat.......................................23.0
Meat, canned, see "Meat spread" and specific listings
Meat, lunch, see "Lunch meat" and specific listings
Meat loaf, refrigerated *(Always Tender),* 5 oz. 14.0
Meat loaf dinner, frozen, 1 pkg.:
(Banquet Extra Helping), 16 oz. 34.0
(Healthy Choice Meal Traditional), 12 oz.................52.0
with mashed potato *(Swanson),* 10¾ oz. 37.0
Meat loaf entree, frozen, 1 pkg.:
(Banquet), 9.5 oz. 23.0
(Stouffer's Homestyle), 9⅞ oz. 28.0
and gravy:
(Boston Market), 9 oz...19.0
(Stouffer's), ⅙ of 33-oz. pkg..............................10.0
with mashed potatoes *(Boston Market),* 16 oz......55.0
with mashed potatoes *(Marie Callender's* Family),
1 patty with gravy, ½ cup potatoes 26.0
with mashed potatoes *(Marie Callender's* Meals), 14 oz. 42.0
with mashed potatoes *(Michelina's),* 8 oz. 20.0
with sour cream mashed potatoes *(Michelina's),*
10.5 oz..25.0
gravy, savory, and *(Banquet* Family Size), 1 patty with gravy 7.0
with mashed potatoes *(Stouffer's Hearty Portions),* 17 oz..........57.0
tomato sauce and:
(Freezer Queen Family Entree), 1 patty and sauce................10.0
(Morton), 9 oz. 24.0
with mashed potatoes *(Freezer Queen* Meal), 9.5 oz.............26.0
with whipped potato *(Lean Cuisine Cafe Classics),* 9⅜ oz. 28.0
Meat loaf seasoning mix *(Adolph's Meal Makers),* 1 tbsp...........5.0
Meat spread:
(Spam), 4 tbsp..1.0
pork and beef, 1 tbsp. 1.8
potted *(Armour),* ¼ cup 0
potted *(Hormel),* 4 tbsp. 0
Meat tenderizer (see also "Marinade"):
(Adolph's Original), ¼ tsp. 0
(Adolph's Original Sodium Free), ½ tsp.....................<1.0
spice-seasoned *(Adolph's),* ¼ tsp...............................0
spice-seasoned *(Adolph's* Sodium Free), ¼ tsp............1.0
Meatball entree, canned *(Dinty Moore),* 1 cup 17.0

Meatball entree, frozen, 1 pkg.:
Italian, in wine sauce *(Michelina's),* 8 oz.............................33.0
mashed potatoes and, with vegetables *(Michelina's),* 8.5 oz. 26.0
noodles with, see "Noodle entree, frozen"
spaghetti and, see "Spaghetti entree, frozen"
Swedish:
    (Lean Cuisine Everyday Favorites), 9⅛ oz......................35.0
    (Marie Callender's Meals), 12.5 oz. 44.0
    (Stouffer's), 11½ oz. 49.0
    gravy with noodles and *(Michelina's),* 10 oz. 37.0
Meatball sandwich/pocket, 1 piece:
Italian style *(Healthy Choice Hearty Handfuls),* 6.1 oz. 51.0
and mozzarella *(Hot Pockets),* 4.5 oz............................41.0
and mozzarella *(Lean Pockets),* 4.5 oz...........................44.0
Melon, see specific melon listings
Melon, mixed, balls, frozen, unthawed, 1 cup 13.7
Menudo, canned *(Juanita's Menudito),* 1 cup 12.0
Menudo spice mix *(Gebhardt),* ¼ tsp. 0
Mexican dinner, frozen, 1 pkg.:
fiesta *(Patio),* 12 oz...53.0
Mexican style *(Patio),* 13.25 oz.....................................59.0
ranchers *(Patio),* 13 oz..55.0
Mexican rice seasoning, see "Rice seasoning mix"
Mexican squash *(Frieda's),* ½ cup, 3 oz........................9.0
Milk, dairy pack or packaged, 1 cup, except as noted:
buttermilk, cultured, low-fat...11.7
buttermilk, low-fat *(Friendship)*......................................12.0
low-fat:
    2%, nonfat milk solids fortified 13.5
    2%, nonfat milk solids and vitamin A fortified 12.2
    2%, protein and vitamin A fortified 13.5
    2%, vitamin A fortified...11.7
    1%, nonfat milk solids and vitamin A fortified 12.2
    1%, protein and vitamin A fortified 13.6
    1%, vitamin A fortified...11.7
    skim...11.9
    skim, nonfat milk solids and vitamin A fortified 12.3
    skim, protein and vitamin A fortified 13.7
    skim, vitamin A fortified 11.9
low-sodium 10.9

whole:

3.25% fat	11.4
3.25% fat, 1 tbsp.	.7
3.7% fat	11.3

Milk, canned:

condensed, sweetened:

(Borden), 2 tbsp.	23.0
(Carnation), 2 tbsp.	22.0
(Eagle/Magnolia Brand), 2 tbsp.	23.0
1 cup	166.5
2 tbsp.	20.8

evaporated:

(Carnation Fat Free), 2 tbsp.	4.0
(Carnation/Carnation Low Fat), 2 tbsp.	3.0
(Pet/Pet Skim), 2 tbsp.	3.0
1 cup	25.3
2 tbsp.	3.2
skim, 1 cup	29.1
skim, 2 tbsp.	3.6
vitamin A fortified, 2 tbsp.	3.2

Milk, chocolate, see "Chocolate milk"

Milk, dry:

buttermilk:

1 oz.	13.9
1 cup	58.9
1 tbsp.	3.2

whole:

1 oz.	10.9
1 cup	49.2
¼ cup	12.3

nonfat (Carnation), ⅓ cup	12.0

nonfat, regular:

1 oz.	14.7
1 cup	62.4
¼ cup	15.6
vitamin A fortified, 1 oz.	14.7
vitamin A fortified, 1 cup	62.4
vitamin A fortified, ¼ cup	15.6

nonfat, instant:

1 oz.	14.8

Milk, dry, nonfat, instant *(cont.)*
3.2-oz. pkt. 47.5
1 cup 35.5
Milk, goat:
(Meyenberg), 1 cup 11.0
1 fl. oz. 1.4
1 cup 10.9
Milk, human:
1 fl. oz. 2.7
1 cup 16.9
Milk, Indian buffalo, 1 cup 12.4
Milk, nondairy, see "Rice beverage" and "Soy beverage"
Milk, sheep, 1 cup 13.1
Milkfish, without added ingredients 0
Millet:
raw, 1 cup 145.7
raw, hulled *(Arrowhead Mills),* ¼ cup 34.0
cooked, 1 cup 41.2
Millet flour *(Arrowhead Mills),* ¼ cup 26.0
Mincemeat, see "Pie filling"
Mint, see "Spearmint"
Mint sauce *(Crosse & Blackwell),* 1 tsp. 1.0
Miso:
barley *(Eden* Organic Mugi), 1 tbsp. 3.0
rice *(Eden* Organic Shiro), 1 tbsp. 5.0
rice, brown *(Eden* Organic Genmai), 1 tbsp. 3.0
soy *(Eden* Organic Hacho), 1 tbsp. 2.0
soy, 1 oz. 7.9
Molasses:
(Grandma's 24 oz.), 1 tbsp. 14.0
(Grandma's 12 oz.), 1 tbsp. 12.0
(Grandma's Mild), 1 tbsp. 14.0
(Grandma's Robust), 1 tbsp. 12.0
1 cup 225.7
1 tbsp. 13.8
blackstrap:
Brer Rabbit), 1 tbsp. 13.0
1 cup 199.4
1 tbsp. 12.2
full- or mild-flavored *(Brer Rabbit),* 1 tbsp. 15.0
Monkfish, without added ingredients 0

Mortadella, 2 oz., except as noted:
(*Boar's Head Cinghiale*)..0
(*Fiorucci*)..0
(*Russer*)..1.0
beef and pork, .5-oz. slice.....................................5
with pistachios (*Boar's Head Cinghiale*)..............3.0
Mothbeans, mature:
raw, 1 cup...120.6
boiled, 1 cup...37.1
Mousse pudding, see "Pudding and pie filling mix"
Muffin, 1 piece, except as noted:
apple (*Awrey's*), 2.5 oz.....................................30.0
apple (*Awrey's*), 1.5 oz.....................................18.0
banana nut:
   (*Awrey's*), 1.5 oz..22.0
   (*Awrey's Grande*), 4 oz...............................48.0
   (*Awrey's Petite*), .85 oz...............................22.0
banana walnut, mini (*Hostess*), 3 pieces, 1.2 oz.....16.0
blueberry:
   (*Awrey's*), 2.5 oz..30.0
   (*Awrey's*), 1.5 oz..19.0
   (*Awrey's Grande*), 4 oz...............................54.0
   (*Awrey's Petite*), .85 oz...............................23.0
   (*Entenmann's Light Fat Free*), 2 oz............27.0
   mini (*Hostess*), 3 pieces, 1.2 oz.................18.0
   mini, 1¼" diam., .4 oz....................................5.3
cheese streusel (*Awrey's*), 4 oz........................52.0
chocolate chip, mini (*Hostess*), 3 pieces, 1.2 oz.....17.0
chocolate chocolate chip (*Awrey's Grande*), 4 oz.....56.0
corn:
   (*Awrey's*), 4 oz...49.0
   (*Awrey's*), 1.25 oz......................................17.0
   (*Entenmann's*), 2 oz....................................30.0
   2 oz...29.0
cranberry-nut (*Awrey's*), 1.5 oz........................19.0
English:
   (*Awrey's*), 2 oz...28.0
   (*Thomas' Original*), 2 oz.............................25.0
   (*Thomas' Original Super Size*)....................38.0
   plain, 2 oz..26.2
   apple cinnamon, 2 oz....................................27.8

Muffin, English *(cont.)*
   blueberry *(Thomas')* 29.0
   cinnamon *(Thomas')* 31.0
   cinnamon raisin *(Thomas')* 30.0
   cranberry *(Thomas')* 30.0
   honey-wheat *(Thomas')* 27.0
   maple French toast *(Thomas')* 30.0
   mixed grain, 2.3 oz. 30.6
   raisin cinnamon, 2 oz. 27.8
   sourdough *(Thomas')* 25.0
   sourdough *(Thomas' Super Size)* 41.0
   sourdough, 2 oz. 26.2
   wheat, 2 oz. 25.5
   whole-wheat, 2.3 oz. 26.7
lemon poppyseed *(Awrey's)*, 4 oz. 45.0
lemon poppyseed *(Awrey's Petite)*, .85 oz. 21.0
oat bran, 2 oz. 27.5
raisin bran:
   (Awrey's), 4 oz. 45.0
   (Awrey's), 2.5 oz. 31.0
   (Awrey's), 1.5 oz. 18.0
Muffin, frozen, 1 piece:
blueberry *(Sara Lee)*, 2.25 oz. 27.0
corn *(Sara Lee)*, 2.25 oz. 30.0
Muffin, mix, 1 piece*, except as noted:
apple cinnamon:
   (Betty Crocker Pouch) 24.0
   ("Jiffy"), ¼ cup 28.0
   (Sweet Rewards Low Fat) 28.0
apple streusel *(Betty Crocker)* 33.0
banana *(Pillsbury Quick Bread & Muffin Mix)* 26.0
banana-nut:
   (Betty Crocker) 27.0
   (Betty Crocker Pouch) 22.0
   ("Jiffy"), ¼ cup 25.0
blueberry:
   (Betty Crocker Twice The Blueberry/Pouch) 25.0
   ("Jiffy"), ¼ cup 28.0
   wild *(Betty Crocker)* 28.0
   wild *(Sweet Rewards Low Fat)* 26.0
bran *(Hodgson Mill)*, ¼ cup, ⅙ pkg. 27.0

bran, with dates *("Jiffy")*, ¼ cup..................................26.0
chocolate, double *(Betty Crocker)*..........................30.0
chocolate chip *(Betty Crocker* Pouch)....................23.0
corn:
    (Hodgson Mill), ¼ cup 28.0
    ("Jiffy"), ¼ cup..28.0
    golden *(Betty Crocker* Pouch) 25.0
cranberry *(Pillsbury* Quick Bread & Muffin Mix) 30.0
cranberry-orange *(Betty Crocker)* 25.0
gingerbread, whole-wheat *(Hodgson Mill)*, ¼ cup, ⅙ pkg..........24.0
lemon poppyseed:
    (Betty Crocker) 29.0
    (Betty Crocker Pouch) 25.0
    (Pillsbury Quick Bread & Muffin Mix) 28.0
nut *(Pillsbury* Quick Bread & Muffin Mix) 24.0
oat bran *(Arrowhead Mills)*, ⅓ cup.........................33.0
raspberry *("Jiffy")*, ¼ cup......................................26.0
whole-grain *(Arrowhead Mills)*, ⅓ cup 26.0
whole-wheat *(Hodgson Mill)*, ¼ cup, ⅙ pkg............27.0
Muffin, toaster, see "Toaster pastry"
Muffin sandwich, see "Breakfast sandwich"
Mulberries, fresh, raw:
untrimmed, 1 lb. 44.5
10 berries, .5 oz. 1.5
1 cup 13.7
Mullet, without added ingredients 0
Mung beans, mature:
raw, 1 cup 129.6
raw, 1 tbsp. 8.1
boiled, 1 cup 38.7
Mung beans, sprouted:
fresh, raw:
    raw *(Jonathan's)*, 1 cup.................................4.0
    raw, 12-oz. pkg...20.2
    raw, 1 cup...6.2
    boiled, drained, 1 cup....................................5.2
    stir-fried, 1 cup...13.1
canned, drained, 1 cup 2.7
Mungo beans, mature:
raw, 1 cup 122.1

Mungo beans *(cont.)*
boiled, 1 cup 33.0
boiled, 2.4 oz. (yield from 1 oz. raw) 12.7
Mushrooms, fresh, raw, except as noted:
whole *(Dole)*, 5 medium, 3 oz. 3.0
whole, 1 cup 3.9
pieces or slices, 1 cup 2.9
boiled, drained, 1 tbsp. 5
boiled, drained, pieces, 1 cup 8.0
brown, Italian or crimini, .5-oz. piece 6
enoki *(Frieda's)*, ¼ pkg., .8 oz. 2.0
enoki, 1 large, .2 oz. 4
enoki, 1 medium, .1 oz. 2
oyster, 1 large, 5.2 oz. 9.2
oyster, 1 small, .5 oz. 9
portobello, 1 oz. 1.4
portobello, caps or slices *(Phillips)*, 2 oz. 2.0
shiitake, cooked, 4 mushrooms, 2.5 oz. 10.3
shiitake, cooked, 1 cup 20.7
Mushrooms, breaded, frozen *(Empire* Kosher),
    7 pieces, 2.9 oz. 16.0
Mushrooms, canned:
all styles *(Green Giant)*, ½ cup 4.0
all styles *(BinB)*, 3 oz. 4.0
drained, 4.6-oz. can 6.5
drained, 1 cup 7.7
straw, drained, .2 oz. 2.6
straw, drained, 1 cup 8.5
Mushrooms, dried:
chanterelle *(Frieda's)*, 2 pieces, .1 oz. 2.0
cloud ear, .2 oz. 3.3
cloud ear, 1 cup 20.4
morel or oyster *(Frieda's)*, 3 pieces, .1 oz. 2.0
oyster or porcini *(Epicurean Specialty)*, ⅓ oz. 2.0
padi straw *(Frieda's)*, 6 pieces, .1 oz. 2.0
porcini *(Frieda's)*, 5 pieces, .1 oz. 4.0
portobello *(Frieda's)*, 7 pieces, .1 oz. 1.0
shiitake:
    (Frieda's), ¼ cup, .1 oz. 3.0
    4 mushrooms, ½ oz. 11.3
    1 mushroom, .1 oz. 2.7

wood ear *(Frieda's)*, 3 pieces, .1 oz. 2.0
Mushrooms, frozen, shiitake *(Seneca)*, ½ cup 4.0
Mushroom batter mix *(Don's Chuck Wagon)*, ¼ cup 21.0
Mushroom pilaf, dried, with vegetables *(AlpineAire)*,
 1¼ cups 66.0
Mushroom gravy, ¼ cup, except as noted:
(Franco-American) 3.0
(Heinz Home Style Rich) 3.0
creamy *(Franco-American)*................................4.0
1 cup 13.0
Mushroom gravy mix *(Loma Linda Gravy Quik)*, 1 tbsp. 3.0
Mushroom pasta sauce, in jar *(Pasta Gusto)*, ⅓ cup 5.0
Mushroom sauce:
carciofi or porcini *(Italia In Tavola)*, 2 tbsp. 2.0
shiitake, regular or hot and spicy *(Annie Chun's)*, 1 tbsp. 3.0
Mushroom sauce mix, dry, except as noted:
1-oz. pkt. 15.5
8 fl. oz.* 12.4
Mussels, blue, meat only:
raw, 4 oz. 4.2
raw, 1 cup 5.5
boiled, poached, or steamed, 4 oz. 8.4
Mussels, canned, in red sauce, drained *(Reese)*, 4-oz-can 4.0
Mussels, smoked *(Ducktrap River* Maine), ¼ cup, 2 oz. 3.0
Mustard, prepared, 1 tsp., except as noted:
(Boar's Head Delicatessen Style)................................0
(French's Classic Yellow/Hearty Brown/Dijon)........................0
(Grey Poupon) ....<1.0
(Gulden's) 0
(Hebrew National Deli) 0
(Kraft Pure) 0
1 tbsp. 1.2
1 tsp. 4
country or spicy brown *(Grey Poupon)* ....<1.0
hot *(Eden* Organic) ....<1.0
Mustard blend, 1 tsp.:
honey:
 (Boar's Head) 2.0
 (French's) 1.0
 (Grey Poupon) 2.0
 (Hellmann's/Best Foods Dressing) 1.0

Mustard blend, honey *(cont.)*
    dressing, see "Salad dressing"
horseradish:
    (French's) 0
    (Grey Poupon Deli) 0
    (Kraft) 0
mayonnaise *(Dijonnaise)* 1.0
sweet onion *(French's)* 2.0
Mustard cabbage *(Frieda's* Gai Choy), 1 cup, 3 oz. 4.0
Mustard greens, fresh:
raw, untrimmed, 1 lb. 20.7
raw, chopped, 1 cup 2.7
boiled, drained, chopped, 1 cup 2.9
Mustard greens, canned, ½ cup:
(Allens/Sunshine) 5.0
(Stubb's Harvest) 5.0
Mustard greens, frozen:
chopped *(Birds Eye* Southern), 1 cup 2.0
unprepared, 10-oz. pkg. 9.7
unprepared, chopped, 1 cup 5.0
boiled, drained, 10-oz. pkg. 6.6
boiled, drained, chopped, ½ cup 2.3
Mustard powder *(Spice Island),* 1 tsp. 3
Mustard seeds, yellow:
(McCormick), ¼ tsp. 2
1 tbsp. 4.0
1 tsp. 1.2
Mustard spinach, see "Spinach, mustard"
Mustard tallow, 1 tbsp. 0

N

Nachos mix *(Taco Bell Home Originals)*, about 12 nachos*.......31.0
Name yam, see "Yam"
Natto:
1 oz. 4.1
1 cup 25.1
Navy beans:
dehydrated *(AlpineAire)*, ½ cup 17.0
dry, 1 cup..126.2
boiled, 1 cup 47.9
Navy beans, canned, ½ cup:
(Allens)...19.0
(Eden Organic) 20.0
with bacon *(Trappey's)*..16.0
with bacon and jalapeños *(Trappey's)*...17.0
Creole style *(Trappey's)*...19.0
Navy beans, sprouted, from mature seeds, raw, 1 cup 13.6
Navy grog drink mix *(Trader Vic's)*, 2 oz. 30.0
Nectarine, fresh, raw:
(Dole), 1 fruit 16.0
untrimmed, 1 lb. 48.6
2½" diam., 4.8 oz. 16.0
sliced, 1 cup 16.3
New Zealand spinach, see "Spinach, New Zealand"
Newburg sauce mix *(Knorr* Classic Sauces), 1 tbsp. 5.0
Noodles, Chinese (see also "Rice pasta"):
(Nasoya), 1 cup 43.0
cellophane or long rice, dry, 2 oz. 48.8
cellophane or long rice, dry, 1 cup...120
chow mein:
   (Annie Chun's Original), 2 oz. 39.0
   (Chun King), ½ cup, 1 oz. 18.0
   1 cup 25.9
   fresh *(Frieda's)*, 4 oz..40.0

Noodles, Chinese, chow mein *(cont.)*
   spinach *(Annie Chun's)*, 2 oz.....................................40.0
crispy *(Frieda's)*, ½ cup, 1 oz. 17.0
Noodles, egg:
dry, 2 oz., except as noted:
   (Creamette/Penn Dutch).......................................39.0
   (Kluski)..40.0
   (Mueller's Old Fashioned)......................................38.0
   four-color *(Hodgson Mill)*.......................................37.0
   spinach *(Nasoya)*, 1 cup.......................................42.0
   whole-wheat *(Pastamania!)*...................................34.0
   whole-wheat, spinach *(Pastamania!)*....................32.0
   yolk-free *(Borden)* 41.0
cooked, 1 cup 39.7
cooked, spinach, 1 cup 38.8
Noodles, Japanese:
(Nasoya), 1 cup...43.0
soba, dry:
   (Annie Chun's), 2 oz...39.0
   (Eden Organic Traditional), ½ cup, ¼ pkg..............38.0
   (Eden Traditional), 2 oz...37.0
   buckwheat *(Eden* 100%), 2 oz...............................41.0
   mugwort or lotus root *(Eden)*, 2 oz........................37.0
   wild yam *(Eden* Jinenjo), 2 oz................................37.0
soba, cooked, 1 cup...24.4
somen, dry, 2 oz. 42.0
somen, dry *(Eden* Organic Traditional), ½ cup, ¼ pkg. 38.0
somen, cooked, 1 cup...48.5
udon, dry:
   (Eden), 2 oz...37.0
   (Eden Organic Traditional), ½ cup, ¼ pkg..............38.0
   brown rice, dry *(Eden)*, 2 oz..................................38.0
Noodles, rice:
dry, 2 oz.:
   (Annie Chun's Hunan/Pad Thai/Original) 50.0
   (A Taste of Thai)..46.0
   basil, Thai *(Annie Chun's/Annie Chun's* Pad Thai) 50.0
   mushroom and roasted garlic *(Annie Chun's)*, ...50.0
cooked, 1 cup 43.8
Noodle dish, mix, ⅔ cup dry, except as noted:
Alfredo *(Lipton* Noodles & Sauce) 39.0

Alfredo broccoli *(Lipton* Noodles & Sauce)................................40.0
beef flavor *(Lipton* Noodles & Sauce) 45.0
butter *(Lipton* Noodles & Sauce) 41.0
butter and herb *(Lipton* Noodles & Sauce) 42.0
cheddar cheese *(Kraft Noodle Classics),* about 1 cup*..............47.0
chicken:
    creamy *(Lipton* Noodles & Sauce) 39.0
    broccoli *(Lipton* Noodles & Sauce) 41.0
    flavor *(Lipton* Noodles & Sauce) 42.0
    savory *(Kraft Noodle Classics),* about 1 cup* 46.0
Parmesan *(Lipton* Noodles & Sauce)................................37.0
sour cream and chives *(Lipton* Noodles & Sauce).....................41.0
Stroganoff *(Lipton* Noodles & Sauce) 37.0
Noodle entree, canned or packaged, 1 cup:
and beef, Stroganoff *(Dinty Moore* Microwave) 16.0
and chicken *(Hormel* Microcup Meals) 20.0
rings, and chicken *(Kid's Kitchen)*.....................................17.0
Noodle entree, frozen, 1 pkg., except as noted:
Alfredo:
    (Michelina's), 8 oz. 40.0
    egg *(Michelina's),* 8 oz. 40.0
    with pepperoni *(Michelina's),* 8 oz...........................40.0
    and vegetable *(Michelina's),* 8 oz. 41.0
Asian, stir-fry *(Amy's),* 10 oz. 41.0
with beef *(Freezer Queen* Family Entree), 1 cup...............33.0
with beef and brown gravy *(Banquet* Family Size), 1 cup 16.0
and cheese, with pepperoni *(Michelina's),* 8 oz. 40.0
and chicken:
    (Michelina's), 8 oz. 38.0
    escalloped *(Marie Callender's* Family), 1 cup 22.0
    escalloped *(Marie Callender's* Meals), 13 oz. 60.0
    home style *(Banquet),* 12 oz. 44.0
    and peas and carrots *(Michelina's),* 8 oz.......................38.0
marinara *(Michelina's),* 8 oz...39.0
and red and green tomatoes *(Michelina's),* 8 oz. 38.0
Romanoff *(Stouffer's),* 12 oz.......................................53.0
Romanoff, with meatballs *(Michelina's),* 10 oz. 46.0
Stroganoff *(Michelina's),* 8 oz. 39.0
and vegetables, with beef *(Michelina's),* 8 oz............................37.0
Nopale:
raw *(Frieda's* Cactus Pads), ¾ cup, 3 oz.............................4.0

Nopale *(cont.)*
raw, sliced, 1 cup...2.9
cooked, 1 pad 9
cooked, 1 cup 4.9
Nori, see "Seaweed"
Nut filling, see "Pastry filling"
Nut topping, see specific nut listings
Nutmeg, ground:
1 tbsp...3.4
1 tsp...1.1
Nuts, see specific listings
Nuts, mixed:
(Nabisco/Nabisco Deluxe/Lightly Salted), 1 oz.............................6.0
(Planters Deluxe/Lightly Salted), 1 oz. 6.0
(River Queen No Peanuts), 3 tbsp., 1 oz.......................................6.0
(River Queen Salt or Unsalted), 3 tbsp., 1 oz................................5.0
cinnamon *(Sweet Roasts),* 1 oz. 9.0
dry-roasted *(River Queen),* 1 oz...7.0
dry-roasted, with peanuts, salted or unsalted, 1 cup.................34.7
honey-roasted *(Planters),* 1 oz...9.0
oil-roasted:
    with peanuts, salted or unsalted, 1 cup.................................30.4
    with peanuts, salted or unsalted, 1 tbsp................................1.9
    without peanuts, salted or unsalted, 1 cup............................32.1
sesame *(Planters),* 1 oz. 9.0
vanilla *(Sweet Roasts),* 1 oz... 10.0

O

FOOD AND MEASURE   **CARBOHYDRATE GRAMS**

Oat (see also "Cereal"):
whole-grain, 1 cup 103.4
steel-cut *(Arrowhead Mills)*, ¼ cup................................29.0
Oat beverage, plain or vanilla *(Westbrae Natural Oat Plus)*,
    8 fl. oz. 26.0
Oat bran (see also "Cereal":
(Arrowhead Mills), ⅓ cup 23.0
raw, 1 cup 62.2
cooked, 1 cup 25.1
Oat bran flour:
(Hodgson Mill), ¼ cup 23.0
(Hodgson Mill Organic), ¼ cup.......................................24.0
blend *(Hodgson Mill)*, scant ¼ cup.................................24.0
Oat flakes, rolled *(Arrowhead Mills)*, ⅓ cup 23.0
Oat flour *(Arrowhead Mills)*, ⅓ cup...............................20.0
Oat groats *(Arrowhead Mills)*, ¼ cup.............................29.0
Oatmeal, see "Oat" and "Cereal"
Oaxacan chili, see "Pepper, chili"
Oca *(Frieda's)*, ½ cup, 3 oz...15.0
Ocean perch, fresh, without added ingredients.................0
Ocean perch entree, frozen, battered *(Van de Kamp's)*,
    2 fillets...18.0
Octopus, meat only:
raw, 4 oz. 2.5
boiled, poached, or steamed, 4 oz. 5.0
Oheloberries, fresh, raw:
10 berries, .4 oz. 8
1 cup 9.6
Oil, all varieties..0
Okra, fresh:
raw, 8 pods, 3" long, 3.4 oz. 7.2
raw, 1 cup 7.2
boiled, drained, 8 pods, 3" long 6.1
boiled, drained, sliced, ½ cup...5.8

Okra, canned, ½ cup:
cut *(Allens/Trappey's)*..6.0
Creole gumbo *(Trappey's)*..6.0
and tomatoes *(Allens/Trappey's)*...5.0
and tomatoes and corn *(Allens/Trappey's)*............................6.0
Okra, frozen:
whole:
    (Birds Eye/Freshlike), 9 pods...5.0
    unprepared, 10-oz. pkg. 18.9
    boiled, drained, 10-oz. pkg..14.7
    boiled, drained, sliced, ½ cup 5.3
cut *(Birds Eye/Freshlike),* ¾ cup 5.0
and tomatoes *(Birds Eye* Deluxe), ¾ cup...............................4.0
Okra, pickled, in jars:
(Talk o' Texas), 2 pieces, .8 oz. 2.0
cocktail, hot *(Trappey's),* 1.1 oz. 2.0
Olives, pickled:
Atalanti *(Peloponnese),* 3 pieces...2.0
black, see "ripe," below
green, cracked *(Krinos),* 2 pieces 2.0
green, Italian *(Rienzi),* 2 pieces, .6 oz. 2.0
green, with pits:
    10 giant 9
    10 large 5
    10 small 4
    Spanish *(Early California),* 2 pieces, .5 oz. 1.0
green, pitted, 1 oz. 4
green, pitted, Spanish *(Early California),* 5 pieces, .5 oz..............1.0
Ionian *(Peloponnese),* 3 pieces...2.0
kalamata *(Krinos),* 3 pieces...2.0
kalamata *(Peloponnese),* 5 pieces..1.0
mixed *(Peloponnese),* 4 pieces 1.0
Nafplion *(Peloponnese),* 4 pieces...2.0
ripe, pitted:
    (Black Pearls), 2 colossal, 3 jumbo, 4 large, 5 medium,
      or 6 small, .5 oz. 1.0
    (Early California), 1 super colossal, 2 colossal, 3 jumbo,
      4 large, 5 medium, or 6 small, .5 oz............................1.0
    (Lindsay), 3 extra large, 4 large, 5 medium, or 6 small 1.0
    (Orbetti), 2 colossal, 3 extra large, or 5 medium 1.0
    1 super colossal 1.0

1 jumbo... .5
1 large 3
chopped *(Black Pearls)*, 1⅓ tbsp. 1.0
chopped, regular or jalapeño flavor *(Early California)*,
   1⅓ tbsp. 1.0
sliced *(Black Pearls)*, 2 tbsp. 1.0
sliced, regular or jalapeño flavor *(Early California)*, 2 tbsp......1.0
ripe, Greek:
   (Krinos), 2 pieces 2.0
   10 extra large 2.3
   10 medium 1.7
   pitted, 1 oz. 2.5
salad, Spanish *(Early California)*, 2 tbsp. 1.0
stuffed:
   with anchovy *(Reese)*, 4 pieces, .5 oz. ....<1.0
   queen *(Goya)*, 1 olive 1.0
   queen, with garlic or capers *(Early California)*, 2 pieces,
     .5 oz...1.0
   Spanish *(Early California)*, 4 pieces, .5 oz. 1.0
   Spanish queen *(Early California)*, 2 pieces, .6 oz. 1.0
Olive salad, drained *(Progresso)*, 2 tbsp. 1.0
Olive sauce, green *(Italia In Tavola)*, 2 tbsp.....................0
Olive spread, in jars *(Peloponnese* Kalamata), 1 tsp. 0
Olives and jalapeños *(D.L. Jardine's* Texas Caviar), ½ oz. 0
Onion, fresh:
raw:
   (Frieda's Boiler/Cipolline), 3 onions, 3 oz. 7.0
   (Frieda's Maui), ⅓ cup, 1.1 oz.............................3.0
   (Frieda's Pearl), ⅔ cup, 3 oz. 7.0
   untrimmed, 1 lb...35.2
   chopped *(Dole* Vidalia), ½ cup 7.0
   chopped, 1 cup..13.8
   sliced, 1 cup...9.9
boiled, drained, chopped, 1 cup................................21.3
boiled, drained, chopped, 1 tbsp..............................1.5
Onion, canned or in jar:
whole *(Hanover* O&C), ½ cup....................................6.0
whole, small *(S&W)*, ½ cup.......................................8.0
2.2-oz. onion...2.6
chopped or diced, ½ cup..4.5

Onion, canned or in jar *(cont.)*

boiled, white *(Twin Tree Gardens)*, 1 oz. 1.0
french-fried *(French's)*, 2 tbsp. 3.0
in sauce *(Boar's Head Sweet Vidalia)*, 1 tbsp. 2.0

Onion, dried:

dehydrated, chopped *(AlpineAire)*, ½ cup.......................17.0
flakes, ¼ cup...11.7
flakes, 1 tbsp...4.2
minced, with green onion *(Lawry's)*, ¼ tsp...........................0

Onion, frozen (see also "Onion rings"):

whole:

    unprepared, 10-oz. pkg. 22.7
    boiled, drained, 1 cup...14.1
    small *(Birds Eye)*, 7 pieces...7.0

chopped:

    (Ore-Ida), ¾ cup..6.0
    unprepared, chopped, 10-oz. pkg. 19.3
    boiled, drained, ½ cup 6.9
    boiled, drained, 1 tbsp. 1.0

diced *(Birds Eye Southern)*, ⅔ cup.......................................6.0
pearl, in cream sauce *(Birds Eye)*, ½ cup 8.0

Onion, green (scallion), fresh, raw:

untrimmed, 1 lb. 32.0

chopped:

    (Andy Boy), ¼ cup 2.0
    (Dole), ¼ cup 2.0
    1 cup 7.3
    1 tbsp. 4

Onion, Welsh, fresh, 1 oz. 1.8

Onion dip, 2 tbsp.:

creamy green *(Kraft Premium Sour Cream)* 2.0

French:

    (Breakstone's Free)...4.0
    (Dean's Dips for One)..2.0
    (Dean's Dips for One Lite) 4.0
    (Frito-Lay) 4.0
    (Knudsen Free) 4.0
    (Kraft Premium Sour Cream) 2.0
    (Kraft Free) 4.0

French or green *(Kraft)* 4.0
French or toasted *(Breakstone's)* 2.0
Onion dip mix, chive *(Knorr)*, ½ tsp. ....<1.0
Onion gravy, zesty *(Heinz)*, ¼ cup................................3.0
Onion gravy mix *(Loma Linda Gravy Quik)*, 1 tbsp. 3.0
Onion powder:
1 tbsp. 5.2
1 tsp. 1.7
Onion relish, Vidalia, in jars:
sweet *(Best of the South)*, 1 tbsp. 4.0
zesty *(Braswell's)*, 1 tbsp. 7.0
Onion ring batter mix, ¼ cup:
(Don's Chuck Wagon) 21.0
(Hodgson Mills Vidalia Sweet Onion)...............................21.0
Onion rings, frozen, breaded:
(Mrs. Paul's), 4 rings 22.0
(Ore-Ida Onion Ringers), 6 pieces, 3.2 oz.......................25.0
(Ore-Ida Vidalia O's), 5 pieces, 3.2 oz............................20.0
partially fried:
    unprepared, 16-oz. pkg. 138.6
    unprepared, 9-oz. pkg. 77.9
    oven-heated, 10 large rings, 3"–4" diam................27.1
    oven-heated, 1 cup 18.3
Onion sprouts *(Jonathan's)*, 1 cup................................5.0
Opo squash *(Frieda's)*, ⅔ cup, 3 oz.............................3.0
Opossum, without added ingredients 0
Orange, fresh, raw:
(Dole), 1 fruit 13.0
all common varieties:
    3¹⁄₁₆" diam. 21.6
    sections, 1 cup 21.2
blood *(Frieda's)*, 5 oz. 16.0
California:
    navel, 2⅞" diam. 16.3
    navel, sections without membrane, 1 cup..................19.2
    Valencia, 2⅝" diam. 14.4
    Valencia, sections without membrane, 1 cup 21.4
Florida, 2⅝" diam. 16.3
Florida, sections without membrane, 1 cup 21.3
Seville *(Frieda's)*, 3 oz. 10.0

Orange, mandarin, see "Tangerine"
Orange drink, 8 fl. oz.:
(Snapple Orangeade) 29.0
(Snapple Tropic)...30.0
(Turkey Hill)...30.0
frozen*, with pulp 28.3
mix* *(Tang)* 23.0
Orange drink blend, 8 fl. oz., except as noted:
(WhipperSnapple Orange Dream), 10 fl. oz. 36.0
apricot, canned 31.8
carrot *(Snapple* Diet) 3.0
cranberry *(Tropicana Twister),* 10 fl. oz. 40.0
mango *(R.W. Knudsen)*...30.0
pineapple *(Kool-Aid Bursts Oh Yeah Orange-Pineapple),*
    1 bottle 24.0
pineapple apple *(Welch's)* 35.0
punch *(Hawaiian Punch Orange Ocean)*......................29.0
strawberry banana:
    (Chiquita)...30.0
    (Crystal Light) 0
    (Tropicana Twister), 10 fl. oz. 40.0
    (Tropicana Twister Light), 10 fl. oz. 11.0
tangerine *(Snapple Hydro)* 24.0
mix*:
    pineapple *(Kool-Aid Oh Yeah Orange-Pineapple)* 25.0
    pineapple *(Kool-Aid Oh Yeah Orange-Pineapple* Sugar
        Sweetened)..16.0
    pineapple *(Tang)*...24.0
Orange drink mix:
(Kool-Aid), 8 fl. oz.* 25.0
(Kool-Aid Sugar Sweetened), 8 fl. oz.* 16.0
3 heaping tsp. powder or .8-oz. pkt. 22.0
8 fl. oz.* 29.3
Orange juice, 8 fl. oz., except as noted:
fresh...25.6
canned, dairy pack, or bottled:
    (Juicy Juice Punch)...29.0
    (Juicy Juice Punch), 8.45-fl.-oz. box.................31.0
    (Juicy Juice Punch), 4.23-fl.-oz. box.................15.0
    (Mott's), 10-fl.-oz. bottle 29.0

    (Mott's 16 oz.)..21.0
    (R.W. Knudsen)...23.0
    (Season's Best Regular/Homestyle/Calcium)...........27.0
    (Snapple Grove), 12 fl. oz.........................44.0
    (Tropicana Pure Premium)...........................26.0
frozen*, unsweetened...26.8
Orange juice blend, 8 fl. oz.:
kiwi–passion fruit *(Tropicana Pure Tropics)*.............26.0
peach-mango *(Dole)*...28.0
peach-mango *(Tropicana Pure Tropics)*...................28.0
pineapple or strawberry banana *(Tropicana Pure Tropics)*..........27.0
strawberry-banana *(Dole)*...................................28.0
tropical *(Tropicana Pure Premium)*......................25.0
Orange peel, fresh, raw:
1 tbsp..1.5
1 tsp... .5
Orange roughy, see "Roughy"
Orangeade, see "Orange drink"
Oregano, dried:
ground, 1 tbsp. 3.0
ground, 1 tsp. 1.0
Oriental sauce, see "Stir-fry sauce" and specific listings
Orzo pasta dish mix, mint garlic *(Casbah)*, ¾ cup.................40.0
Oysters, meat only:
Eastern:
    wild, raw, 6 medium, 3 oz. 3.3
    wild, raw, 1 cup..9.7
    wild, baked, broiled, or microwaved, 6 medium, 2.1 oz.........2.8
    wild, boiled, poached or steamed, 6 medium, 1.5 oz..............3.3
    wild, breaded, fried, 6 medium, 3.1 oz. 10.2
    farmed, raw, 6 medium, 3 oz. 4.6
    farmed, baked, broiled, or microwaved, 6 medium,
        2.1 oz...4.3
Pacific, raw, 1 medium, 1¾ oz. 2.5
Pacific, boiled, poached or steamed, 1 medium, .9 oz.............2.5
Oysters, canned:
(Bumble Bee Fancy), 2 oz. 3.0
Eastern, undrained, 1 cup.....................................9.7
Eastern, drained, 1 cup.......................................6.2

Oysters, smoked, canned, 2 oz.:
(Bumble Bee) 6.0
(Reese) 6.0
Oyster plant, see "Salsify"
Oyster sauce, 1 tbsp. 4
Oyster stew, see "Soup, canned, condensed"

FOOD AND MEASURE	CARBOHYDRATE GRAMS

Pad Thai sauce *(A Taste of Thai)*, 2 tbsp. 20.0
Palm, hearts of, canned:
1 piece, 1.2 oz...1.5
1 cup 6.7
Pancake, frozen, 3 cakes, except as noted:
(Aunt Jemima Homestyle)...40.0
(Aunt Jemima Low Fat)...33.0
(Hungry Jack Original) 51.0
blueberry or buttermilk *(Aunt Jemima)*.............................40.0
buttermilk *(Kellogg's Eggo)*...44.0
mini *(Aunt Jemima)*, 13 cakes 46.0
regular or buttermilk, 4"-diam. cake, 1.3 oz. 15.7
Pancake, refrigerated, ready-to-eat:
blueberry *(Mama Mary's)*, 2.75-oz. cake........................30.0
buttermilk *(Mama Mary's)*, 2.75-oz. cake 29.0
Pancake batter, frozen, ½ cup:
(Aunt Jemima Homestyle)...50.0
blueberry *(Aunt Jemima)* 54.0
buttermilk *(Aunt Jemima)* 51.0
Pancake mix, dry, except as noted:
(Aunt Jemima Complete Regular), ⅓ cup.........................32.0
(Aunt Jemima Original), ⅓ cup..34.0
(Betty Crocker Original Complete Box), ⅓ cup mix, 3 cakes* 39.0
(Betty Crocker Original Pouch), 3 cakes*..........................39.0
(Bisquick Shake 'n Pour Original), ½ cup mix, 3 cakes* 39.0
(Estee), 6 tbsp..40.0
(Hungry Jack Extra Light & Fluffy), ⅓ cup mix, 3 cakes*, 4" 33.0
(Hungry Jack Extra Light & Fluffy Complete), ⅓ cup mix,
    3 cakes*, 4"..30.0
(Hungry Jack Original), ⅓ cup mix, 3 cakes*, 4"...............32.0
4" cake* 11.0
complete, 4" cake* 13.9
all purpose *(Don's Chuck Wagon* Batter Mix), ¼ cup 20.0
blueberry *(AlpineAire)*, 6 cakes*, 4".................................63.0

blueberry *(Bisquick Shake 'n Pour)*, ½ cup mix, 3 cakes* 41.0
buckwheat:
    (Arrowhead Mills), ⅓ cup 25.0
    (Aunt Jemima), ¼ cup...23.0
    (Don's Chuck Wagon), ⅓ cup 33.0
    (Hodgson Mill), ⅓ cup 36.0
    ("Jiffy" Complete), ⅓ cup 32.0
buttermilk:
    (Arrowhead Mills), ⅓ cup 25.0
    (Aunt Jemima Complete), ⅓ cup 31.0
    (Aunt Jemima Complete Reduced Calorie), ⅓ cup...............28.0
    (Betty Crocker Complete Box), ⅓ cup mix, 3 cakes* 39.0
    (Betty Crocker Complete Pouch), ½ cup mix, 3 cakes* 37.0
    (Bisquick Shake 'n Pour), ½ cup mix, 3 cakes*....................38.0
    4" cake* 11.0
    complete, 4" cake* 13.9
corn, blue *(Arrowhead Mills)*, ⅓ cup 28.0
gluten-free *(Arrowhead Mills)*, ¼ cup 24.0
kamut *(Arrowhead Mills)*, ¼ cup 26.0
multigrain *(Arrowhead Mills)*, ¼ cup 24.0
multigrain, 5 grains *(AlpineAire)*, 2 cakes*, 4"............................18.0
oat bran *(Arrowhead Mills)*, ⅓ cup 25.0
whole-grain *(Arrowhead Mills)*, ¼ cup...24.0
whole-wheat:
    (Aunt Jemima), ¼ cup...26.0
    (Hodgson Mill), ⅓ cup 28.0
    4" cake* 12.9
wild rice *(Arrowhead Mills)*, ⅓ cup..30.0
Pancake syrup (see also "Maple syrup" and specific syrup
    listings), ¼ cup, except as noted:
(Aunt Jemima Butter Rich) 52.0
(Aunt Jemima Butterlite/Country Rich Lite) 26.0
(Aunt Jemima Country Rich/Pancake & Waffle) 53.0
(Golden Griddle)...60.0
(Karo)...63.0
(Log Cabin Lite) 25.0
(Log Cabin Original) 53.0
(Mrs. Butterworth's Original) 54.0
(Vermont Maid)..53.0
(Vermont Maid Lite)...26.0
cinnamon apple *(Mrs. Butterworth's)* 50.0

cinnamon flavor *(Golden Griddle)*, 4 tbsp. 60.0
maple-flavored *(Estee)* 20.0
maple-flavored *(Featherweight Lite)* 20.0
strawberry *(Mrs. Butterworth's)* 55.0
Pancreas, without added ingredients 0
Papa John's Pizza:
original crust, 1 slice, ⅛ of 14" pie:
    All the Meats, cheese, pepperoni, or sausage 37.0
    Garden Special 39.0
    The Works 38.0
thin crust, 1 slice, ⅛ of 14" pie:
    All the Meats, cheese, pepperoni, or sausage 22.0
    Garden Special 24.0
    The Works 23.0
side items:
    bread sticks, 1 stick 26.0
    cheese sticks, 2 sticks 20.0
    garlic sauce or nacho cheese sauce, 1 tbsp. 0
    pizza sauce 1.0
Papaya, fresh, pulp:
(Dole), ½ cup 7.0
(Frieda's), 1 cup, 5 oz. 14.0
2 cup 13.6
mashed, 1 cup 22.6
Papaya, dried:
(Frieda's), ⅓ cup, 1.4 oz. 29.0
(Sonoma), 8 pieces, 1.4 oz. 26.0
Papaya drink blend *(Rocket Juice Papaya Ginseng)*,
    16 fl. oz. 66.0
Papaya juice, creamed, concentrate* *(R.W. Knudsen)*,
    8 fl. oz. 10.0
Papaya nectar, 8 fl. oz., except as noted:
(After the Fall Pele's Papaya Nectar) 25.0
(Libby's), 11.5-fl.-oz. can 51.0
(R.W. Knudsen) 34.0
(Santa Cruz Organic) 28.0
canned 36.3
Paprika:
1 tbsp. 3.8
1 tsp. 1.2

Parsley, fresh:

raw, 1 cup 3.8

raw, 1 tbsp. 2

Parsley, dried:

1 tbsp. 7

1 tsp. 2

freeze-dried, ¼ cup 6

freeze-dried, 1 tbsp. 2

Parsley root, raw:

(Frieda's), ⅔ cup, 3 oz. 2.0

untrimmed, 1 lb. 10.4

1 oz. 7

Parsnip, fresh:

raw, sliced, ½ cup 12.1

boiled, drained, 9"-long parsnip 31.3

boiled, drained, sliced, ½ cup 15.2

Passion fruit, fresh, raw:

(Frieda's), 5 oz. 33.0

purple, 1 cup 55.2

purple, trimmed, 1 fruit, .6 oz. 4.2

Passion fruit, frozen, chunks *(Goya),* ⅓ pkg. 13.0

Passion fruit drink blend:

orange *(Fruit Works),* 12 fl. oz. 43.0

mix*, pineapple *(Crystal Light),* 8 fl. oz. ....<1.0

Passion fruit juice, fresh, 8 fl. oz.:

purple...33.6

yellow...35.7

Passion fruit juice blend *(After the Fall Passion*

of the Islands), 8 fl. oz. 26.0

Passion fruit syrup *(Trader Vic's),* 2 tbsp. 21.0

Pasta, dry, uncooked (see also "Macaroni," and "Noodles"),

2 oz., except as noted:

all varieties:

(Creamette/Prince) 42.0

(Mueller's Classic/Italian Style)..42.0

(Mueller's Hearty) 38.0

alphabets, vegetable *(Eden* Organic) 40.0

bows, vegetable *(Westbrae Natural),* ½ cup 40.0

corn..44.9

dumplings *(Mueller's)* 42.0

elbows, plain or hot pepper *(Eden* Organic), ½ cup 41.0

extra fine *(Eden* Organic) 40.0
finbows, parsley garlic *(Eden* Organic) 41.0
fettuccine:
    durum wheat, durum wheat and spinach, pesto,
        or garlic and parsley *(Pastamania!)* 38.0
    with Jerusalem artichoke or mushroom *(Pastamania!)* 41.0
    lemon and pepper *(Pastamania!)* 40.0
    spinach *(Pastamania!)* 37.0
fusilli, tri-color with tomato and spinach *(Pastamania!)* 40.0
kamut *(Eden* Organic) 33.0
kamut quinoa *(Eden* Organic Twisted Pair), ½ cup....................40.0
kuzu, and sweet potato or kiri *(Eden)* 47.0
lasagna *(Westbrae Natural),* 20" piece, 1.8 oz.............................36.0
lasagna, spinach *(Westbrae Natural),* 20" piece, 1.8 oz. 35.0
linguine, thin *(Pastamania!)* 38.0
linguine or cavatappi, pesto *(Mueller's Savory Collection)*..........41.0
mung bean *(Eden)* 47.0
oat bran *(Pastamania!)* 41.0
penne or spaghetti, lemon pepper *(Mueller's Savory*
    Collection) 42.0
pennette, sun-dried tomato, and basil *(Mueller's Savory*
    Collection) 41.0
ribbons:
    all varieties, except spinach and thick kluski
        (Eden Organic)...40.0
    spinach or thick kluski *(Eden* Organic)...............................41.0
    whole-wheat *(Westbrae Natural),* 1 cup 38.0
    yolkless *(Pastamania!)* 34.0
rice *(Eden* Bifun) 44.0
rice, penne, rotini, or spaghetti *(Lundberg)* 44.0
rotelle, roasted garlic and herb *(Mueller's Savory Collection)*.....41.0
rotelle or seashell mix *(Pastamania!)*..40.0
shapes *(Pastamania!* Pot Pourri) 40.0
shells, vegetable (Eden Organic)..40.0
spaghetti:
    (Eden Organic) 40.0
    corn *(Westbrae Natural)* 46.0
    parsley garlic *(Eden* Organic) 41.0
    plain...42.3
    protein-fortified 38.3
    spinach..42.4

spinach *(Pastamania!)*..35.0
spinach *(Westbrae Natural)*..38.0
whole-grain *(Eden* Organic), ½ cup, 1/7 pkg. 40.0
whole-wheat 42.5
spirals:
    (Westbrae Natural), 1 cup 43.0
    sesame rice *(Eden* organic)...37.0
    sesame rice *(Westbrae Natural)*, 1 cup 38.0
    spinach *(Eden* Organic) 41.0
    vegetable *(Eden* Organic) 40.0
taglierini, tomato spinach and durum wheat *(Pastamania!)*........40.0
tubes, endless *(Eden* Organic) 41.0
twists, pesto *(Eden* Organic) 40.0
veggie, four-color, all varieties *(Hodgson Mill)* 41.0
whole-wheat, all varieties, except spinach spaghetti
    (Pastamania!)..34.0
Pasta, dry, cooked, 1 cup:
corn..39.1
spaghetti:
    plain...39.7
    protein-fortified 44.3
    spinach 36.6
    whole-wheat 37.2
spinach...36.6
whole-wheat..37.2
Pasta, refrigerated (see also specific pasta listings), plain:
uncooked, 2 oz. 31.0
uncooked, spinach, 2 oz. 31.6
cooked, 4 oz...28.3
cooked, spinach, 4 oz. 28.4
Pasta dinner, see specific listings
Pasta dish, frozen (see also "Pasta entree, frozen," and specific
    pasta listings):
cheddar *(Freshlike Pasta Combo's* Classic), 2 cups....................24.0
cheddar, white *(Birds Eye Pasta Secrets)*, 2 cups.......................30.0
cheese, three *(Birds Eye Pasta Secrets)*, 2 cups.........................31.0
garlic, zesty *(Birds Eye Pasta Secrets)*, 2 cups 31.0
garlic herb *(Freshlike Pasta Combo's)*, 2 cups............................33.0
herb, Italian *(Freshlike Pasta Combo's)*, 2⅓ cups.......................32.0
pepper, roasted *(Freshlike Pasta Combo's)*, 1 cup 32.0

peppercorn *(Freshlike Pasta Combo's)*, 2¼ cups.........................33.0
pesto, Italian *(Birds Eye Pasta Secrets)*, 2⅓ cups 32.0
primavera *(Birds Eye Pasta Secrets)*, 2⅓ cups............................26.0
primavera, creamy *(Freshlike Pasta Combo's)*, 2¼ cups 27.0
ranch *(Birds Eye Pasta Secrets)*, 2⅓ cups...................................29.0
Pasta dish, mix (see also specific pasta listings):
Alfredo *(Bowl Appétit!)*, 1 bowl...51.0
Alfredo, garlic *(Pasta Roni)*, about 1 cup* 50.0
broccoli or broccoli au gratin *(Pasta Roni)*, about 1 cup* 41.0
butter and herb *(Lipton* Pasta & Sauce), ¾ cup, 1 cup* 40.0
cheddar:
    broccoli *(Lipton* Pasta & Sauce), ⅔ cup...............................46.0
    mild *(Lipton* Pasta & Sauce), ¾ cup 38.0
    mild *(Pasta Roni)*, about 1 cup* 41.0
    zesty *(Lipton* Pasta & Sauce), ¾ cup 42.0
cheese, nacho *Knorr Forkfulls)*, 1 bowl......................................60.0
cheese, triple or zesty *(Knorr Forkfulls)*, 1 bowl 59.0
chicken:
    (Pasta Roni), about 1 cup* 41.0
    (Pasta Roni Homestyle), about 1 cup*..................................39.0
    creamy *(Knorr Forkfulls)*, 1 bowl...54.0
    and garlic *(Pasta Roni* Low Fat), about 1 cup* 39.0
    herb Parmesan *(Lipton* Pasta & Sauce), ½ cup, 1 cup* 43.0
    quesadilla *(Knorr Forkfulls)*, 1 bowl 58.0
    stir-fry *(Lipton* Pasta & Sauce), ½ cup, 1 cup* 43.0
garlic:
    creamy *(Fantastic Foods Ready, Set Pasta!* Cup),
      2.2 oz..42.0
    creamy *(Lipton* Pasta & Sauce), ⅔ cup 47.0
    roasted, chicken flavor *(Lipton* Pasta & Sauce), ¾ cup 40.0
    roasted, and oil, with tomatoes *(Lipton* Pasta & Sauce),
      ¾ cup, 1 cup* 42.0
herb and butter *(Pasta Roni)*, about 1 cup*................................42.0
herb with garlic, savory *(Lipton* Pasta & Sauce), ½ cup,
    1 cup* 52.0
mushroom, creamy *(Lipton* Pasta & Sauce), ¾ cup...................43.0
Parmesan, smoke *(Fantastic Foods Ready, Set Pasta!* Cup),
    2.1 oz. 42.0
Parmesano *(Pasta Roni)*, about 1 cup* 49.0
pizza flavor *(Knorr Forkfulls)*, 1 bowl 60.0
Romanoff *(Pasta Roni)*, about 1 cup* 48.0

Pasta dish, mix *(cont.)*
salad:
    Caesar *(Suddenly Salad)*, ¾ cup* 31.0
    Caesar, creamy *(Kraft)*, about ¾ cup* 31.0
    classic *(Suddenly Salad)*, ¾ cup* 38.0
    garden primavera *(Kraft)*, about ¾ cup* 35.0
    herb and garlic *(Kraft)*, about ¾ cup* 34.0
    Italian *(Kraft 97% Fat Free)*, about ¾ cup* 35.0
    Italian, garden *(Suddenly Salad)*, ½ cup mix 28.0
    Parmesan, creamy *(Suddenly Salad)*, ¾ cup* 30.0
    Parmesan-peppercorn *(Kraft)*, about ¾ cup* 29.0
    ranch, with bacon *(Kraft)*, about ¾ cup* 32.0
    ranch and bacon *(Suddenly Salad)*, ¾ cup* 31.0
    roasted garlic Parmesan *(Suddenly Salad)*, ¾ cup* ...33.0
Stroganoff *(Pasta Roni)*, about 1 cup* 49.0
Thai, spicy *(Fantastic Foods Ready, Set Pasta! Cup)*, 1.9 oz. 40.0
tomato, spicy *(Near East)*, 1 cont. 48.0
Pasta entree, canned (see also specific pasta listings), 1 cup:
with meatballs, in tomato sauce *(Franco-American Garfield)*......31.0
twists, with meat sauce, hearty *(Franco-American Superiore)*....41.0
Pasta entree, dried *(AlpineAire Pasta Roma)*, 1 cup 53.0
Pasta entree, frozen (see also "Pasta dish, frozen," and
    specific pasta listings), 1 pkg., except as noted:
Alfredo, and vegetable *(Amy's)*, 1 cup 27.0
Alfredo primavera *(Lean Cuisine Everyday Favorites)*, 10 oz. 46.0
cheddar *(Stouffer's)*, 11 oz. 44.0
cheese, three, with broccoli *(Cedarlane)*, 9 oz. 43.0
pizza *(Michelina's)*, 8.5 oz. 39.0
primavera *(Amy's)*, 9.5 oz. 39.0
and Stroganoff sauce with meatballs *(Freezer Queen*
    Deluxe Family Entree), 1 cup...............................30.0
stuffed, trio *(Marie Callender's Meals)*, 10.5 oz. 40.0
with tomato Parmesan sauce *(Michelina's)*, 8 oz. 41.0
with vegetables, cheese *(Amy's Country Cheddar)*, 1 cup 27.0
wheels and cheese *(Michelina's)*, 8 oz. 43.0
Pasta flour, see "Wheat flour"
Pasta salad, see "Pasta dish, mix"
Pasta sauce (see also specific listings), tomato base,
    canned or in jar, ½ cup, except as noted:
(Aunt Millie's Traditional) 17.0

(Del Monte Traditional) 15.0
(Eden Organic Pizza/Spaghetti) 12.0
(Healthy Choice Traditional) 11.0
(Prego Extra Chunky Tomato Supreme)..................22.0
(Prego No Salt) 11.0
(Prego Traditional) 23.0
(Progresso Spaghetti) 12.0
(Ragú Old World Style Traditional)....................10.0
Alfredo, see "Alfredo sauce"
balsamic roasted onion *(Muir Glen* Organic) 10.0
beef, sautéed, onion and garlic *(Ragú Robusto!)* 10.0
cheese (see also "Cheese sauce, cooking"):
    four *(Classico* Di Parma) 8.0
    four *(Del Monte)*..15.0
    three *(Prego)*...18.0
    six *(Ragú Robusto!)*......................................9.0
garden combination *(Prego* Extra Chunky) 19.0
garden combination *(Ragú Chunky Gardenstyle)*.........18.0
garlic *(Prego* Extra Chunky Supreme)...................23.0
garlic, super *(Ragú Chunky Gardenstyle)*................17.0
garlic, roasted:
    (Classico Di Sorrento) 9.0
    (Healthy Choice Garlic Lovers') 11.0
    (Muir Glen Organic)...................................10.0
    (Ragú Robusto!)...11.0
    and herb *(Prego)* 17.0
    Parmesan *(Prego* Extra Chunky) 23.0
    primavera *(Ragú* Light) 12.0
    and Romano *(Healthy Choice* Mediterranean Harvest)...........11.0
    and sun-dried tomato *(Healthy Choice* Garlic Lovers')..........11.0
garlic and herb:
    (Del Monte Chunky) 11.0
    (Healthy Choice)..10.0
    (Hunt's)...8.0
garlic mushroom *(Amy's)* 10.0
garlic and mushroom *(Healthy Choice* Garlic Lovers')..............10.0
garlic and onion:
    (Del Monte) 16.0
    (Muir Glen Organic)....................................10.0
    (Healthy Choice Garlic Lovers') 9.0
    oven-roasted *(Five Brothers)*...........................10.0

Pasta sauce *(cont.)*

green pepper and mushrooms *(Del Monte)*................................16.0
hamburger *(Prego)* 17.0
herb:
    Italian *(Del Monte Chunky)*..12.0
    Italian *(Muir Glen Organic)*...10.0
    7, tomato *(Ragú Robusto!)*...9.0
marinara:
    (Amy's Family)...8.0
    (Prego) 12.0
    (Progresso) 8.0
    (Progresso Authentic) 12.0
    (Ragú Old World Style) 9.0
    with Burgundy *(Healthy Choice Mediterranean Harvest)*.......11.0
    cabernet *(Muir Glen Organic)*..10.0
    mushroom *(Muir Glen Organic)* 10.0
    with pizza paste *(Aunt Millie's)*.......................................10.0
    sweet basil *(Classico Di Campania)*..................................11.0
with meat:
    (Del Monte) 14.0
    (Prego) 21.0
    (Ragú Old World Style) 9.0
meat-flavored:
    (Aunt Millie's)...17.0
    (Hunt's) 10.0
    (Progresso) 12.0
mushroom:
    (Aunt Millie's)...17.0
    (Del Monte) 14.0
    (Healthy Choice Super Chunky)..9.0
    (Hunt's) 9.0
    (Prego) 23.0
    (Prego Extra Chunky Supreme).......................................21.0
    (Ragú Old World Style) 10.0
    and diced tomato *(Prego Extra Chunky)*...........................19.0
    with extra spice *(Prego Extra Chunky)* 19.0
    portobello *(Classico Di Toscana)* 11.0
    portobello *(Muir Glen Organic)*.......................................10.0
    sautéed *(Five Brothers)* 10.0
    super *(Ragú Chunky Gardenstyle)*...................................19.0
mushroom and garlic *(Prego)*...20.0

mushroom and garlic, chunky (Ragú Light) 13.0
mushroom and green pepper (Prego Extra Chunky)...................18.0
mushroom and green pepper or roasted garlic (Ragú Chunky
 Gardenstyle) 18.0
mushroom and olives, ripe (Classico Di Sicilia)...............11.0
mushroom Parmesan (Prego)...............23.0
mushroom and sweet pepper (Healthy Choice Super Chunky).....9.0
olive, green (Muir Glen Organic)...............10.0
olive and tomato (Pasta Gusto), ⅓ cup 7.0
onion:
   diced, and garlic (Prego)...............18.0
   sautéed, and garlic (Aunt Millie's) 17.0
   sautéed, and garlic (Ragú Robusto!)...............10.0
   sautéed, and mushroom (Ragú Robusto!)...............9.0
Parmesan (Prego)...............23.0
Parmesan and Romano (Ragú Robusto!)...............10.0
pepper, green, and mushroom (Muir Glen Organic) 10.0
pepper, red:
   roasted (Muir Glen Organic)...............10.0
   roasted, and garlic (Five Brothers) 13.0
   roasted, and garlic (Prego)...............18.0
   roasted, and onion (Classico Di Salerno) 9.0
   roasted, and onion (Ragú Chunky Gardenstyle) 18.0
   spicy (Classico Di Roma Arrabbiata) 7.0
   spicy (Ragú Robusto!) 10.0
pepper, sweet, and onion (Muir Glen Organic)...............8.0
pepper and tomato (Pasta Gusto), ⅓ cup...............7.0
pepperoni (Prego)...............18.0
pesto, see "Pesto sauce"
red wine and herbs (Ragú Robusto!)...............10.0
Romano:
   cheese (Muir Glen Organic)...............14.0
   Pecorino, and herb (Classico Di Palermo)...............8.0
   with garlic (Five Brothers) 10.0
sausage:
   flavored (Aunt Millie's) 17.0
   Italian, and garlic (Prego) 16.0
   Italian, with green peppers and onions
    (Classico D'Abruzzi)...............8.0
   sweet, and cheese (Ragú Robusto!) 9.0
spinach and cheese Florentine (Classico Do Firenze) 8.0

Pasta sauce *(cont.)*
tomato:
    Alfredo *(Five Brothers)* 13.0
    chopped, olive oil and garlic *(Ragú Robusto!)* 9.0
    fire-roasted, and garlic *(Classico Di Siena)* 10.0
    garlic and onion *(Ragú Chunky Gardenstyle)* 19.0
    herb, chunky *(Muir Glen Organic)* 10.0
    mushroom, and garlic *(Healthy Choice Super Chunky)* 10.0
    onion, and garlic *(Prego Extra Chunky)* 19.0
    roasted, Mediterranean *(Five Brothers)* 12.0
    spicy, and pesto *(Classico Di Genoa)* 9.0
    spinach and cheese *(Ragú Chunky Gardenstyle)* 18.0
    sun-dried *(Classico Di Capri)* 8.0
    sun-dried *(Muir Glen Organic)* 10.0
    sun-dried, and herb *(Healthy Choice Mediterranean
      Harvest)* 12.0
tomato and basil:
    (Amy's) 11.0
    (Classico Di Napoli) 9.0
    (Del Monte) 16.0
    (Muir Glen Organic) 12.0
    (Prego) 19.0
    (Ragú Light) 11.0
    (Ragú Light No Sugar) 9.0
    and Italian cheese *(Ragú Chunky Gardenstyle)* 17.0
    summer *(Five Brothers)* 10.0
vegetable:
    (Prego Extra Chunky Supreme) 18.0
    garden *(Muir Glen Organic)* 10.0
    garden, primavera *(Five Brothers)* 11.0
    Italian style *(Healthy Choice)* 9.0
    primavera *(Healthy Choice Super Chunky)* 9.0
    primavera, super *(Ragú Chunky Gardenstyle)* 17.0
Pasta sauce, mix, dry, 2 tbsp., except as noted:
(Hain Spaghetti Sauce), 1 tbsp. 4.0
Alfredo, carbonara, or creamy cheddar *(Knorr)* 7.0
cheese, four *(Knorr)* 4.0
garlic herb *(Knorr)* 8.0
with mushrooms, 1.4-oz. pkt. 19.1
Parma rosa *(Knorr)* 8.0
pesto, see "Pesto sauce mix"

Pasta sauce, refrigerated, ½ cup, except as noted:
cream, plum tomato *(Di Giorno)*.....................................8.0
cream, roasted red pepper *(Di Giorno)*, ¼ cup 8.0
Pasta sauce, refrigerated *(cont.)*
marinara:
   (Contadina Buitoni)..9.0
   (Di Giorno) 15.0
   garlic, roasted *(Contadina Buitoni)* 10.0
   mushroom *(Contadina Buitoni)* 11.0
Parmesan, tomato herb *(Contadina Buitoni)*...................12.0
pesto, see "Pesto sauce, refrigerated"
tomato, plum, and mushroom *(Di Giorno)* 13.0
vegetable, garden *(Contadina Buitoni)* 9.0
Pasta sauce seasoning mix:
(Lawry's Spatini), 2 tsp. 3.0
(Lawry's Spices & Seasonings Extra Rich & Thick), 1 tbsp..........6.0
(Lawry's Spices & Seasonings Original Style), 1½ tbsp. 6.0
Pastrami (see also "Turkey pastrami"), 2 oz., except as noted:
(Boar's Head First Cut)..2.0
(Boar's Head Round)...1.0
(Carl Buddig Lean), 2.5-oz. pkg. 1.0
(Healthy Choice)...2.0
(Healthy Choice Savory Selections), 6 slices, 1.9 oz. 2.0
(Hebrew National), 4 slices, 2 oz. 1.0
(Russer) 1.0
1-oz. slice... .9
Pastry, see specific listings
Pastry filling (see also "Pie filling"), canned, 2 tbsp.:
almond:
   (Baker Brand) 23.0
   (Solo) 23.0
   paste, see "Almond paste"
apple *(Baker* Brand) 20.0
apple, Dutch *(Solo)*..20.0
apricot:
   (Baker Brand) 17.0
   (Bohemian Kitchen) 17.0
   (Solo) 17.0
blueberry *(Baker* Brand) 17.0
blueberry, wild *(Solo)* 17.0
cherry *(Baker* Brand)...20.0

cherry *(Solo)* 20.0
date *(Baker* Brand) 22.0
date *(Solo)* 22.0
nut *(Baker* Brand) 25.0
nut *(Solo* Fancy) 25.0
pecan *(Solo)* 24.0
pineapple:
   (Baker Brand) 19.0
   (Bohemian Kitchen) 19.0
   (Solo) 19.0
poppyseed *(Baker* Brand) 24.0
poppyseed *(Solo)* 24.0
prune *(Bohemian Kitchen* Povidla) 18.0
prune *(Simon Fischer* Lekvar) 21.0
prune plum *(Baker* Brand) 18.0
prune plum *(Solo)* 18.0
raspberry:
   (Baker Brand) 19.0
   (Bohemian Kitchen) 19.0
   red *Solo* 19.0
strawberry:
   (Baker Brand) 18.0
   (Bohemian Kitchen) 18.0
   (Solo) 18.0
Pastry shell, frozen:
baked, 8.6-oz. sheet 112.0
puff pastry sheet *(Pepperidge Farm)*, ⅙ sheet 14.0
puff pastry shell *(Pepperidge Farm)*, 1.7 oz. 16.0
shell, 1.7 oz. 21.1
tart *(Pet-Ritz)*, 3" 13.0
Paté, liver (see also "Liverwurst"):
chicken liver, 1 tbsp. 9
duck and pork mousse with truffles *(Marcel & Henri)*, 2 oz. ......<1.0
glazed, with truffles *(Tour Eiffel Campagnard Française)*,
  2 oz. 2.0
goose liver, smoked, 1 tbsp. 6
Pea pod, Chinese, see "Peas, edible-podded"
Peach, fresh:
(Dole), 2 fruits 19.0
(Frieda's Donut/Frieda's Late Season), 5 oz. 16.0

2¾" diam., approx. 2½ per lb. 17.4
sliced, 1 cup...18.9
Peach, canned:
(Del Monte Fruitrageous Pie Peaches), 4-oz. cup 21.0
(Dole FruitBowls), 4-oz. bowl...16.0
in water:
    halves, 1 half with liquid...6.0
    halves or slices, 1 cup..14.9
in juice:
    halves or sliced *(Libby's* Lite), ½ cup 13.0
    halves or slices, 1 cup..28.7
    slices *(S&W* Natural Style), ½ cup..............................19.0
    diced *(Del Monte* Fruit Naturals Snack Cup), 4-oz. cup.........13.0
    pear and peach juices, slices *(Del Monte* Fruit Naturals),
      ½ cup 15.0
in extra light syrup:
    halves or slices *(Del Monte* Lite Cling), ½ cup.....................15.0
    halves or slices, 1 cup..27.4
    slices *(Del Monte* Lite Freestone), ½ cup...................14.0
    diced *(Del Monte* Lite Snack Cup), 4-oz. cup 13.0
in light syrup:
    halves, 1 half with liquid...14.3
    halves or slices, 1 cup..36.5
    slices *(Del Monte* Orchard Select), ½ cup..............................20.0
    banana-berry *(Del Monte* Fruit-to-Go), 4-oz. cup 17.0
    peach-flavored *(Del Monte* Fruit-to-Go), 4-oz. cup................17.0
    raspberry-flavored *(Del Monte* Fruit Pleasures), ½ cup 20.0
    raspberry-flavored *(Del Monte* Fruitrageous), 4-oz. cup 20.0
    raspberry-flavored, slices *(Del Monte)*, ½ cup.....................20.0
    spiced, slices *(Del Monte)*, ½ cup.............................21.0
    sweet cinnamon, chunky cut *(Del Monte)*, ½ cup.................20.0
in heavy syrup:
    halves *(Del Monte/Del Monte* Melba), ½ cup 24.0
    halves *(S&W)*, ½ cup 24.0
    halves, 1 half with liquid...19.5
    halves or slices, 1 cup..52.2
    slices *(Del Monte)*, ½ cup...24.0
    diced *(Del Monte* Snack Cup), 4-oz. cup 20.0
    spiced, whole *(Del Monte)*, ½ cup 24.0
    spiced, whole, 1 cup..48.6
in extra heavy syrup, halves or slices, 1 cup 68.3

Peach, dehydrated:
sulfured, uncooked, 1 cup...96.5
sulfured, stewed, 1 cup...82.6
Peach, dried:
(Sonoma Organic), 4 pieces, 1.4 oz.............................31.0
halves, sulfured:
    uncooked, 1 half, .5 oz.......................................8.0
    uncooked, 1 cup..98.1
    stewed, 1 cup..50.8
    stewed, with sugar, 1 cup..................................71.8
freeze-dried *(AlpineAire)*, .38 oz................................9.0
Peach, frozen, sliced:
sweetened, 10 slices..37.2
sweetened, thawed, 1 cup..60.0
Peach drink *(Snapple* Summer Peach), 8 fl. oz............30.0
Peach drink blend:
berry St. John's wort *(R.W. Knudsen Simply Delicious),*
    8 fl. oz..33.0
blackberry *(Rocket Juice Peach Berry Clarity),* 16 fl. oz....52.0
mango *(WhipperSnapple),* 10 fl. oz............................39.0
papaya *(Fruitworks),* 12 fl. oz...................................46.0
Peach juice *(Dole* Orchard), 8 fl. oz........................34.0
Peach juice blend *After the Fall Georgia Peach),* 8 fl. oz....27.0
Peach nectar:
(Goya), 6 fl. oz..27.0
(Libby's), 11.5-fl.-oz. can...49.0
(Libby's), 8 fl. oz..34.0
(Libby's), 5.5-fl.-oz. can..23.0
(R.W. Knudsen), 8 fl. oz...30.0
canned, 8 fl. oz...34.7
Peach and pear, canned, in light syrup *(Del Monte*
    Fruit-to-Go Wild Berry Jumble), 4-oz. cup..............20.0
Peanuts, shelled, except as noted:
(Beer Nuts Classic), 1 oz..7.0
(Frito-Lay Salted), 3 tbsp., 1.1 oz..............................5.0
(Little Debbie Salted), 1 oz......................................5.0
(Planters Cocktail Lightly Salted), 1 oz.......................5.0
(Planters Cocktail Salted/Unsalted), 1 oz....................6.0
(Planters Salted), 1 oz..5.0
(River Queen), 3 tbsp., 1 oz.....................................5.0
(River Queen Pub Nuts), ¼ cup................................10.0

in shell, boiled, salted, 1 cup (edible yield 2.2 oz.) 14.4
all varieties, raw, 1 cup 23.6
all varieties, salted, 1 cup..38.3
Cajun *(River Queen),* 3 tbsp., .9 oz. 5.0
honey-roasted:
    (Planters), 1 oz. 8.0
    .*(River Queen),* 3 tbsp., .9 oz. 7.0
    (Weight Watchers), 1 pouch..7.0
hot:
    (D.L. Jardine's Texacali), ¼ cup, 1 oz. 5.0
    (Frito-Lay), 3 tbsp., 1.1 oz. 6.0
    (Planters Heat), 1 oz. 6.0
dry-roasted:
    (Planters Lightly Salted), 1 oz. 5.0
    (Planters Salted/Unsalted), 1 oz. 6.0
    (River Queen), 1 oz. 6.0
    salted, 1 peanut...2
    salted, 1 oz. 6.1
oil-roasted, salted, 1 oz. 5.4
oil-roasted, salted, 1 cup...27.3
roasted, in shell *(Planters* Salted in the Shell), 1 oz. 5.0
Spanish:
    (Planters), 1 oz. 5.0
    (River Queen), 3 tbsp., 1 oz. 5.0
    raw, 1 cup...23.1
    oil-roasted, salted or unsalted, 1 oz. 4.9
    oil-roasted, salted or unsalted, 1 cup 25.7
Valencia:
    raw, 1 cup...30.5
    oil-roasted, salted or unsalted, 1 oz. 4.6
    oil-roasted, salted or unsalted, 1 cup 23.5
Virginia:
    raw, 1 cup...24.1
    oil-roasted, salted, 1 oz. 5.6
    oil-roasted, salted, 1 cup..28.4
and cashews, see "Peanut and cashew mix"
Peanut butter, 2 tbsp., except as noted:
(Estee)..7.0
chunky:
    (Reese's) 8.0
    (Skippy Reduced Fat) 14.0

Peanut butter, chunky *(cont.)*
1 cup 55.7
chunky or creamy:
   (Adam's)...7.0
   (Arrowhead Mills Easy Spread) 7.0
   (Arrowhead Mills/Arrowhead Mills Organic Valencia) 6.0
   (Jif)...7.0
   (Laura Scudder's)...6.0
   (Peter Pan/Peter Pan Plus 8)................................6.0
   (Skippy)...7.0
   (Smucker's) 7.0
   (Teddie/Teddie Old Fashioned)..............................7.0
   roast honey nut, super *(Skippy)*.............................7.0
creamy:
   (Laura Scudder's Reduced Fat) 12.0
   (Peter Pan Whipped) 5.0
   (Reese's) 7.0
   (Skippy Reduced Fat) 15.0
   (Smucker's Reduced Fat) 12.0
   (Teddie Spread Reduced Fat)................................13.0
   1 cup 49.7
pouch *(AlpineAire)*, 1.5 oz..9.0
pourable *(Reese's)* 7.0
Peanut butter baking chips:
(Reese's), 1 tbsp. 7.0
(Reese's Bits for Baking), 1 tbsp................................10.0
1 oz. 12.7
1 cup 75.4
Peanut butter and jelly *(Goober's)*, 2 tbsp...................24.0
Peanut butter and jelly sandwich, grape or strawberry
   (Smucker's Uncrustables), 1 piece 27.0
Peanut butter snack, see "Cookie" and "Cracker"
Peanut butter sprinkles, see "Chocolate sprinkles"
Peanut butter topping *(Smucker's Magic Shell)*, 2 tbsp.............12.0
Peanut and cashew mix, 1 oz.:
honey *(Sweet Roasts)*...10.0
honey-roasted *(Planters)*...10.0
Peanut flour:
defatted, 1 cup 20.8
low-fat, 1 cup 18.8

Peanut sauce, Thai, 2 tbsp.:
(Annie Chun's) 10.0
(San-J Cooking Sauce) 7.0
(A Taste of Thai Satay) 5.0
Peanut sauce mix, Thai *(A Taste of Thai),* ¼ pkt. 7.0
Peanut seasoning and coating mix, Thai, spicy *(A Taste of*
   Thai Peanut Bake), ¼ pkt. 7.0
Peanut topping *(Teddie),* 2 tbsp. 7.0
Pear, fresh:
(Dole), 1 fruit 25.0
1 large, approx. 2 per lb. 31.6
sliced, 1 cup 24.9
Pear, Asian, fresh, raw:
(Frieda's), 5 oz. 15.0
1 pear, 3⅜" x 3" diam., 9⅔ oz. 29.3
1 pear, 2¼" x 2½" diam., 4.3 oz. 13.0
Pear, cactus, see "Prickly pear"
Pear, canned:
in water, halves, 1 half with liquid 5.5
in water, halves, 1 cup 19.1
in juice:
   halves *(Del Monte),* ½ cup 15.0
   halves, 1 half with liquid 9.8
   halves, 1 cup 32.1
   halves, Bartlett *(S&W* Natural Style), ½ cup 21.0
   halves or slices *(Libby's* Lite), ½ cup 13.0
in extra light syrup:
   halves, 1 half with liquid 9.3
   halves, 1 cup 30.1
   halves or slices *(Del Monte* Lite), ½ cup 15.0
   diced *(Del Monte* Lite Snack Cup), 4-oz. cup 13.0
in light syrup:
   halves, 1 half with liquid 11.5
   halves, 1 cup 38.1
   halves, Bartlett *(Del Monte* Orchard Select), ½ cup 20.0
   diced *(Del Monte* Snack Cup), 4-oz. cup 20.0
   cinnamon-flavored, halves *(Del Monte),* ½ cup 21.0
in heavy syrup:
   halves *(Del Monte),* ½ cup 24.0
   halves, 1 half with liquid 14.6
   halves, 1 cup 51.0

Pear, canned, in honey syrup *(cont.)*
halves, Bartlett *(S&W),* ½ cup 22.0
in extra heavy syrup, halves, 1 half with liquid 19.9
in extra heavy syrup, halves, 1 cup....................................67.2
ginger flavor, halves *(Del Monte),* ½ cup...........................22.0
Pear, dried:
(Sonoma Organic), 4 pieces, 1.4 oz...................................32.0
halves, sulfured:
uncooked, 1 half..12.5
uncooked, 1 cup..125.5
stewed, 1 cup..86.2
stewed, with sugar, halves, 1 cup....................................104.0
Pear butter *(Sonoma),* 2 tbsp...11.0
Pear juice, 8 fl. oz.:
(After the Fall Special Harvest)..22.0
(R.W. Knudsen Organic)..30.0
Pear juice blend *(After the Fall Rogue River Pear),* 8 fl. oz.........24.0
Pear nectar:
(Goya), 12-fl.-oz. can 59.0
(Libby's), 11.5-fl.-oz. can 51.0
(Libby's), 8 fl. oz...36.0
(Libby's), 5.5-fl.-oz. can 25.0
(Natural Country), 8 fl. oz. 38.0
(Santa Cruz Organic), 8 fl. oz...28.0
canned, 8 fl. oz...39.4
Peas, baked, see "Baked beans"
Peas, black-eyed, see "Black-eyed peas"
Peas, butter, frozen *(Birds Eye* Deluxe), ½ cup 20.0
Peas, cream, canned, fresh shell *(East Texas Fair),* ½ cup 17.0
Peas, crowder, canned, fresh shell *(Allens/East Texas Fair),*
½ cup 19.0
Peas, crowder, frozen *(Birds Eye* Deluxe), ½ cup 22.0
Peas, edible-podded, fresh (see also "Edamame"):
raw:
(Dole Sugar), ½ cup, 2.5 oz..5.0
(Frieda's Snow Peas), 1 cup, 3 oz. 6.0
(Frieda's Sugar Snap), ⅔ cup, 3 oz..................................6.0
whole *(Mann's* Stringless Sugar Snap), 4 oz......................9.0
whole, 1 cup..4.8
chopped, 1 cup..7.4
boiled, drained, 1 cup 11.3

Peas, edible-podded, frozen:
(Birds Eye Sugar Snap), ½ cup 7.0
(Freshlike Snow Peas), 1 cup..6.0
(Freshlike Sugar Snap), ⅔ cup 6.0
(Green Giant Sugar Snap), ¾ cup..7.0
Peas, edible-podded, frozen *(cont.)*
(La Choy Snow Peas), 3 oz..4.0
(Seneca Snap), ⅔ cup 8.0
unprepared, 10-oz. pkg. 20.4
unprepared, ½ cup 5.2
boiled, drained, 10-oz. pkg..22.8
boiled, drained, 1 cup 14.4
Peas, edible-podded, combination:
fresh, and carrots *(Mann's),* 3 oz. 8.0
frozen *(Birds Eye* Farm Fresh Stir-Fry), ¾ cup...........................5.0
frozen, pods and water chestnuts *(Freshlike),* 1¼ cups...............7.0
Peas, edible-podded, pickled, in jar *(Hogue Farms*
    Snappers), ¼ cup, 1 oz. 3.0
Peas, field, canned:
fresh shell *(Sunshine),* ½ cup...21.0
fresh shell, with snaps *(Allens/East Texas Fair),* ½ cup 21.0
mature, with bacon *(Trappey's),* ½ cup 15.0
mature, with bacon and snaps *(Trappey's),* ½ cup 19.0
Peas, field, frozen, with snaps *(Birds Eye* Southern),
    ⅔ cup..24.0
Peas, green, fresh:
raw *(Frieda's),* ⅓ cup, 3 oz. 22.0
raw, 1 cup 21.0
boiled, drained, 1 cup 25.0
Peas, green, canned or in jar, ½ cup:
(Del Monte)..13.0
(Del Monte No Salt) 11.0
(Del Monte Very Young Small)...10.0
(Green Giant Sweet)..11.0
(Greene's Farm Garden) 10.0
(Hain)..10.0
(LeSueur Early) 12.0
(Twin Tree Gardens Garden)..13.0
(Walnut Acres Organic Farms Sweet) 10.0
drained...10.7

Peas, green, canned or in jar *(cont.)*
mature *(Crest Top* Early June) 20.0
seasoned 10.5
Peas, green, freeze-dried *(AlpineAire),* ½ cup........................14.0
Peas, green, frozen:
(Birds Eye), ½ cup...13.0
(Birds Eye Baby Sweet), ⅔ cup 12.0
(Birds Eye Tiny Tender), ½ cup...11.0
(Freshlike Garden/Tiny), ⅔ cup 12.0
(Green Giant Sweet), ⅔ cup 13.0
(Green Giant/LeSueur Baby Sweet), ⅔ cup 13.0
(Seabrook Farms/Seabrook Farms Petite), ⅔ cup 12.0
(Seneca), ⅔ cup 14.0
unprepared, 10-oz. pkg..39.0
unprepared, ½ cup...9.9
boiled, drained, 10-oz. pkg...36.1
boiled, drained, ½ cup..11.4
in butter sauce *(Green Giant/LeSueur* Baby Sweet), ¾ cup........14.0
Peas, green, combination, canned or in jar:
and carrots:
    (Del Monte), ½ cup...11.0
    (Twin Tree Gardens), 4.5 oz...16.0
    1 cup 21.6
and onions, 1 cup 10.3
Peas, green, combination, frozen:
and carrots:
    (Birds Eye Southern), ⅔ cup 9.0
    (Seneca), ⅔ cup..9.0
    unprepared, 10-oz. pkg...31.7
    unprepared, ½ cup..7.8
    boiled, drained, 10-oz. pkg..28.1
    boiled, drained, ½ cup 8.1
and carrots, corn *(Birds Eye/Freshlike* Baby Blend), ¾ cup..........7.0
and carrots, sugar snap peas *(Birds Eye),* ½ cup........................9.0
and onions:
    (Birds Eye Baby), ⅔ cup 12.0
    (Seneca), ⅔ cup..12.0
    unprepared, 10-oz. pkg. 38.4
    unprepared, ½ cup..9.3
    boiled, drained, 1 cup...15.5
    pearl onions *(Birds Eye),* ⅔ cup 18.0

and potatoes, in cream sauce *(Birds Eye)*, ½ cup 13.0
Peas, pepper, canned, fresh shell *(East Texas Fair)*, ½ cup.......22.0
Peas, purple hull, canned, fresh shell
   (Allens/East Texas Fair), ½ cup 21.0
Peas, purple hull, frozen *(Birds Eye Southern)*, ½ cup..............21.0
Peas, snow or Chinese, see "Peas, edible-podded"
Peas, split, see "Split peas"
Peas, sprouted, mature seeds:
1 cup...33.9
boiled, drained, 1 oz...6.2
Peas, sugar snap, see "Peas, edible-podded"
Peas, sweet, see "Peas, green"
Peas, white acre, canned, fresh shell *(East Texas Fair)*,
   ½ cup...17.0
Peas and carrots or onions, see "Peas, green, combination"
Pecans, shelled:
halves *(Planters)*, 2-oz. pkg. 9.0
dry-roasted, salted or unsalted, 1 oz. 3.8
oil-roasted, salted or unsalted, 15 halves, 1 oz.........................3.7
oil-roasted, salted or unsalted, 1 cup......................................14.3
Pecans, in syrup *(Smucker's)*, 2 tbsp. 20.0
Pecan filling, see "Pastry filling"
Pecan flour, 1 oz. 14.4
Pectin, see "Fruit pectin"
Penne, plain, see "Pasta"
Penne dish, mix:
and black beans *(Marrakesh Express Pasta & Sauce)*,
   ¼ cup, 1 cup* 32.0
rigate, Italian herb butter sauce *(Land O Lakes International
   Pasta Collection)*, 2.5 oz...45.0
with sausage-flavored tomato sauce *(Classico It's Pasta
   Anytime)*, 15.25-oz. cont..100.0
with sun-dried tomato Parmesan sauce *(Knorr)*, ½ cup.............50.0
with tomato and mushroom sauce *(Classico It's Pasta
   Anytime)*, 15.25-oz. cont...98.0
tomato Parmesan *(Bowl Appétit!)*, 1 bowl 57.0
Penne entree, frozen, 1 pkg., except as noted:
(Lean Cuisine Everyday Favorites), 10 oz. 47.0
and chicken bake *(Stouffer's)*, 11½ oz.....................................37.0
marinara, with Italian sausage *(Michelina's)*, 8 oz. 36.0

Penne entree *(cont.)*

with meat sauce *(Freezer Queen* Homestyle), 9 oz. 40.0
and meatballs *(Marie Callender's* Skillet Meals), ½ of
    24-oz. pkg. 53.0
with mushroom sauce *(Michelina's)*, 8 oz. 42.0
with mushrooms *(Michelina's)*, 8 oz. 39.0
pollo *(Michelina's)*, 8.5 oz. 39.0
primavera *(Michelina's)*, 8.5 oz. 40.0
Pepeao:
raw, .2-oz. piece 4
raw, sliced, 1 cup 6.7
dried, 1 cup 19.4
Pepper, seasoning, 1 tsp., except as noted:
black:
    whole, 1 tsp. 1.9
    ground, 1 tbsp. 4.1
    ground, 1 tsp. 1.4
chili, 1 tsp. 1.2
red or cayenne, 1 tbsp. 3.0
red or cayenne, 1 tsp. 1.0
seasoned *(Lawry's)*, ¼ tsp. ....<1.0
white, 1 tbsp. 4.9
white, 1 tsp. 1.6
Pepper, ancho, dried, .6-oz. pepper...................................8.7
Pepper, banana, fresh, raw:
1 small, 1.2 oz. 1.8
1 cup 6.6
mild *(Trappey's)*, 1 oz. 1.0
Pepper, bell, see "Pepper, sweet"
Pepper, cherry, mild *(Trappey's)*, 1.1 oz. 2.0
Pepper, chili (see also specific listings), fresh:
all varieties *(Frieda's)*, 1 oz. 3.0
green or red, 1.6-oz. pepper 4.3
green or red, chopped or diced, 1 cup.....................................7.1
Pepper, chili, canned or in jar:
(Trappey's Tabasco), 1 oz...1.0
green:
    whole *(Chi-Chi's)*, ¾ pepper, 1 oz. 1.0
    whole *(Ortega)*, 1 pepper...3.0
    chopped *(Ortega)*, 2 tbsp. 2.0
    diced *(Chi-Chi's)*, 2 tbsp...1.0

green or red:

2.6-oz. pepper 3.7

1 cup 6.4

chopped or diced, ½ cup 3.5

Pepper, chili, dried:

1 pepper.. .4

1 cup 25.8

Pepper, Hungarian, fresh, raw, 1-oz. pepper 1.8

Pepper, Hungarian, powdered, see "Paprika"

Pepper, jalapeño, fresh:

.5-oz. pepper.. .8

sliced, 1 cup..5.3

Pepper, jalapeño, canned or in jar:

whole *(Chi-Chi's)*, 2½ peppers, 1 oz.................2.0

whole *(Ortega)*, 2 peppers 2.0

chopped, 1 cup 6.4

diced *(Ortega)*, 2 tbsp....................................2.0

diced, marinated, or pickled *(La Victoria)*, 1.1 oz. 2.0

sliced:

(Trappey's), 1 oz. ....<1.0

1 cup 4.9

nacho *(La Victoria)*, 1.1 oz. ....<1.0

wheels *(Chi-Chi's)*, 19 wheels, 1 oz. 2.0

Pepper, pasilla, dried, ¼-oz. pepper.........................3.6

Pepper, poblano *(Herdez)*, 3.5 oz.............................5.0

Pepper, roasted, see "Pepper, sweet, canned or in jar"

Pepper, seasoned, see "Pepper" and specific listings

Pepper, serrano, fresh, raw:

.2-oz. pepper.. .4

chopped, 1 cup 7.0

Pepper, stuffed, entree, frozen:

(Stouffer's), 10-oz. pkg. 25.0

(Stouffer's), ½ of 15½-oz. pkg. 20.0

(Stouffer's), ¼ of 32-oz. pkg. 21.0

Pepper, sweet, fresh:

green or red:

raw *(Dole)*, 1 medium, 5.3 oz......................7.0

raw, sliced, 1 cup 5.9

raw, chopped, 1 cup 9.6

boiled, drained, 1 pepper, 2.6 oz. 4.9

boiled, drained, 1 tbsp. 8

Pepper, sweet, green or red *(cont.)*

boiled, drained, strips, 1 cup 9.0
yellow, raw, 1 large, 5" x 3" diam. 11.8
yellow, raw, 10 strips, 1.8 oz. 3.3

Pepper, sweet, canned or in jar:

green or red, halves, 1 cup 5.5
green or red, ½ cup 2.7
pickled *(Hogue Farms* Sweet Bells), ¼ cup 6.0
red, antipasto, in oil and vinegar *(Victoria)*, ¼ cup 2.0
red, roasted:
   (Krinos), 1.7-oz. piece 3.0
   (Peloponnese Florina), 1 oz. 2.0
   (Progresso), 2 pieces, 1 oz. 3.0
   in olive oil *(Haddon House)*, 2 tbsp. 5.0
salad, drained *(Progresso)*, 2 tbsp. 1.0

Pepper, sweet, dried:

dehydrated, combination *(AlpineAire)*, ½ cup 1.0
freeze-dried, ¼ cup 1.1
freeze-dried, 1 tbsp. 3

Pepper, sweet, frozen:

(Birds Eye Farm Fresh Stir-Fry), 1 cup 5.0
green, diced *(Birds Eye* Southern), ¾ cup 4.0
green or red, unprepared, chopped, 10-oz. pkg. 12.6
red *(Seneca)*, ¾ cup 4.0

Pepper, sweet, and onion, frozen, stir-fry
   (Seabrook Farms), 1 cup 5.0
Pepper, torrido *(Trappey's* Sante Fe Grande), 2.1 oz. 3.0
Pepper dip, red, roasted *(Victoria)*, ¼ cup 12.0
Pepper jelly, see "Jelly, hot"
Pepper loaf, see "Lunch meat loaf"
Pepper relish, hot or sweet *(Cains)*, 1 tbsp. 5.0
Pepper salad, see "Pepper, sweet, canned or in jar"
Pepper sauce (see also "Chili sauce" and "Hot sauce"), 2 tbsp.:
cracked *(San-J)* 8.0
lemon, peanut, or tomato *(San-J)* 9.0
Pepper seasoned salt, red or black *(Lawry's)*, ¼ tsp. 0
Pepper spread, sweet, in jar *(Peloponnese)*, 1 tbsp. 0
Pepper steak, see "Beef entree"
Peppercorn sauce mix *(Knorr* Classic Sauces), 2 tsp. 3.0
Pepperoncini *(Trappey's* Tempero), 1 oz. 1.0

Pepperoni:
(Pillow Pack), 5 slices, 1 oz. 0
(Sara Lee Sandwich), 7 slices, 1.1 oz. 1.0
(Sara Lee Sandwich Deli), 7 slices, .9 oz. 0
chunk or sliced *(Hormel),* 1 oz...................................0
pork and beef, 1 sausage, 10¼" long, approx. 9 oz. 7.1
pork and beef, 1-oz. slice..1.3
Perch, without added ingredients 0
Persimmon, fresh:
(Dole), 1 medium..8.0
(Frieda's), 5 oz. 26.0
Japanese, 2½" diam., 5.9 oz. 31.2
native, trimmed, .9 oz. 8.4
Persimmon, dried:
(Sonoma), 7 pieces, 1.4 oz. 35.0
fuyu *(Frieda's),* ⅓ cup, 1.4 oz. 35.0
Japanese, trimmed, 1.2 oz. 25.0
Pesto sauce, in jar, ¼ cup, except as noted:
(Christopher Ranch)..12.0
(Pasta Gusto), ⅓ cup..6.0
basil and garlic *(Christopher Ranch)*........................4.0
black *(Cora* Gourmet)..5.0
creamy *(Five Brothers)*..3.0
Genovese *(Italia In Tavola),* 2 tbsp..........................4.0
green *(Cora* Gourmet) 2.0
red *(Cora* Gourmet), 2 tbsp..................................3.0
tomato, dried *(Sonoma)*..6.0
white *(Cora* Gourmet) 1.0
Pesto sauce, mix, dry, 2 tbsp.:
(Knorr)..2.0
creamy *(Knorr)*..3.0
red bell pepper *(Knorr)* 4.0
sun-dried tomato *(Knorr)*......................................6.0
Pesto sauce, refrigerated, ¼ cup:
basil:
 (Contadina Buitoni)..12.0
 (Contadina Buitoni Reduced Fat)..............................11.0
 (Di Giorno) 2.0
garlic *(Di Giorno)* 3.0
with sun-dried tomatoes *(Contadina Buitoni)* 10.0
Pheasant, without added ingredients 0

Phyllo pastry, see "Fillo pastry"
Picante sauce (see also "Salsa"), 2 tbsp.:
all varieties *(Chi-Chi's)* 2.0
all varieties *(Pace)* 2.0
green chili, medium or mild *(Ortega)* 2.0
hot or medium *(Shotgun Willie's* Texas) 2.0
with jalapeño, medium *(La Victoria* All Natural) 3.0
medium or mild *(Muir Glen* Organic) 2.0
medium or mild *(Taco Bell Home Originals)* 3.0
Pickle, cucumber:
bread and butter *(B&G),* 6 pieces, 1 oz. 7.0
bread and butter *(Mrs. Fanning's Bread'n Butter),* 1 oz. ...6.0
cornichon *(Dessaux),* 5 pieces, .6 oz. 0
dill:
    (Claussen Super Spices for Burgers), .8-oz. slice 1.0
    (Del Monte), 1½ pickles 1.0
    (Del Monte Tiny Kosher), 1½ pickles 1.0
    (Hebrew National Kosher Plastic Pack), 1 pickle 4.0
    all varieties *(B&G),* 1 oz. 0
    whole *(Claussen),* ½ pickle, 1 oz. 1.0
    halves *(Del Monte),* ¼ pickle 1.0
    sliced, 1 cup, approx. 23 slices 6.4
    chips *(Del Monte),* 5½ chips, 1 oz. 0
    chopped or diced, 1 cup 5.9
sour, 1 large, 4" long, 4¾ oz. 3.0
sweet:
    (Del Monte), 1-oz. pickle 10.0
    (Del Monte Gherkins), 2 pickles 10.0
    (Del Monte Midget), 3 pickles 10.0
    (Vlasic Gherkins), 1 oz., about 3 pickles 8.0
    sliced, 1 cup 54.1
    chips *(Del Monte),* 5 chips, 1 oz. 10.0
    chopped, 1 cup 50.9
Pickle relish, cucumber (see also specific listings):
(Crosse & Blackwell Branston), 1 tbsp. 6.0
hamburger:
    (Del Monte), 1 tbsp. 6.0
    ½ cup 42.1
    1 tbsp. 5.2
hot dog:
    (Del Monte), 1 tbsp. 4.0

½ cup	28.5
1 tbsp.	3.5
India *(Heinz)*, 1 tbsp.	5.0
sweet:	
(Del Monte), 1 tbsp.	5.0
1 cup	85.9
1 tbsp.	5.3

Pickled vegetables, see "Vegetables, mixed, pickled" and specific vegetable listings

Pico de gallo, see "Salsa"

Pie:

apple *(Entenmann's* Homestyle), ⅙ pie	55.0
apple, ⅛ of 9" pie	42.5
blueberry, ⅛ of 9" pie	43.6
cherry, ⅛ of 9" pie	49.8
chocolate creme, ¼ of 6" pie	33.3
coconut creme, ⅙ of 7" pie	23.8
coconut custard *(Entenmann's)*, ⅕ pie	35.0
coconut custard, ⅙ of 8" pie	31.4
custard, ⅙ of 8" pie	21.8
lemon *(Entenmann's)*, ⅙ pie	47.0
lemon meringue, ⅙ of 8" pie	53.3
peach, ⅙ of 8" pie	38.5
pecan, ⅙ of 8" pie	63.7
pumpkin *(Entenmann's)*, ⅕ pie	38.0
pumpkin, ⅙ of 8" pie	29.8
sweet potato *(Entenmann's)*, ⅙ pie	39.0

Pie, frozen:

apple:

(Amy's), 4 oz.	37.0
(Mrs. Smith's 10"), 1/12 pie	45.0
(Mrs. Smith's 9"), ⅛ pie	46.0
(Sara Lee Homestyle), ⅛ pie	46.0
(Sara Lee 45% Reduced Fat), ⅙ pie	51.0
Dutch *(Mrs. Smith's* 10"), 1/10 pie	49.0
Dutch *(Mrs. Smith's* 9"), ⅛ pie	52.0
Dutch *(Sara Lee* Homestyle), ⅛ pie	53.0
blueberry *(Mrs. Smith's* 9"), ⅛ pie	43.0
blueberry *(Sara Lee* Homestyle), ⅛ pie	54.0
cappuccino *(Mrs. Smith's* 10"), 19 pie	44.0

Pie, frozen *(cont.)*
cherry:
    (Mrs. Smith's 10"), 1/12 pie 49.0
    (Mrs. Smith's 9"), 1/8 pie 49.0
    (Sara Lee Homestyle), 1/8 pie 42.0
cherry-berry *(Mrs. Smith's* 10"), 1/12 pie 43.0
chocolate cream *(Mrs. Smith's* 8"), 1/3 pie 54.0
chocolate mint cream *(Mrs. Smith's* 9"), 1/6 pie 52.0
chocolate silk *(Sara Lee Supreme),* 1/5 pie 49.0
coconut cream *(Sara Lee),* 1/5 pie......................................47.0
coconut custard *(Mrs. Smith's* 9"), 1/8 pie 30.0
cookies and cream *(Mrs. Smith's* 9"), 1/6 pie 51.0
French silk *(Mrs. Smith's* 10"), 1/9 pie................................48.0
lemon cream *(Mrs. Smith's* 8"), 1/3 pie 49.0
lemon meringue *(Sara Lee),* 1/6 pie....................................59.0
lemonade *(Mrs. Smith's* 9"), 1/6 pie 46.0
lime, Key *(Mrs. Smith's* 10"), 1/9 pie 56.0
mince *(Mrs. Smith's* 9"), 1/8 pie 53.0
mince *(Sara Lee* Homestyle), 1/8 pie..................................56.0
peach:
    (Sara Lee), 1/8 pie..46.0
    (Mrs. Smith's 10"), 1/12 pie 42.0
    (Mrs. Smith's 9"), 1/8 pie 40.0
peanut butter silk *(Mrs. Smith's* 10"), 1/9 pie 51.0
pecan:
    (Mrs. Smith's 10"), 1/8 pie 75.0
    (Mrs. Smith's 8"), 1/5 pie 75.0
    (Sara Lee Homestyle), 1/8 pie 70.0
pumpkin:
    (Sara Lee Homestyle), 1/8 pie 37.0
    custard *(Mrs. Smith's* 10"), 1/10 pie 41.0
    custard *(Mrs. Smith's* 9"), 1/8 pie 36.0
    custard *(Mrs. Smith's* Hearty 9"), 1/8 pie 39.0
raspberry *(Mrs. Smith's* 9"), 1/8 pie....................................44.0
raspberry *(Sara Lee* Homestyle), 1/8 pie 48.0
S'mores cream *(Mrs. Smith's* 9"), 1/6 pie 54.0
strawberry-banana *(Mrs. Smith's* 9"), 1/6 pie 45.0
sweet potato custard *(Mrs. Smith's* 9"), 1/8 pie..................45.0
Pie, mix, chocolate silk, *(Jell-O* No Bake), 1/6 pie.............37.0
Pie, snack:
apple *(Drake's),* 2 pieces, 5 oz. 60.0

apple *(Hostess)*, 4.5 oz. 67.0
cherry *(Hostess)*, 4.5 oz..65.0
cherry or lemon, fried, 4.5 oz. 54.5
pecan *(Little Debbie* Singles), 3 oz...46.0

Pie crust:

(Nilla Wafer), ⅙ crust, 1 oz...18.0
chocolate *(Oreo)*, ⅙ crust, 1 oz. 18.0
graham cracker:
  (Honey Maid), ⅙ crust, 1 oz. 18.0
  (Ready Crust), ⅛ crust...12.0
  (Ready Crust Reduced Fat), ⅛ crust 14.0
  (Ready Crust 2 Extra Servings), ⅒ crust 17.0
  chocolate *(Ready Crust)*, ⅛ crust 14.0
  tart *(Ready Crust* Single Serve), 1 crust................................15.0
frozen, ⅛ of 9" crust 7.9
shortbread *(Ready Crust)*, ⅛ crust 12.0

Pie crust, frozen or refrigerated:

(Mrs. Smith's 19.5 oz.), ⅛ crust..10.0
(Mrs. Smith's 18 oz., ⅛ crust 9.0
(Pillsbury), ⅛ crust..13.0

Pie crust mix:

(Betty Crocker), ⅛ of 9" crust* 9.0
("Jiffy"), ¼ cup 19.0
(Pillsbury), ⅛ of 9" crust* 10.0

Pie filling canned:

apple:
  (Comstock More Fruit), ⅓ cup 20.0
  (Lucky Leaf/Lucky Leaf Premium), ⅐ can, 3 oz......................22.0
  (Lucky Leaf Lite), ⅐ can, 3 oz...7.0
  ⅛ of 21-oz. can 19.4
apricot *(Lucky Leaf)*, ⅐ can, 3 oz. 22.0
berry, triple *(Crosse & Blackwell)*, ⅓ cup 30.0
blackberry *(Crosse & Blackwell)*, ⅓ cup..................................26.0
blueberry:
  (Comstock More Fruit), ⅓ cup 21.0
  (Lucky Leaf), ⅐ can, 3 oz. 22.0
  (Lucky Leaf Lite), ⅐ can, 3 oz...14.0
  (Lucky Leaf Premium), ⅐ can, 3 oz. 24.0
cherry:
  (Comstock Lite), ⅓ cup...15.0
  (Comstock Original), ⅓ cup 23.0

Pie filling, cherry *(cont.)*
   (Lucky Leaf Lite), 1/7 can, 3 oz. 8.0
   (Lucky Leaf/Lucky Leaf Premium), 1/7 can, 3 oz. 24.0
   1/8 of 21-oz. can 20.7
   red tart, in water *(Oregon)*, 2/3 cup 14.0
lemon *(Comstock)*, 1/3 cup 28.0
lemon *(Lucky Leaf)*, 1/7 can, 3 oz. 30.0
mincemeat *(Lucky Leaf)*, 1/8 can, 3 oz. 33.0
mincemeat, regular or rum and brandy *(Crosse & Blackwell)*,
   1/4 cup 43.0
peach *(Comstock* More Fruit)*, 1/3 cup 19.0
peach *(Lucky Leaf)*, 1/7 can, 3 oz. 21.0
pumpkin *(Comstock)*, 1/3 cup 24.0
pumpkin, 1 cup 71.3
raisin *(Lucky Leaf)*, 1/7 can, 3 oz. 22.0
strawberry *(Lucky Leaf)*, 1/7 can, 3 oz. 20.0
Pie filling mix, see "Pudding mix"
Pie glaze, see "Strawberry pie glaze"
Pie shell, see "Pie crust"
Pierogi, frozen:
"cheddar," nondairy, and potato *(Tofutti)*, 4 pieces, 5.3 oz. 35.0
cheese, American *(Mrs. T's)*, 3 pieces, 4.25 oz. 32.0
jalapeño and cheddar *(Mrs. T's)*, 3 pieces, 4.25 oz. 35.0
jalapeño and cheddar, mini *(Mrs. T's)*, 7 pieces, 3 oz. 25.0
potato and cheddar, mini *(Mrs. T's)*, 7 pieces, 3 oz. 24.0
potato and cheese *(Empire* Kosher), 1/2 of 10.5-oz. pkg. 44.0
potato and cheese *(Mrs. T's)*, 3 pieces, 4.25 oz. 34.0
potato and onion *(Empire* Kosher), 1/2 of 10.5-oz. pkg. 47.0
potato and onion *(Mrs. T's)*, 3 pieces, 4.25 oz. 34.0
potato and roasted garlic *(Mrs. T's)*, 3 pieces, 4.25 oz. 41.0
sauerkraut *(Mrs. T's)*, 3 pieces, 4.25 oz. 32.0
sweet potato *(Mrs. T's)*, 3 pieces, 4.25 oz. 34.0
Pigeon peas:
immature:
   raw, 10 pigeon peas 1.0
   raw, 1 cup 36.8
   boiled, drained, 1 cup 29.8
mature, raw, 1 cup 128.7
mature, boiled, 1 cup 39.1
Pig's feet, pickled (see also "Pork, pickled"):
(Hormel), 2 oz. 0

cured, 1 lb..<.1
Pignolia nuts, see "Pine nuts"
Pike, without added ingredients 0
Pili nuts, shelled:
dried, 1 oz. 1.1
dried, 1 cup 4.8
Pimiento, canned:
1 cup 9.8
1 tbsp. 6
Piña colada drink *(AriZona)*, 8 fl. oz. 34.0
Piña colada drink mixer:
canned or bottled:
   (Daily's), 3 fl. oz. 37.0
   (Goya), ⅓ cup 20.0
   (Mr & Mrs T), 4.5 fl. oz. 43.0
   (Roland), 3 fl. oz. 17.0
frozen *(Bacardi)*, 2 fl. oz............................35.0
Pine nuts, dried:
(Frieda's), ¼ cup, 1.1 oz. 4.0
pignolia:
   (Progresso), 1-oz. jar 2.0
   1 oz. 4.0
   1 cup 10.3
   1 tbsp. 1.2
pinyon, 1 oz. 5.5
pinyon, 10 kernels 2
Pineapple, fresh, raw:
(Dole), 2 slices 16.0
(Frieda's Baby Sugar Loaf), 3 oz. 17.0
1-lb. pineapple 58.5
diced, 1 cup 19.2
Pineapple, candied, slices *(S&W)*, 1 piece 45.0
Pineapple, canned:
in water, slices, 1 slice with liquid.....................3.9
in water, slices, chunks or crushed, 1 cup 20.4
in juice:
   (Dole Fun Shapes), ½ cup...........................20.0
   chunks *(Dole)*, ½ cup 15.0
   chunks or crushed *(Del Monte)*, ½ cup 17.0
   crushed *(Dole)*, ½ cup 17.0
   slices *(Del Monte)*, 2 slices 16.0

Pineapple, canned, in juice *(cont.)*

slices *(Dole)*, 2 slices, 4 oz..15.0
slices, 1 slice with liquid..7.4
slices, chunks or crushed, 1 cup..39.1
spears, tidbits, or wedges *(Del Monte)*, ½ cup....................17.0
tidbits *(Del Monte* Snack Cup), 4-oz. cup............................15.0
tidbits *(Dole)*, ½ cup 15.0

in syrup:

chunks or crushed *(Dole)*, ½ cup 24.0
slices *(Dole)*, 2 slices, 4.1 oz..23.0
tidbits *(Dole)*, ½ cup 24.0

in light syrup, slices, 1 slice with liquid 6.3
in light syrup, slices, chunks, or crushed, 1 cup 33.9

in heavy syrup:

chunks or crushed *(Del Monte)*, ½ cup 24.0
slices *(Del Monte)*, 2 slices 23.0
slices, 1 slice with liquid 9.9
slices, chunks, or crushed, 1 cup.......................................51.3

in extra heavy syrup, slices, chunks, or crushed, 1 cup 55.9

Pineapple, dried:

(Sonoma Organic), ¼ cup, 1.4 oz......................................25.0
freeze-dried, chunks *(AlpineAire)*, .38 oz. 10.0

Pineapple, frozen, sweetened, chunks, 1 cup 54.4

Pineapple drink blend, 8 fl. oz., except as noted:

coconut *(R.W. Knudsen)*..32.0
coconut *(Rocket Juice Spirulina Smoothie)*, 16 fl. oz. 60.0
guava nectar *(Goya)*...37.0
guava smoothie *(Rocket Juice Pacific Protein)*, 16 fl. oz...........54.0
orange *(WhipperSnapple)*, 10 fl. oz. 41.0
orange-banana *(Chiquita)*..29.0
passion fruit nectar *(Goya)*, 6 fl. oz....................................28.0
piña-pineapple, mix* *(Kool-Aid)*...25.0
piña-pineapple, mix* *(Kool-Aid* Sugar Sweetened).................17.0

Pineapple filling, see "Pastry filling"

Pineapple juice, 8 fl. oz., except as noted:

canned or bottled:

(Del Monte From Concentrate)...32.0
(Del Monte From Concentrate), 6 fl. oz..................................20.0
(Del Monte Not From Concentrate) 29.0
(Dole) 29.0
(Dole), 6-fl.-oz. can 22.0

(Goya), 6 fl. oz...21.0
nectar *(R.W. Knudsen)* 34.0
unsweetened 34.5
frozen*, unsweetened 31.9
Pineapple juice blend:
apple *(Snapple* Vitamin Supreme), 8 fl. oz.............44.0
grapefruit:
    (Dole), 6-fl.-oz. can...............................24.0
    pink *(Dole)*, 8 fl. oz.............................32.0
    pink *(Dole)*, 6-fl.-oz. can......................25.0
orange *(Dole)*, 8 fl. oz. 27.0
orange *(Dole)*, 6-fl.-oz. can.........................24.0
orange-banana *(Dole)*, 8 fl. oz.....................29.0
orange-banana *(Dole)*, 6-fl.-oz. can 25.0
orange-strawberry *(Dole)*, 8 fl. oz................32.0
Pineapple topping, 2 tbsp.:
(Kraft)..28.0
(Smucker's)..28.0
Pineapple-apricot sauce *(Sable & Rosenfeld)*, 2 tbsp.........20.0
Pink beans:
mature, raw, 1 cup....................................134.8
mature, boiled, 1 cup 47.2
Pinto beans, mature:
dry *(Arrowhead Mills)*, ¼ cup.....................27.0
dry, 1 cup...122.4
boiled, 1 cup 43.9
Pinto beans, canned, mature, ½ cup, except as noted:
(Allens/Brown Beauty) 20.0
(Eden Organic)..18.0
(Goya), ½ of 15-oz. can...........................31.0
(Hain)...18.0
(Joan of Arc)...20.0
(Progresso)...18.0
(Westbrae Natural)..................................16.0
with bacon *(Trappey's)* 20.0
with bacon and jalapeños *(Trappey's* Jalapinto).......22.0
spicy *(Eden* Organic)................................24.0
Pinto beans, dehydrated *(AlpineAire)*, ½ cup.........14.0
Pinto beans, frozen, immature:
10-oz. pkg. 92.3
⅓ of 10-oz. pkg. 30.6

Pinto beans, frozen *(cont.)*
boiled, drained, 10-oz. pkg..87.7
boiled, drained, ⅓ of 10-oz. pkg...................................29.0
Pinto beans, sprouted, boiled, drained, 4 oz. 4.6
Pinto bean salsa, see "Salsa"
Pistachio nuts, shelled, except as noted:
  (AlpineAire Raging Flame), 2.5 oz....................................22.0
  (AlpineAire Wild West), 2.5 oz. 20.0
  (Sonoma), ¼ cup, 1.1 oz...9.0
  natural, in shell *(River Queen),* ¼ cup 8.0
  raw, 1 oz., 47 kernels...8.3
  raw, 1 cup..37.4
  dried, in shell, 1 oz..3.0
  dry-roasted:
    (Planters), 1 oz..7.0
    (Planters In Shell), 2.25-oz. pkg...................................8.0
    unsalted, 1 cup...35.8
    unsalted, 1 oz..7.1
    salted, 1 cup...34.7
    salted, 1 oz..7.8
Pita, see "Bread"
Pitanga, fresh, raw:
trimmed, 1 fruit, ¼ oz. 5
1 cup...13.0
Pizza, frozen:
bacon cheeseburger *(Jack's Great Combinations* 12"), ¼ pie.....31.0
bacon cheeseburger *(Jack's Naturally Rising Pizza* 12"),
  ⅙ pie...35.0
Canadian bacon:
  (Jack's Naturally Rising Pizza 12"), ⅙ pie 34.0
  (Jack's Original 12"), ¼ pie..31.0
  (Tombstone Original 12"), ¼ pie.....................................36.0
cheese:
  (Amy's), ⅓ pie...38.0
  (Celeste Large), ¼ pie 33.0
  (Celeste for One), 1 pie 43.0
  (Empire Kosher), 4-oz. pie...37.0
  (Empire Kosher 10 oz.), ⅓ pie...38.0
  (Jack's Naturally Rising Pizza 12"), ⅙ pie 35.0
  (Jack's Naturally Rising Pizza 9"), ⅓ pie 38.0
  (Jack's Original 12"), ⅓ pie...41.0

(Kid Cuisine Munchers Fire Chief), 1 pie 44.0
(Michelina's Singles), 1 pie 38.0
(Michelina's That'za Pizza!), 1 pie 39.0
(Tombstone For One ½ Less Fat), 1 pie 43.0
double *(Jack's Great Combinations* 12"), ¼ pie 32.0
double *(Jack's Great Combinations* 9"), ½ pie 38.0
extra *(Tombstone* Original 12"), ¼ pie 35.0
extra *(Tombstone* Original 9"), ½ pie 40.0
extra *(Tombstone For One)*, 1 pie 41.0
four *(Celeste* for One Original), 1 pie 41.0
four *(Celeste* for One Zesty), 1 pie 43.0
four *(Celeste* Rising Crust), ⅙ pie 42.0
four *(Di Giorno Rising Crust* 12"), ⅙ pie 39.0
four *(Di Giorno Rising Crust* 8"), ⅓ pie 33.0
three *(Tombstone* Thin Crust), ¼ pie 25.0
three *(Tombstone* Oven Rising Crust), ⅙ pie 34.0
two *(Tombstone* Double Top), ⅕ pie 29.0
"cheese," soy *(Amy's* Cheeze), ⅓ pie 37.0
"cheese," soy *(Tofutti* Pizza Piazzaz), 1 slice 24.0
chicken supreme *(Celeste* for One Zesty), 1 pie 38.0
chicken supreme *(Di Giorno Rising Crust* 8"), ⅓ pie 33.0
combination:
  (Michelina's Singles), 1 pie 37.0
  the works *(Jack's Naturally Rising Pizza* 12"), ⅙ pie 34.0
  the works *(Jack's Naturally Rising Pizza* 9"), ¼ pie 29.0
deluxe:
  (Celeste Large), ¼ pie 34.0
  (Celeste for One), 1 pie 46.0
  (Tombstone Original 12"), ⅕ pie 29.0
  (Tombstone Original 9"), ⅓ pie 27.0
hamburger:
  (Jack's Original 12"), ¼ pie 28.0
  (Tombstone Original 12"), ⅕ pie 29.0
  (Tombstone Original 9"), ⅓ pie 27.0
meat:
  four *(Tombstone* Thin Crust), ¼ pie 26.0
  three *(Celeste* Rising Crust), ⅙ pie 42.0
  three *(Di Giorno Rising Crust* 12"), ⅙ pie 40.0
  three *(Di Giorno Rising Crust* 8"), ⅓ pie 33.0
  three *(Tombstone* Oven Rising Crust), ⅙ pie 34.0
mushroom and olive *(Amy's)*, ⅓ pie 33.0

Pizza, frozen *(cont.)*

pesto, with tomato and broccoli *(Amy's)*, ⅓ pie 40.0
pepperoni:
(Banquet Meal), 6.75-oz. pkg. 56.0
(Celeste Large), ½ pie 43.0
(Celeste for One), 1 pie 46.0
(Celeste Rising Crust), ⅙ pie 42.0
(Di Giorno Rising Crust 12"), ⅙ pie 40.0
(Di Giorno Rising Crust 8"), ⅓ pie 33.0
(Jack's Great Combinations 12"), ¼ pie 42.0
(Jack's Naturally Rising Pizza 12"), ⅙ pie 35.0
(Jack's Naturally Rising Pizza 9"), ⅓ pie 38.0
(Jack's Original 12"), ¼ pie 31.0
(Jack's Original 9"), ½ pie 37.0
(Kid Cuisine Munchers Poolside), 1 pie 44.0
(Michelina's Singles), 1 pie 38.0
(Michelina's That'za Pizza!), 1 pie 38.0
(Tombstone Original 12"), ¼ pie 35.0
(Tombstone Original 9"), ⅓ pie 27.0
(Tombstone Thin Crust), ¼ pie 25.0
(Tombstone Double Top), ⅙ pie 24.0
(Tombstone For One), 1 pie 41.0
(Tombstone Oven Rising Crust), ⅙ pie 34.0
supreme *(Jack's Naturally Rising Pizza* 12"), ⅙ pie 34.0
pepperoni and mushroom *(Jack's Great Combinations* 12"), ¼ pie 32.0
pepperoni and sausage *(Jack's Great Combinations* 9"), ½ pie 36.0
pepperoni and sausage *(Tombstone* Original 9"), ⅓ pie 27.0
sausage:
(Celeste for One), 1 pie 45.0
(Jack's Great Combinations 12"), ¼ pie 40.0
(Jack's Naturally Rising Pizza 12"), ⅙ pie 34.0
(Jack's Naturally Rising Pizza 9"), ⅓ pie 38.0
(Jack's Original 12"), ¼ pie 28.0
(Jack's Original 9"), ½ pie 36.0
(Tombstone Original 12"), ⅕ pie 29.0
(Tombstone Original 9"), ⅓ pie 27.0
(Tombstone Double Top), ⅙ pie 25.0
Italian *(Di Giorno Rising Crust* 12"), ⅙ pie 40.0
Italian *(Di Giorno Rising Crust* 8"), ⅓ pie 33.0

Italian *(Tombstone* Thin Crust), ¼ pie..............................26.0
Italian *(Tombstone Oven Rising* Crust), ⅙ pie 35.0
Italian, spicy *(Jack's Naturally Rising Pizza* 12"), ⅙ pie 34.0
Italian, spicy *(Jack's Original* 12"), ¼ pie.............................29.0
sausage and mushroom *(Jack's Great Combinations* 12"),
   ¼ pie 29.0
sausage and mushroom *(Tombstone* Original 12"), ⅕ pie..........29.0
sausage and pepperoni:
   (Celeste for One), 1 pie 43.0
   (Jack's Great Combinations 12"), ¼ pie 29.0
   (Tombstone Original 12"), ⅕ pie..............................29.0
   (Tombstone Double Top), ⅙ pie..............................25.0
   combination with *(Jack's Naturally Rising Pizza* 12"),
     ⅙ pie 34.0
   combination with *(Jack's Naturally Rising Pizza* 9"),
     ¼ pie..29.0
spinach *(Amy's),* ⅓ pie 40.0
spinach *(Di Giorno Rising Crust* 8"), ⅓ pie......................33.0
supreme:
   (Celeste Rising Crust), ⅙ pie..................................41.0
   (Celeste Suprema for One), 1 pie 48.0
   (Di Giorno Rising Crust 12"), ⅙ pie 40.0
   (Di Giorno Rising Crust 8"), ⅓ pie............................34.0
   (Jack's Great Combinations 12"), ¼ pie 30.0
   (Michelina's Singles), 1 pie 38.0
   (Tombstone Original 12"), ⅕ pie 29.0
   (Tombstone Original 9"), ⅓ pie 27.0
   (Tombstone Thin Crust), ¼ pie..................................26.0
   (Tombstone Double Top), ⅙ pie..............................25.0
   (Tombstone For One), 1 pie.....................................42.0
   (Tombstone Light), ⅕ pie.......................................30.0
   (Tombstone Oven Rising Crust), ⅙ pie......................34.0
taco, supreme *(Tombstone* Thin Crust), ¼ pie......................27.0
vegetable:
   (Amy's Veggie Combo), ⅓ pie 34.0
   (Celeste for One), 1 pie 45.0
   (Di Giorno Rising Crust 12"), ⅙ pie 41.0
   (Di Giorno Rising Crust 8"), ⅓ pie............................33.0
   (Tombstone For One ½ Less Fat), 1 pie.....................48.0
   (Tombstone Light), ⅕ pie.......................................31.0
   roasted *(Amy's),* ⅓ pie..43.0

Pizza, bagel, frozen, cheese, 1 piece:
(Empire Kosher) 14.0
nondairy *(Tofutti)* 15.0
Pizza, English muffin, frozen, cheese *(Empire* Kosher),
   3-oz. piece 15.0
Pizza, French bread, frozen, 1 piece:
cheese:
  (Healthy Choice) 51.0
  (Lean Cuisine Everyday Favorites) 48.0
  (Marie Callender's) 50.0
  (Stouffer's) 43.0
  extra *(Stouffer's)* 49.0
  five *(Stouffer's)* 48.0
deluxe *(Lean Cuisine Everyday Favorites)* 43.0
deluxe *(Stouffer's)* 48.0
meat, three *(Stouffer's)* 50.0
pepperoni:
  (Healthy Choice) 49.0
  (Lean Cuisine Everyday Favorites) 43.0
  (Marie Callender's) 50.0
  (Stouffer's) 48.0
pepperoni and mushroom *(Stouffer's)* 49.0
sausage *(Healthy Choice)* 48.0
sausage *(Stouffer's)* 48.0
sausage and pepperoni *(Stouffer's)* 47.0
sun-dried tomato *(Lean Cuisine Everyday Favorites)* ... 48.0
supreme *(Healthy Choice)* 51.0
supreme *(Marie Callender's)* 50.0
vegetable *(Healthy Choice)* 44.0
vegetable, grilled *(Stouffer's)* 48.0
white *(Stouffer's)* 45.0
Pizza crust, refrigerated *(Pillsbury)*, ⅕ pkg. 27.0
Pizza crust mix:
(Betty Crocker Pouch), ¼ crust 33.0
("Jiffy"), ⅓ cup 31.0
Italian herb *(Betty Crocker* Pouch), ¼ crust 32.0
Pizza Hut:
The Big New Yorker pizza, 1 slice:
  cheese 42.4
  pepperoni 41.9
  supreme 44.4

Pizza Hut (cont.)

hand-tossed pizza, 1 slice of medium pie:

    cheese 43.0

    beef 44.0

    ham 43.0

    Italian sausage, pork topping, or *Meat Lover's*....................44.0

    pepperoni or *Pepperoni Lover's* 43.0

    super supreme 45.0

    supreme or chicken supreme..44.0

    taco 34.0

    taco, beef, chicken, or meatless..35.0

    Veggie Lover's 45.0

The New Edge pizza, 1 slice of medium pie:

    the works, *Veggie Lover's,* or chicken supreme 9.0

    Meat Lover's...8.0

pan pizza, 1 slice of medium pie:

    cheese 44.0

    beef 45.0

    ham 44.0

    Italian sausage, pork topping, or *Meat Lover's*....................45.0

    pepperoni or *Pepperoni Lover's* 44.0

    super supreme 46.0

    supreme or chicken supreme..45.0

    taco, all varieties...36.0

    Veggie Lover's 46.0

Personal Pan Pizza, 1 pie:

    cheese 110.0

    pepperoni or supreme 111.0

    taco 90.0

Sicilian pizza, 1 slice of medium pie:

    cheese 32.0

    beef 31.0

    ham 30.0

    Italian sausage, pork topping, or *Meat Lover's*....................31.0

    pepperoni or *Pepperoni Lover's* 31.0

    supreme, chicken supreme, or super supreme 32.0

    Veggie Lover's 32.0

stuffed crust pizza, 1 slice of medium pie:

    cheese, beef, or Italian sausage 46.0

    chicken supreme 47.0

    ham or pepperoni..45.0

Pizza Hut, *stuffed crust pizza (cont.)*

     pork topping, *Meat Lover's* or *Pepperoni Lover's* 46.0

     super supreme 46.0

     supreme 47.0

     Veggie Lover's 48.0

Thin n' Crispy pizza, 1 slice of medium pie:

     beef 28.0

     cheese, ham, or pepperoni 27.0

     chicken supreme 29.0

     Italian sausage, pork topping, or *Meat Lover's* 28.0

     Pepperoni Lover's 28.0

     supreme or super supreme 29.0

     taco or meatless taco 27.0

     taco, beef 29.0

     taco, chicken 26.0

     Veggie Lover's 30.0

pasta, 1 serving:

     Cavatini 66.0

     Cavatini Supreme 73.0

     spaghetti with marinara sauce 91.0

     spaghetti with meat sauce 98.0

     spaghetti with meatballs 120.0

sandwiches, 1 serving:

     ham and cheese 57.0

     supreme 62.0

appetizers:

     bread stick 20.0

     bread stick dipping sauce 5.0

     Buffalo wings, hot, 4 pieces 4.0

     Buffalo wings, mild, 5 pieces ....<1.0

     garlic bread, 1 slice 16.0

desserts, 1 slice:

     apple dessert pizza 48.0

     cherry dessert pizza 47.0

Pizza roll, see "Pizza snack"

Pizza pocket, 1 piece:

(Ken & Robert's Veggie Pockets), 4.5 oz. 41.0

cheese:

     (Amy's), 4.5 oz. 42.0

     double *(Toaster Breaks),* 2.2 oz. 21.0

     double *(Toaster Breaks Pizza Mini's),* 3.1 oz. 35.0

pepperoni:
    (Croissant Pockets), 4.5 oz. 40.0
    (Deli Stuffs), 4.5 oz. 41.0
    (Hot Pockets), 4.5 oz. 43.0
    (Lean Pockets Deluxe), 4.5 oz. 45.0
    (Toaster Breaks), 2.2 oz. 22.0
    (Toaster Breaks Pizza Mini's), 3.1 oz. 33.0
pepperoni and sausage *(Hot Pockets)*, 4.5 oz. 39.0
pepperoni and sausage *(Toaster Breaks Pizza Mini's)*, 3.1 oz. 34.0
pepperoni style *(Morningstar Farms* Stuffed Sandwich),
    4.5 oz. 42.0
sausage *(Hot Pockets)*, 4.5 oz. 40.0
sausage and pepperoni *(Toaster Breaks)*, 2.2 oz. 21.0
supreme *(Croissant Pockets)*, 4.5 oz. 41.0
vegetarian *(Amy's)*, 4.5 oz. 39.0
Pizza sauce, ¼ cup:
(Contadina/Contadina Pizza Squeeze) 6.0
(Muir Glen Organic) 6.0
(Prince) 4.0
(Ragú Pizza Quick Traditional) 5.0
cheese, four *(Contadina)* 6.0
garlic and basil *(Ragú Pizza Quick)* 5.0
mushroom, chunky *(Ragú Pizza Quick)* 6.0
pepperoni-flavored *(Contadina)* 5.0
pepperoni-flavored *(Ragú Pizza Quick)* 5.0
tomato, chunky *(Ragú Pizza Quick)* 7.0
Pizza snack, frozen:
(Kid Cuisine Munchers Backpacking), 6 pieces 23.0
cheese:
    (Amy's), ½ pkg., 5-6 pieces 22.0
    (Banquet Munchers), 6 pieces............................24.0
    (Jack's Pizza Bursts Supercheese), 6 pieces, 3 oz. 25.0
pepperoni *(Banquet Munchers)*, 6 pieces 23.0
pepperoni and sausage *(Banquet Munchers)*, 6 pieces 24.0
rolls:
    cheese, hamburger, or pepperoni *(Michelina's)*,
      6 rolls, 3 oz. 23.0
    combination or four-meat *(Michelina's)*, 6 rolls, 3 oz. 22.0
    nacho cheese *(Michelina's)*, 6 rolls, 3 oz. 25.0
wedges, 1 cup:
    cheese, three *(Kid's Kitchen)* 44.0

Pizza snack, wedges *(cont.)*
 cheeseburger *(Kid's Kitchen)*......................................41.0
 pepperoni *(Kid's Kitchen)*...38.0
pepperoni or sausage *(Jack's Pizza Bursts)*, 6 pieces, 3 oz. 25.0
sausage and pepperoni combination *(Jack's Pizza Bursts)*,
 6 pieces, 3 oz. 26.0
supreme *(Jack's Pizza Bursts)*, 6 pieces, 3 oz. 26.0
Plantain, fresh:
raw:
 (Frieda's), 3 oz...27.0
 1 medium, 6.3 oz. 57.1
 sliced, 1 cup..47.2
cooked, sliced, 1 cup...48.0
cooked, mashed, 1 cup...62.3
Plantain, frozen, fried *(Goya Tostones)*, 2 medium pieces 37.0
Plum, fresh, raw:
(Dole), 2 fruits..17.0
2⅛"-diam. fruit, 2⅓ oz..8.6
sliced, 1 cup...21.5
Plum, canned, purple:
in water, 1 plum with liquid..5.1
in water, pitted, 1 cup...27.5
in juice, 1 plum with liquid..7.0
in juice, pitted, 1 cup...38.2
in light syrup, 1 plum with liquid 7.5
in light syrup, pitted, 1 cup.......................................41.0
in heavy syrup:
 (Oregon Purple), ½ cup 25.0
 1 plum with liquid...10.7
 pitted, 1 cup 60.0
in extra heavy syrup, pitted, 1 cup 68.7
Plum butter *(Sonoma)*, 2 tbsp...................................13.0
Plum dipping sauce, 2 tbsp.:
Asian *(Sonoma)* 15.0
Oriental style *(Trader Vic's)*.....................................16.0
Plum pudding *(Crosse & Blackwell)*, ⅓ pkg......................87.0
Plum sauce, 1 tbsp. 8.1
Poi, fresh:
1 oz..7.7
1 cup...65.4
Poblano chili, see "Pepper, chili"

Pocket sandwich, see specific listings
Poke greens, canned *(Allens),* ½ cup 5.0
Pokeberry shoots:
raw, 1 cup 5.9
boiled, drained, 1 cup 5.1
boiled, drained, 1 tbsp. 3
Polenta, dry, see "Cornmeal"
Polenta, canned *(Greene's Farm),* ½ cup 17.0
Polenta, refrigerated:
plain *(Frieda's),* 4 oz. 21.0
plain or basil and garlic *(San Gennaro),* 2 slices, ½" 15.0
sun-dried tomato *(San Gennaro),* 2 slices, ½"...............16.0
Polenta dish, mix, 1 cont.:
cheese, three *(Fantastic Foods* Cup), 1.8 oz. 37.0
Mediterranean *(Fantastic Foods* Cup), 1.8 oz.............36.0
Mexicana, spicy *(Fantastic Foods* Cup), 1.8 oz. 39.0
Santa Fe *(Fantastic Foods* Cup), 1.9 oz....................40.0
Polenta mix (see also "Cornmeal") *(Fantastic*
    Foods Fantastica), 1 cup* 46.0
Polish sausage (see also "Kielbasa"):
(Johnsonville), 3-oz. link, grilled.............................1.0
(Russer Loaf), 2 oz. 7.0
1 sausage, 10" long, 8 oz. 3.1
smoked *(Johnsonville),* 2.7-oz. link 2.0
smoked *(Johnsonville* Light), 2.3-oz. link 3.0
Pollock, without added ingredients 0
Pollock dinner, frozen, fish and chips, battered
    (Swanson), 10 oz. 59.0
Pomegranate, fresh:
(Dole), 1 medium...26.0
(Frieda's), 5 oz. 24.0
3⅜"-diam. fruit...26.4
Pomegranate juice *(R.W. Knudsen),* 8 fl. oz. 37.0
Pomegranate syrup, see "Grenadine syrup"
Pommello, see "Pummelo"
Pompano, without added ingredients.............................0
Popcorn, unpopped:
(Act II Corn on the Cob), 3 tbsp., 3½ cups popped.............17.0
(Act II 96% Fat Free), 3 tbsp., 3½ cups popped...................26.0
(Arrowhead Mills), ¼ cup 36.0
(Orville Redenbacher's Smart Pop!), 1.1 oz................20.0

(Pop•Secret Homestyle), 3 tbsp...17.0
(Weight Watchers), 1 bag 20.0
butter/butter flavor:
    (Act II Butter Lovers), 3 tbsp., 3½ cups popped..................17.0
    (Act II Butter Lovers Reduced Fat), 3 tbsp.,
      3½ cups popped...23.0
    (Act II Butter/Extreme Butter), 3 tbsp., 3½ cups popped......19.0
    (Act II Light), 3 tbsp., 3½ cups popped.............................24.0
    (Act II Pop N' Serve Theater Butter Tub), 3 tbsp.,
      3½ cups popped...19.0
    (American's Best 94% Fat Free), 2 tbsp., 5 cups popped......23.0
    (Jolly Time Blastobutter), 2 tbsp., 3½ cups popped 19.0
    (Jolly Time Blastobutter Light), 2 tbsp., 4 cups popped 21.0
    (Jolly Time Butter-Licious), 2 tbsp., 4 cups popped 18.0
    (Jolly Time Butter-Licious Light), 2 tbsp., 5 cups popped 21.0
    (Jolly Time Healthy Pop), 2 tbsp., 5 cups popped 23.0
    (Jolly Time White & Buttery), 2 tbsp., 4 cups popped 16.0
    (Orville Redenbacher's Microwave), 1.1 oz. 14.0
    (Orville Redenbacher's Microwave Light), 1.1 oz. 18.0
    (Pop•Secret Light), 3 tbsp..23.0
    (Pop•Secret 94% Fat Free), 3 tbsp..................................26.0
    (Pop•Secret Jumbo Pop), 3 tbsp.....................................18.0
    (Pop•Secret Land O Lakes/Rev It Up/Movie Theater/
      Homestyle Extra Butter), 3 tbsp...................................17.0
    (Weaver), ⅓ bag, 1.2 oz...19.0
    (Weaver Light), ⅓ bag, 1 oz...18.0
    extra *(Weaver)*, ⅓ bag, 1.2 oz.......................................17.0
butter or natural flavor *(Healthy Choice)*, 3 tbsp.......................26.0
cheddar cheese flavor *(Act II)*, 3 tbsp., 3½ cups popped...........19.0
cheddar cheese flavor *(Jolly Time)*, 2 tbsp., 3 cups popped.......17.0
natural flavor:
    (Act II), 3 tbsp., 3½ cups popped 19.0
    (Jolly Time Crispy 'n White), 2 tbsp., 4 cups popped 16.0
    (Jolly Time Crispy 'n White Light), 2 tbsp., 5 cups popped ..20.0
    (Orville Redenbacher's Microwave), 1.1 oz. 15.0
    (Orville Redenbacher's Microwave Light), 1.1 oz. 18.0
    (Pop•Secret), 3 tbsp..17.0
    (Pop•Secret 94% Fat Free), 3 tbsp..................................26.0
    (Weaver), ⅓ bag, 1.2 oz..18.0
yellow or white *(Jolly Time)*, 2 tbsp., 5 cups air-popped 24.0

Popcorn, popped:
(Bearitos Lite 50% Less Oil), 3½ cups 20.0
(Bearitos Lite No Salt/Oil), 4¼ cups..............................24.0
(Bearitos Microwave No Oil), 5 cups 23.0
(Boston's Gourmet Super Premium), 2 cups 13.0
(Boston's Lite), 4 cups 19.0
(Boston's Lite), 1 oz. 18.0
(Little Bear 50% Less Oil), 3½ cups 20.0
air-popped, 1 cup...6.2
butter/butter flavor:
   (Bearitos Buttery), 2½ cups 14.0
   (Bearitos Buttery Lite), 3½ cups 19.0
   (Chester's), 3 cups 15.0
   (Chester's Microwave), 5 cups 22.0
   (Healthy Choice), 1 cup 4.0
   (Weight Watchers), 1 pkg.......................................14.0
   golden *(Smartfood* Reduced Fat), 3⅓ cups 21.0
butter toffee *(Cracker Jack* Fat Free), ¾ cup 26.0
butter toffee *(Weight Watchers),* 1 pkg............................21.0
caramel:
   (Boston's), ⅔ cup 23.0
   (Little Bear Fat Free) 1 cup....................................27.0
   (Weaver 97% Fat Free), ½ cup................................28.0
   (Weight Watchers), 1 pkg.......................................22.0
   with peanuts *(Cracker Jack* Fat Free), ¾ cup 26.0
   with peanuts *(Cracker Jack* Original), ½ cup 23.0
   with peanuts *(Estee),* 1 cup 26.0
   with peanuts *(Weaver),* ⅔ cup.................................23.0
cheese:
   cheddar *(Chester's),* 3 cups...................................17.0
   cheddar, white *(Bearitos),* 2⅓ cups..........................14.0
   cheddar, white *(Boston's* 40% Less Fat), 2¾ cups 17.0
   cheddar, white *(Smartfood)*.....................................17.0
   cheddar, white *(Smartfood* Reduced Fat), 3 cups 19.0
   cheddar, white *(Weight Watchers),* 1 pkg...................12.0
natural flavor *(Healthy Choice),* 1 cup..............................4.0
oil-popped, 1 cup...6.3
Popcorn cake:
plain *(Hain),* .3-oz. cake 8.0
plain, mini *(Hain),* 8 cakes, .5 oz...................................11.0
barbecue flavor, mini *(Hain),* 6 cakes, .5 oz. 11.0

Popcorn cake *(cont.)*

barbecue flavor, mini *(Orville Redenbacher's)*, .5 oz. 11.0
butter flavor:
   (Hain), .3-oz. cake 10.0
   (Orville Redenbacher's), .5 oz. 12.0
   mini *(Hain)*, 7 cakes, .5 oz. 10.0
butterscotch *(Orville Redenbacher's Clusters)*, 1.1 oz. 28.0
caramel flavor:
   (Hain), .45-oz. cake 11.0
   (Orville Redenbacher's), .5 oz. 14.0
   mini *(Hain)*, 6 cakes, .5 oz. 12.0
   mini *(Orville Redenbacher's)*, .5 oz. 13.0
caramel apple *(Quaker)*, .5 oz. 12.0
caramel chocolate chip *(Quaker)*, .5 oz. 13.0
cheddar:
   mild or white, mini *(Hain)*, 6 cakes, .5 oz. 10.0
   white *(Orville Redenbacher's)*, .5 oz. 11.5
   white, mild, grain *(Quaker)*, .4 oz. 8.0
chocolate *(Orville Redenbacher's)*, .5 oz. 13.0
nacho cheese, mini *(Orville Redenbacher's)*, .5 oz. 12.0
nuts *(Orville Redenbacher's Clusters)*, 1.1 oz. 25.0
peanut, mini *(Orville Redenbacher's)*, .5 oz. 10.5
rice *(Lundberg Organic)*, 1 cake 16.0
Poppyseed:
1 tbsp. 2.1
1 tsp. 7
Poppyseed filling, see "Pastry filling"
Porgy, see "Scup"
Pork (see also "Ham"):
fresh, without added ingredients, 4 oz. 0
cured:
   arm (picnic), roasted, 4 oz. 0
   blade roll, lean with fat, roasted, 4 oz. 4
   shoulder, blade roll, lean and fat, unheated, 13.3 oz.
     (yield from 1 lb. unheated) 1.4
Pork, pickled, hocks or tidbits *(Hormel)*, 2 oz. 0
Pork, refrigerated, 4 oz.:
all cuts, unseasoned *(Always Tender)* 0
loin filet and roast:
   honey mustard *(Always Tender)* 4.0
   lemon garlic *(Always Tender)* 1.0

mesquite barbecue *(Always Tender)*..................2.0
salsa *(Always Tender)*....................2.0
roast, au jus *(Always Tender)*.....................0
shoulder roast, boneless, country roast *(Always Tender)*............1.0
shoulder roast, onion garlic *(Always Tender)*...................2.0
tenderloin, peppercorn *(Always Tender)* 2.0
tenderloin, teriyaki *(Always Tender)* 4.0
Pork belly, raw, 1 oz...................0
Pork ear:
simmered, 1 ear, 3.9 oz. 2
frozen, raw, 1 ear, 4 oz................... .7
Pork dinner, frozen, 1 pkg.:
boneless rib, shaped, in sauce *(Swanson Hungry-Man),*
   14.1 oz. 74.0
boneless riblet *(Banquet Extra Helping),* 15.25 oz. 62.0
Pork entree, canned, chow mein *(Chun King Bi-Pack),* 1 cup.....9.0
Pork entree, frozen, 1 pkg.:
chop, country-fried *(Marie Callender's Meals),* 15 oz. 50.0
chop suey, with rice *(Michelina's Yu Sing),* 8.5 oz...................50.0
cutlet *(Banquet),* 10.25 oz...................38.0
cutlet, breaded *(Stouffer's Homestyle),* 10 oz. 35.0
fried rice, see "Rice dish, frozen"
honey-roasted *(Lean Cuisine Cafe Classics),* 9½ oz. 32.0
patty, herb-breaded *(Healthy Choice Entree),* 8 oz...................38.0
rib, boneless *(Banquet),* 10 oz. 40.0
and roasted potatoes *(Stouffer's Hearty Portions),* 15⅜ oz........70.0
Pork and beans, see "Baked beans" and specific bean listings
Pork gravy, ¼ cup:
(Franco-American Golden) 3.0
(Heinz Home Style) 3.0
Pork gravy mix, roasted *(Knorr Gravy Classics),* 1 tbsp.,
   ¼ cup* 4.0
Pork lunch meat:
canned, ¾-oz. slice................... .4
fresh roast *(Hansel 'n Gretel Healthy Deli),* 2 oz. 1.0
oven-roasted *(Sara Lee),* 2 oz...................1.0
Pork rinds, all varieties *(Baken-ets),* ½ oz...................<1.0
Pork sandwich, frozen, 1 piece:
barbecued *(Hormel Quick Meal),* 4.3 oz...................38.0
barbecued, rib-shaped *(Hormel Quick Meal),* 4.8 oz...................40.0

Pork seasoning and coating mix, ⅛ pkt.:

(Shake 'n Bake Original Recipe)...8.0

barbecue, honey mustard, or tangy honey *(Shake 'n Bake*
    Glazes)..9.0

extra crispy *(Oven Fry)*..11.0

hot and spicy *(Shake 'n Bake)*......................................7.0

Italian, classic *(Shake 'n Bake)*....................................7.0

Pot pie, see specific entree listings

Potato, fresh:

raw, with skin:

    (Dole), 1 medium, 5.3 oz................................26.0

    (Frieda's Baby/Fingerling/*Princess* La Ratte/Purple/Red/
      Yellow Finnish/Yukon Gold), ½ cup, 3 oz. 15.0

    1 large, 3"-4¼" diam., 6.5 oz...........................33.1

    1 long type, 2⅓" diam. x 4¾", 7.1 oz. 36.3

raw, skin only, from 1 potato, 1.3 oz. 4.7

baked:

    with skin, 2⅓" x 4¾", 7.1 oz.............................51.0

    with skin, ½ cup...15.4

    without skin, 1 potato, 2⅓" x 4¾", 5.5 oz. 33.6

    without skin, ½ cup..13.1

boiled in skin, peeled, 2½" diam., 4.8 oz. 27.4

boiled in skin, peeled, ½ cup 15.7

boiled, skin only, from 1 potato, 1.2 oz............................5.9

boiled without skin, 2½" diam......................................27.0

boiled without skin, ½ cup...15.7

microwaved in skin:

    unpeeled, 2½" diam., 7.1 oz..............................48.7

    peeled, 1 potato, 2⅓" X 4¾", 5.5 oz. 36.3

    peeled, ½ cup..18.1

    skin only, 2 oz. 17.2

au gratin, 1 cup..27.6

hash-browned, 1 cup 33.3

mashed, with whole milk, with butter or margarine, 1 cup.........35.1

scalloped, 1 cup...26.4

Potato, canned:

16-oz. can...44.9

drained, 1 cup...24.5

whole:

    (Butterfield), 2½ pieces, 5.6 oz........................20.0

(Del Monte), 2 medium, with liquid......................................13.0
   1 cup 29.7
   drained, 1.2-oz. potato 4.8
sliced *(Butterfield)*, ½ cup 22.0
sliced *(Del Monte)*, ⅔ cup 13.0
diced *(Butterfield)*, ⅔ cup 22.0
Potato, dehydrated, diced *(AlpineAire)*, ½ cup..........16.0
Potato, dried, see "Potato dish, mix"
Potato, frozen (see also "Potato dish, frozen"):
whole *(Birds Eye* Southern), 3 pieces 13.0
whole, baby *(Birds Eye)*, 7 pieces, 4 oz. 21.0
whole, unprepared, 1 cup 31.8
french-fried, crinkle-cut *(Empire* Kosher), 3 oz............21.0
french-fried:
   unprepared, 9-oz. pkg. 62.0
   unprepared, 10 pieces, 2.3 oz. 15.8
   oven-heated, 9-oz. pkg. 61.8
   oven-heated, 10 pieces, 1¾ oz..............................15.6
french-fried, partially fried:
   cottage-cut, unprepared, 9-oz. pkg. 61.1
   cottage-cut, unprepared, 10 pieces, 2.3 oz. 15.6
   cottage-cut, oven-heated, 9-oz. pkg. 67.4
   cottage-cut, oven-heated, 10 pieces, 1¾ oz. 17.0
   extruded, unprepared, 9-oz. pkg. 76.9
   extruded, unprepared, 10 pieces, 2.3 oz. 19.6
   extruded, oven-heated, 9-oz. pkg. 78.6
   extruded, oven-heated, 10 pieces., 1¾ oz.............19.8
fried:
   (Ore-Ida Deep Fries), 3 oz. 23.0
   (Ore-Ida Oven Chips), 7 pieces, 3 oz...................22.0
   (Ore-Ida Waffle Fries), 3 oz., approx. 9 pieces 21.0
   (Ore-Ida Wedges), 8 pieces, 3 oz. 18.0
   (Ore-Ida Crispy Crunchies!)*, 3 oz., approx. 13 pieces 20.0
   (Ore-Ida Fast Food Fries), 3 oz., approx. 35 pieces...............22.0
   (Ore-Ida Golden Crinkles), 3 oz., approx. 13 pieces.............19.0
   (Ore-Ida Golden Fries), 3 oz., approx. 13 pieces 20.0
   (Ore-Ida Golden Twirls), 3 oz., approx. 17 pieces 22.0
hash browns:
   (Ore-Ida Toaster), 2 patties, 3.6 oz.....................25.0
   unprepared, 12-oz. pkg. 60.2
   unprepared, ½ cup...18.6

Potato, frozen, hash browns *(cont.)*
    prepared, 1 oval patty, 3" x 1½" x ½" 8.1
    prepared, ½ cup 21.9
    with butter sauce, unprepared, 6-oz. pkg. 31.1
    Southern style *(Ore-Ida)*, ⅔ cup 16.0
mashed *(Boston Market)*, ½ cup 23.0
O'Brien hash browns *(Ore-Ida)*, ¾ cup 14.0
patty *(Ore-Ida Golden Patties)*, 2.2-oz. patty..............14.0
puffs:
    (Ore-Ida Tater Tots), 9 pieces, 3 oz. 21.0
    unprepared, 1 cup 31.1
    prepared, 1 cup 39.0
    prepared, 1 puff 2.1
    onion *(Ore-Ida Tater Tots)*, 9 pieces, 3 oz. 21.0
Potato, stuffed, see "Potato dish, frozen"
Potato, sweet, see "Sweet potato"
Potato and cheddar pocket, frozen *(Ken & Robert's Veggie Pockets)*, 4.5-oz. piece 42.0
Potato chips and crisps, 1 oz., except as noted:
(Air Crisps)...21.0
(Barbara's/Barbara's No Salt/Ripple) 15.0
(Hain Baked Crisps Original) 23.0
(Harry's Hampton Recipe).......................................12.0
(Harry's Hampton Recipe), 1¼-oz. pkg. 19.0
(Herr's)...16.0
(Lay's Baked Original) 23.0
(Lay's Classic/Limon/Wavy Original) 15.0
(Lay's Deli Style Original/Unsalted) 16.0
(Lay's Wow Original)..18.0
(Little Bear) 15.0
(Ruffles Baked) 24.0
(Ruffles Buffalo Style) 16.0
(Ruffles Original/The Works) 14.0
(Ruffles Reduced Fat Regular) 18.0
(Ruffles Wow Original) 17.0
(Sun Chips Original)..19.0
(Tastee Yukon Gold)..19.0
(Terra Yukon Gold Original)......................................19.0
(Westbrae Natural Organic No Salt) 15.0
barbecue:
    (Air Crisps)...21.0

(Andy Capp Fries)...19.0
(Lay's/Ruffles KC Masterpiece)................................15.0
(Terra Yukon Gold) 19.0
baked (Lay's KC Masterpiece)................................22.0
and cheddar (Ruffles Flavor Rush)..........................15.0
Louisiana (Hain Baked Crisps) 23.0
mesquite (Lay's Wow)..17.0
spicy (Lay's)..16.0
cheddar:
(Andy Capp Fries)..17.0
(Sun Chips Harvest) 19.0
white (Andy Capp Steak Fries), 1.75-oz. bag............30.0
cheddar and sour cream:
(Ruffles) 14.0
(Ruffles Baked)..25.0
(Ruffles Wow) 16.0
cheese (Lay's Cracker Barrel)....................................16.0
hot:
(Andy Capp Fries)..18.0
(Chester's Fries Flamin' Hot) 17.0
(Lay's Flamin' Hot) 16.0
(Ruffles Flamin' Hot) 15.0
onion, French (Ruffles) 15.0
onion, French (Sun Chips) 18.0
onion and cheese, toasted (Lay's).............................14.0
onion and garlic (Terra Yukon Gold) 19.0
ranch (Air Crisps), 1.1 oz..21.0
salsa (Andy Capp Fries) 18.0
salsa (Chester's Fries Flamin' Hot) 18.0
salt and pepper (Terra Yukon Gold) 19.0
salt and vinegar:
(Lay's)..15.0
(Terra Yukon Gold) 20.0
sour cream and chive (Lay's Wow)............................17.0
sour cream and onion:
(Air Crisps)..21.0
(Lay's)...12.0
(Ruffles Flavor Rush Zesty) 15.0
baked (Lay's)...21.0
sticks:
(Butterfield), 1 cup, 1.7 oz. 26.0

346 *Corinne T. Netzer*

Potato chips and crisps, sticks *(cont.)*
   (Butterfield), ⅔ cup, 1 oz...................................16.0
   (French's), .6 oz...11.0
sweet potato:
   (Harry's Hampton Recipe).............................15.0
   (Tastee)...17.0
   (Terra Chips Original No Salt)........................18.0
   cinnamon nutmeg *(Tastee)*.............................17.0
   jalapeño or mesquite barbecue *(Terra Chips)*......18.0
   salsa *(Terra Chips)*.......................................20.0
   spiced *(Terra Chips)*......................................16.0
tomato basil *(Harry's Hampton Recipe)*.................15.0
tomato basil *(Harry's Hampton Recipe)*, 1¼-oz. pkg....19.0
yogurt and green onion *(Barbara's)*.......................15.0
yogurt and green onion *(Terra* Yukon Gold)............19.0
Potato dish, canned or packaged:
au gratin, with *Cure 81* ham *(Dinty Moore American
   Classics)*, 1 bowl..29.0
scalloped, with ham *(Hormel* Microcup Meals), 1 cup....20.0
Potato dish, frozen, 1 pkg., except as noted:
au gratin:
   (Marie Callender's Skillet Meals), ⅔ cup.........19.0
   (Stouffer's Side Dish), ½ cup.........................15.0
   ham and broccoli *(Banquet* Family Size), ⅔ cup....16.0
baby blend *(Birds Eye)*, 2.6 oz............................9.0
cheddar, deluxe *(Lean Cuisine Everyday Favorites)*, 10⅜ oz....37.0
cheddar-broccoli *(Healthy Choice* Entree), 10.5 oz....53.0
mashed, with beef or chicken gravy *(Larry's* Classic),
   4.46-oz. pkg..21.0
pancakes, see "Potato pancake"
pot pie, cheesy, and broccoli with ham *(Banquet)*, 7 oz....40.0
roasted, with broccoli *(Lean Cuisine Everyday Favorites)*,
   10¼ oz...39.0
roasted, with ham *(Healthy Choice* Bowl), 8.5 oz....26.0
scalloped *(Stouffer's* 40 oz.), ½ cup...................19.0
scalloped *(Stouffer's* Side Dish 11½ oz.), ½ cup....18.0
stuffed, cheddar or onion, sour cream and chives
   (OhBoy!), 1 piece...22.0
whipped, with bacon and cheese or cheese *(Ore-Ida)*,
   5-oz. pkg..23.0

Potato dish, mix:

Alfredo *(Knorr Skillet Potatoes)*, ½ cup 20.0

au gratin:

    (Betty Crocker), ½ cup* 22.0

    (Betty Crocker 9 oz.), ½ cup* 23.0

    ⅙ of 5.5-oz. pkg., prepared with water, milk, butter 17.6

broccoli au gratin *(Betty Crocker)*, ½ cup* 21.0

broccoli and cheddar *(Fantastic Foods
Stuffed-Mashed Cup)*, 1.7 oz 35.0

butter, sweet creamery *(Fantastic Foods
Stuffed-Mashed Cup)*, 1.8 oz 36.0

and cheddar *(Fantastic Foods Stuffed-Mashed)*, ¼ cup 20.0

and cheddar, with chives *(AlpineAire)*, 1 cup 39.0

cheddar:

    (Betty Crocker Homestyle), ½ cup* 21.0

    (Fantastic Foods Stuffed-Mashed), ¼ cup 21.0

    (Fantastic Foods Stuffed-Mashed Cup), 1.7 oz 35.0

    flavor, cheesy *(Knorr Skillet Potatoes)*, ½ cup 19.0

cheddar and bacon *(Betty Crocker)*, ½ cup* 21.0

cheddar and bacon, twice-baked *(Betty Crocker)*, ⅔ cup* 22.0

cheddar and sour cream *(Betty Crocker)*, ½ cup* 25.0

cheese, three *(Betty Crocker)*, ½ cup* 23.0

chicken, creamy, and vegetable *(Betty Crocker)*, ⅔ cup* 24.0

garlic, roasted *(Knorr Skillet Potatoes)*, ⅔ cup 23.0

garlic and herbs *(Fantastic Foods Stuffed-Mashed)*, ¼ cup 22.0

garlic and herbs *(Fantastic Foods
Stuffed-Mashed Cup)*, 1.7 oz 37.0

hash browns:

    (Betty Crocker), ½ cup* 30.0

    cheesy *(Knorr Skillet Potatoes)*, ⅓ cup 22.0

    onion *(Knorr Skillet Potatoes)*, ⅓ cup 20.0

    with peppers and tomato *(AlpineAire Reds & Greens)*,
    1¼ cups 44.0

jalapeño jack cheese *(Fantastic Foods
Stuffed-Mashed Cup)*, 1.8 oz 36.0

julienne *(Betty Crocker)*, ½ cup* 21.0

mashed:

    (Betty Crocker Potato Buds), ½ cup* 19.0

    (Hungry Jack), ½ cup* 18.0

    (Pillsbury Idaho), ½ cup* 20.0

    flakes, without milk, unprepared *(Barbara's)*, ⅓ cup 17.0

Potato dish, mix, mashed *(cont.)*

   flakes, prepared with milk and butter, 1 cup 31.5

   granules, without milk, prepared with milk and butter,
     1 cup..30.2

   granules, with milk, prepared with water and margarine,
     1 cup..27.5

   butter, creamy *(Betty Crocker)*, ½ cup* 20.0

   butter and herb *(Betty Crocker)*, ½ cup* 20.0

   cheddar, white *(Nile Spice* Chef Express), 1 cont. 29.0

   cheddar, white, creamy *(Near East)*, 1 cont.......................49.0

   cheddar and bacon *(Betty Crocker)*, ½ cup*.......................20.0

   cheese, four *(Betty Crocker)*, ½ cup* 20.0

   chicken and herb *(Betty Crocker)*, ½ cup*..........................21.0

   red, roasted garlic and rosemary *(Near East)*, 1 cont...........34.0

   roasted garlic *(Betty Crocker)*, ½ cup* 19.0

   roasted garlic and rosemary *(Nile Spice* Chef
     Express), 1 cont..32.0

   sour cream and chives *(Betty Crocker)*, ½ cup* 21.0

  mashed, and gravy:

   beef gravy, hearty *(Betty Crocker)*, ¾ cup* 24.0

   brown gravy *(Hungry Jack)*, ⅓ flakes, 1 tbsp. mix 20.0

   chicken gravy *(Hungry Jack)*, ⅓ flakes, 1 tbsp. mix 21.0

   chicken gravy, roasted *(Betty Crocker)*, ¾ cup*..................25.0

  ranch *(Betty Crocker)*, ½ cup*...25.0

  scalloped:

   (Betty Crocker), ½ cup*..23.0

   ⅙ of 5.5-oz. pkg., prepared with water, milk, and butter 17.5

   cheesy *(Betty Crocker* Homestyle), ½ cup* 21.0

   creamy, cheese and bacon *(Knorr* Skillet Potatoes),
     ½ cup 18.0

  sour cream and chives:

   (Betty Crocker), ½ cup* 22.0

   (Fantastic Foods Stuffed-Mashed), ¼ cup..........................21.0

   (Fantastic Foods Stuffed-Mashed Cup), 1.7 oz..................37.0

  Southwestern style *(Knorr* Skillet Potatoes), ½ cup 25.0

Potato flour, 1 cup..132.9

Potato knish, refrigerated *(Joshua's Coney Island)*, 1 piece 59.0

Potato pancake, frozen:

(Dr. Praeger's Homestyle), 1.5-oz. cake 10.0

(Empire Kosher), 2-oz. cake...15.0

(Ratner's), 1.5-oz. cake 12.0

(Tofutti), 1.33-oz. cake 10.0
mini *(Empire* Kosher), 12 cakes, 3 oz. 19.0
Potato salad, refrigerated:
(Blue Ridge Farms), ½ cup..22.0
(Chef's Express), 4 oz. 16.0
Potato seasoning mix:
cheddar, crispy *(Shake 'n Bake)*, ⅙ pkt. 2.0
herb and garlic *(Shake 'n Bake)*, ⅙ pkt............................5.0
home fries *(Shake 'n Bake)*, ⅙ pkt....................................5.0
Potato seasoning mix *(cont.)*
Parmesan peppercorn *(Shake 'n Bake)*, ⅙ pkt...................3.0
savory onion *(Shake 'n Bake)*, ⅙ pkt.................................5.0
Potato sticks, see "Potato chips and crisps"
Poultry, see specific listings
Poultry salad spread, 1 tbsp...1.0
Poultry seasoning:
1 tbsp..2.4
1 tsp..1.0
Pout, ocean, without added ingredients.............................0
Praline sauce, pecan *(Trader Vic's)*, 2 tbsp. 21.0
Preserves, see "Jam and preserves"
Pretzel:
(Air Crisps Fat Free), 23 pieces, 1 oz. 23.0
(Air Crisps Original), 1 oz. 22.0
(Estee Unsalted), 23 pieces...25.0
(Pepperidge Farm Goldfish), 43 pieces, 1.1 oz. 22.0
cheese, cheddar *(Combos)*, 1.8-oz. bag 35.0
cheese, cheddar, twists *(Rold Gold* Tiny), 1 oz. 22.0
cheese, nacho *(Combos)*, 1.8-oz. bag.............................34.0
Dutch *(Estee)*, 2 pieces 26.0
honey mustard:
    (Harry's), ½ cup, 1 oz. 23.0
    (Harry's), 1.5-oz. pkg. 35.0
    twists *(Rold Gold* Tiny), 1 oz.............................22.0
honey wheat *(Harry's)*, .85-oz. piece..............................20.0
honey wheat *(Harry's Whole Wheat Honeys)*, .85-oz. piece........24.0
mini *(Harry's)*, 1 oz. 24.0
pizza flavor *(Combos* Pizzeria), 1.8-oz. bag 35.0
rods *(Bachman)*, 1.1 oz...24.0
rods *(Rold Gold)*, 1 oz. 22.0

Pretzel *(cont.)*
sourdough:

(Harry's), .9-oz. piece	23.0
(Harry's), 1.65-oz. pkg.	25.0
(Harry's Everything), .85-oz. piece	23.0
hard *(Rold Gold)*, 1 oz.	21.0
nuggets *(Harry's)*, 14 pieces, 1.1 oz.	25.0
nuggets *(Harry's)*, 1.5-oz. pkg.	38.0
nuggets *(Rold Gold)*, 1 oz.	23.0

sticks:

(Bachman Stix), 1 oz.	20.0
(Harry's), 1 oz.	24.0
(Rold Gold Classic/Thin), 1 oz.	23.0

twists:

(Bachman),	22.0
(Rold Gold Classic/Tiny)	23.0
10 twists, 2.1 oz.	47.6
mini *(Little Debbie)*, 1.5 oz.	33.0

Pretzel, soft:

(Act II Big Softy), 2.3-oz. piece	35.0
(Superpretzel), 2¼-oz. piece	36.0
bites *(Superpretzel)*, 5 bites, 1.9 oz.	32.0
cheddar-filled *(Superpretzel)*, 2 pieces, 1.8 oz.	24.0

Prickly pear, fresh, raw:

(Frieda's Cactus Pear), 5 oz.	13.0
trimmed, 1 prickly pear, 3.6 oz.	9.9
1 cup	14.3

Prosciutto *(Boar's Head)*, 1 oz. | 0

Prunes, canned:

(Sonoma Organic), 3–4 prunes, 1.4 oz.	26.0
in heavy syrup, 5 prunes with 2 tbsp. liquid	23.9
in heavy syrup, 1 cup	65.1

Prunes, dehydrated:

uncooked, 1 cup	117.6
stewed, 1 cup	83.2

Prunes, dried:

pitted *(Dole)*, ¼ cup	26.0
pitted *(Sonoma* Organic), ¼ cup, 1.4 oz.	29.0
uncooked, .3 oz.	5.3
uncooked, pitted, 1 cup	106.6
stewed, pitted, 1 cup	69.6

stewed, with sugar, pitted, 1 cup 81.5
Prune juice, 8 fl. oz.:
(R.W. Knudsen Organic) 45.0
(Sunsweet)...42.0
canned 44.7
Prune filling, see "Pastry filling"
Pudding, ready-to-eat, 4-oz. cont., except as noted:
all flavors (Jell-O Free Fat Free Snacks) 23.0
banana:
   (Kozy Shack) 22.0
   (Kraft Handi-Snacks), 3.5-oz. cont. 22.0
   5-oz. can...30.1
   cream (Swiss Miss), 3.5-oz. cont...20.0
butterscotch (Kraft Handi-Snacks), 3.5-oz. cont. 22.0
butterscotch (Swiss Miss)...23.0
chocolate:
   (Jell-O Snacks) 28.0
   (Kozy Shack) 24.0
   (Kozy Shack No Sugar) 17.0
   (Kraft Handi-Snacks), 3.5-oz. cont. 23.0
   (Kraft Handi-Snacks Fat Free), 3.5-oz. cont.........................21.0
   (Swiss Miss)..26.0
   (Swiss Miss Fat Free), 3.5-oz. cont. 19.0
   cream (Swiss Miss), 3.5-oz. cont...21.0
   milk (Swiss Miss)..27.0
   5-oz. can...32.4
chocolate-caramel swirl (Swiss Miss).......................................26.0
chocolate fudge (Kraft Handi-Snacks), 3.5-oz. cont...............23.0
chocolate fudge (Swiss Miss Fat Free) 22.0
chocolate-marshmallow (Jell-O Snacks) 27.0
chocolate/vanilla swirls (Jell-O Snacks) 27.0
coconut cream (Swiss Miss), 3.5-oz. cont...............................21.0
flan (Kozy Shack) 25.0
lemon, 5-oz. can..35.5
mocha cream (Swiss Miss), 3.5-oz. cont.................................21.0
plum, see "Plum pudding"
rice, see "Rice pudding"
tapioca:
   (Jell-O Snacks) 26.0
   (Kozy Shack) 25.0
   (Kraft Handi-Snacks), 3.5-oz. cont. 21.0

Pudding, tapioca *(cont.)*

   (Swiss Miss)..24.0
   (Swiss Miss Fat Free), 3.5-oz. cont. 18.0
   5-oz. can...27.5

vanilla:

   (Jell-O Snacks) 25.0
   (Kozy Shack) 22.0
   (Kozy Shack No Sugar) 17.0
   (Kraft Handi-Snacks), 3.5-oz. cont. 22.0
   (Kraft Handi-Snacks Fat Free), 3.5-oz. cont...........21.0
   (Swiss Miss)..24.0
   (Swiss Miss Fat Free), 3.5-oz. cont. 17.0

vanilla/chocolate parfait *(Swiss Miss)* 25.0
vanilla/chocolate parfait *(Swiss Miss* Fat Free), 3.5-oz. cont. 18.0

Pudding, nondairy, ready-to-eat, 3.75-oz. cont.:

banana or butterscotch *(Imagine)*........................28.0
chocolate *(Imagine)* 34.0
lemon *(Imagine)*...31.0

Pudding and pie filling mix, ½ cup*, except as noted:

banana:

   whole milk 25.3
   2% milk 25.5
   instant, whole milk 28.8
   instant, 2% milk 29.1
   skim milk *(Jell-O* Instant Fat/Sugar Free) 12.0

banana cream, 2% milk *(Jell-O* Cook & Serve)...........26.0
banana cream, 2% milk *(Jell-O* Instant)....................29.0
butterscotch, 2% milk *(Jell-O* Cook & Serve) 30.0
butterscotch, 2% milk *(Jell-O* Instant) 29.0
butterscotch, skim milk *(Jell-O* Instant Fat/Sugar Free).............12.0

chocolate:

   whole milk 25.6
   2% milk *(Jell-O* Cook & Serve) 28.0
   2% milk *(Jell-O* Cook & Serve Sugar Free) 13.0
   2% milk *(Jell-O* Instant) 31.0
   2% milk 28.0
   instant, 2% milk 27.8
   skim milk *(Jell-O* Cook & Serve Fat Free)..............29.0
   skim milk *(Jell-O* Instant Fat Free) 31.0
   skim milk *(Jell-O* Instant Fat/Sugar Free) 14.0

chocolate, milk, 2% milk *(Jell-O* Cook & Serve) 28.0

chocolate, white, skim milk *(Jell-O* Instant Fat Free) 29.0
chocolate, white, skim milk *(Jell-O* Instant Fat/Sugar Free) 12.0
chocolate fudge:
   2% milk *(Jell-O* Cook & Serve) 28.0
   2% milk *(Jell-O* Instant) 31.0
   skim milk *(Jell-O* Instant Fat/Sugar Free) 14.0
coconut cream, 2% milk *(Jell-O* Cook & Serve) 24.0
coconut cream, 2% milk *(Jell-O* Instant) 27.0
coconut creme:
   whole milk 24.8
   2% milk 24.9
   instant, whole milk 28.1
   instant, 2% milk 28.2
custard:
   whole milk 23.4
   2% milk *(Jell-O Americana)* 25.0
   2% milk 23.5
   chocolate *(Junket* Rennet), ½ cup dry 12.0
   raspberry or strawberry *(Junket* Rennet), ½ cup dry.............10.0
devil's food, skim milk *(Jell-O* Instant Fat Free) 31.0
flan:
   (Goya Spanish Style Custard), .5 oz. mix 13.0
   2% milk *(Jell-O* Cook & Serve) 26.0
   caramel, whole milk..25.4
   caramel, 2% milk..25.5
lemon:
   2% milk *(Jell-O* Cook & Serve) 29.0
   2% milk *(Jell-O* Instant) 29.0
   instant, whole milk 29.5
   instant, 2% milk 29.7
pistachio, 2% milk *(Jell-O* Instant)..29.0
raspberry or strawberry *(Junket Danish Dessert),* ½ cup dry 33.0
rennet, see "Rennet dessert mix"
rice, see "Rice pudding mix"
tapioca:
   whole milk 27.6
   2% milk *(Jell-O Americana)* 28.0
   2% milk 27.8
vanilla:
   whole milk 25.9
   2% milk *(Jell-O* Cook & Serve) 26.0

Pudding and pie filling mix, vanilla *(cont.)*

2% milk *(Jell-O Cook & Serve Sugar Free)*	11.0
2% milk *(Jell-O Instant)*	29.0
2% milk	26.2
skim milk *(Jell-O Cook & Serve Fat Free)*	28.0
skim milk *(Jell-O Instant Fat Free)*	29.0
skim milk *(Jell-O Instant Fat/Sugar Free)*	12.0
French, 2% milk *(Jell-O Instant)*	29.0

Pudding bar, frozen *(Eskimo Pie Variety Pack),*
1.75-fl.-oz. bar ... 15.0

Puff pastry, see "Pastry shell"

Pummelo, fresh, raw:

(Frieda's), 5 oz.	13.0
1 medium, 5½" diam., 2.4 lbs.	58.6
trimmed, 1 pummelo, 1⅓ lbs.	58.6
sections, 1 cup	18.3

Pumpkin, fresh:

raw, cubed, 1 cup	7.5
boiled, drained, mashed, 1 cup	12.0
mini *(Frieda's),* ¾ cup, 3 oz.	6.0

Pumpkin, canned, ½ cup:

(Comstock)	10.0
(Libby's)	15.0
(Shari Ann's Organic)	10.0
(Stokely)	10.0

Pumpkin flower, fresh:

raw, 1 cup	1.1
raw, 1 flower	<.1
boiled, drained, 1 cup	4.4

Pumpkin leaf, fresh:

raw, 1 cup	.9
boiled, drained, 1 cup	2.4

Pumpkin pie spice:

1 tbsp.	3.9
1 tsp.	1.2

Pumpkin and squash seeds:

dried, 1 oz.	5.0
dried, 1 cup	24.6
roasted, in shell, salted or unsalted, 1 cup	34.4
roasted, in shell, salted or unsalted, 1 oz. or 85 seeds	15.2

Punch, see "Fruit drink blend" and specific fruit listings
Purslane:
raw, untrimmed, 1 lb...11.8
raw, 1 cup 1.5
boiled, drained, 1 cup 4.1

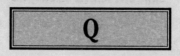

Q

FOOD AND MEASURE	CARBOHYDRATE GRAMS
Quail, without added ingredients	0
Quesadilla, frozen *(Cedarlane),* 3 pieces, ⅓ pkg.	27.0
Quince, fresh, raw:	
(Frieda's), 5 oz.	21.0
trimmed, 1 quince, 3.2 oz.	14.1
Quinoa, uncooked:	
(Eden), ¼ cup	31.0
1 oz.	19.5
1 cup	117.1
Quinoa seeds *(Arrowhead Mills),* ¼ cup	25.0

R

Rabbit, without added ingredients......................................0
Radiatore pasta dish, mix:
Alfredo primavera sauce *(Land O Lakes International
   Pasta Collection),* 2.5 oz.....................................45.0
and mixed beans *(Marrakesh Express* Pasta & Sauce),
   ⅓ cup, 1 cup*...41.0
Radicchio, fresh:
(Frieda's), ⅔ cup, 3 oz...4.0
1 leaf, .3 oz.. .4
shredded, 1 cup 1.8
Radish, fresh, raw:
1 large, 1"–1¼" diam.. .3
sliced, 1 cup..4.2
Radish, black *(Frieda's),* ¾ cup, 3 oz........................3.0
Radish, Oriental:
(Frieda's Daikon), ½ cup, 1.1 oz. 1.0
(Frieda's Korean), ⅔ cup, 3 oz.................................3.0
(Frieda's Lo Bak), ⅔ cup, 3 oz.................................5.0
raw, 7"-long radish, 11.9 oz.......................................13.9
boiled, drained, sliced, 1 cup 5.0
dried, 1 cup...73.5
Radish, white icicle, fresh, raw:
7"-long radish, .6 oz... .4
sliced, ½ cup 1.3
Radish leaves, 1 oz..2.8
Radish sprouts, 1 cup:
(Jonathan's) 3.0
(Jonathan's Gourmet) 4.0
seeds, fresh, raw...1.4
Raisins:
seeded, not packed, 1 cup 113.8
seeded, packed, 1 cup..129.5
seedless:
   (Dole California), ¼ cup 31.0

Raisins, seedless *(cont.)*
(*Sonoma* Organic Monukka/Thompson), ¼ cup, 1.4 oz........31.0
(*Sun•Maid*), ¼ cup 31.0
not packed, 1 cup 114.7
packed, 1 cup 130.6
seedless, golden, not packed, 1 cup 115.3
seedless, golden, packed, 1 cup 131

Raisin filling, see "Pie filling"
Raisin sauce *(Reese),* ¼ cup 36.0
Rambutan, canned, 1 cup:
in syrup...44.7
in syrup, drained 31.3

Ranch dip, 2 tbsp.:
(*Breakstone's Free*) 4.0
(*Knudsen Free*) 4.0
(*Kraft*)..3.0
(*Kraft* Premium Sour Cream) 2.0
(*Kraft Free*) 4.0
Ranch dip mix, cracked pepper *(Knorr),* ½ tsp......................<1.0
Rapini, see "Broccoli rabe"

Raspberries, fresh:
(*Dole*), 1 cup, 3 oz. 10.0
1 pint 36.1
1 cup 14.2

Raspberries, canned, in heavy syrup:
(*Oregon*), ½ cup 30.0
1 cup 59.8

Raspberries, frozen, sweetened:
(*Birds Eye*), ½ cup 22.0
10-oz. pkg. 74.3
unthawed, 1 cup 65.4

Raspberry baking chips, see "Chocolate, baking"
Raspberry drink, 8 fl. oz.:
blue *(Kool-Aid Splash)* 30.0
ice *(Crystal Light)*...0
mix* *(Kool-Aid)*...25.0
mix* *(Kool-Aid* Sugar Sweetened) 17.0

Raspberry drink blend, 8 fl. oz.:
cherry *(R.W. Knudsen Razzleberry)* 33.0
cherry *(R.W. Knudsen Razzleberry* Aseptic)............................29.0
hibiscus tea *(R.W. Knudsen)*...23.0

lemonade *(Santa Cruz Organic)* 24.0
lemonade *(Turkey Hill)* 29.0
peach *(Snapple)* 29.0
nectar *(Santa Cruz Organic)* 30.0
mix*, cranberry *(Kool-Aid Roarin' Raspberry-Cranberry)* 25.0
mix*, cranberry *(Kool-Aid Roarin' Raspberry-Cranberry*
   Sugar Sweetened) 17.0
Raspberry filling, see "Pastry filling"
Raspberry juice *(Dole Country)*, 8 fl. oz. 35.0
Raspberry juice blend:
(Mott's), 11.5-fl.-oz. can 41.0
apple *(Rocket Juice Rockin' Razzberry)*, 16 fl. oz. 63.0
peach *(R.W. Knudsen)*, 8 fl. oz. 31.0
Raspberry syrup, red, ¼ cup:
(Maple Grove Farms) 60.0
(Smucker's) 52.0
red *(Knott's Berry Farm)* 52.0
Raspberry-tamarind dipping sauce *(Helen's Tropical*
   Exotics), 2 tbsp. 11.0
Ratatouille, in jar *(Life in Provence)*, ½ cup 9.0
Ravioli, refrigerated:
artichoke, in lemon parsley pasta *(Cafferata)*, ½ pkg., 4.5 oz.....43.0
beef *(Contadina Buitoni)*, 1 cup 46.0
black bean in fiesta pasta *(Cafferata)*, ½ pkg., 4.5 oz. 37.0
cheese:
   (Contadina Buitoni), 1 cup...38.0
   (Di Giorno Light), 1 cup 40.0
   four *(Contadina Buitoni Light)*, 1 cup................................37.0
   four *(Di Giorno)*, 1 cup 40.0
chicken, roasted, and garlic *(Contadina Buitoni)*, 1¼ cups.........45.0
chicken herb parmigiana *(Contadina Buitoni)*, 1¼ cups 44.0
sausage, Italian, in green bell pepper pasta *(Di Giorno)*,
   1¼ cups 45.0
tomato, sun-dried *(Di Giorno)*, 1⅓ cups...............................48.0
vegetable, garden *(Contadina Buitoni)*, 1 cup 39.0
Ravioli entree, canned or packaged:
beef:
   (Chef Boyardee), 1 cup..37.0
   (Chef Boyardee 99% Fat Free), 1 cup................................41.0
   (Chef Boyardee Overstuffed), 1 cup 47.0
   (Chef Boyardee Mini Ravioli), 1 cup..................................37.0

Ravioli entree, canned or packaged, beef *(cont.)*

    (Dinty Moore American Classics), 1 bowl 34.0

    in meat sauce *(Franco-American* Superiore), 1 cup 41.0

    mini *(Kid's Kitchen)*, 1 cup 35.0

    with pasta, in tomato and cheese *(Franco-American)*,

        1 cup...42.0

    in tomato meat sauce *(Chef Boyardee)*, 1 cup 35.0

    in tomato meat sauce *(Chef Boyardee* Overstuffed),

        1 cup...47.0

cheese *(Chef Boyardee* 99% Fat Free)*, 1 cup 44.0

sausage, Italian *(Chef Boyardee* Overstuffed)*, 1 cup 53.0

tomato sauce *(Hormel* Microcup Meals)*, 1 cup.........................35.0

Ravioli entree, frozen, 1 pkg.:

(Michelina's Ravin' Ravioli)*, 8.5 oz. 48.0

cheese:

    (Lean Cuisine Everyday Favorites), 8½ oz...........................38.0

    (Stouffer's), 10⅝ oz. 58.0

    with Alfredo and broccoli sauce *(Michelina's)*, 8 oz. 42.0

    jumbo *(Michelina's)*, 11 oz. 53.0

    in marinara sauce, with spirals and garlic bread *(Marie

        Callender's* Meals)*, 16 oz..96.0

    parmigiana *(Healthy Choice* Entree)*, 9 oz. 44.0

    with sauce *(Amy's)*, 8 oz. 44.0

    and tomato sauce *(Freezer Queen* Deluxe Family

        Entree)*, 1 cup...47.0

    tomato sauce with peas, carrots, and brownie *(Freezer

        Queen* Meal)*, 7.75-oz. pkg...57.0

meat, with Pomodoro sauce *(Michelina's)*, 8 oz. 41.0

Red beans, canned (see also "Kidney beans"), ½ cup:

(Allens)...19.0

(Joan of Arc)...19.0

(Westbrae Natural)..16.0

small *(Eden* Organic)*..17.0

small *(Goya)*..18.0

Red snapper, without added ingredients 0

Redfish, without added ingredients 0

Refried beans, dried, mixed, with cheese *(AlpineAire)*, 1 cup 27.0

Refried beans, canned, ½ cup:

(Allens)...24.0

(Bearitos Fat Free)*..20.0

(Bearitos Low Fat Traditional)* 23.0

(Chi-Chi's Fiesta/Fat Free)	20.0
(Gebhardt Fat Free)	16.0
(Greene's Farm)	20.0
(Hain Canola Oil)	17.0
(Ortega Traditional)	25.0
(Rosarita Authentic)	15.0
(Rosarita Fat Free)	28.0
(Taco Bell Home Originals)	23.0
(Taco Bell Home Originals Fat Free)	21.0
all varieties *(Shari Ann's* Organic)	20.0

black beans:

(Bearitos Fat Free)	20.0
(Bearitos Low Fat)	22.0
(Greene's Farm)	19.0
(Rosarita Low Fat)	19.0
with green chilies and spices *(Greene's Farm)*	17.0
vegetarian *(Hain)*	18.0

green chilies:

(Bearitos Fat Free)	19.0
(Rosarita)	17.0
and spices *(Greene's Farm)*	19.0
jalapeño *(Gebhardt)*	18.0
mild chilies *(Taco Bell Home Originals* Fat Free)	20.0
pinto beans *(Bearitos* Low Fat No Salt)	23.0
pinto beans, spicy *(Bearitos* Low Fat)	24.0
spicy *(Rosarita)*	16.0
vegetable *(Chi-Chi's)*	18.0

vegetarian:

(Gebhardt)	15.0
(Hain)	16.0
(Rosarita)	18.0
Refried beans, mix *(Fantastic Foods* Instant), ⅓ cup	29.0
Relish, see "Pickle relish" and specific listings	
Relish, Indian (see also specific listings), mixed, hot *(Patak's)*, 1 tbsp.	<1.0
Remoulade sauce *(Zatarain's)*, ¼ cup	9.0
Rennet, tablets:	
(Junket), 1 tablet	0
unsweetened, .35-oz. pkg.	2.0
Rennet dessert mix, ½ cup:	
chocolate, whole milk	18.1

Rennet dessert mix *(cont.)*
chocolate, 2% milk...18.4
vanilla, whole milk..16.2
vanilla, 2% milk...16.4
Rhubarb, fresh:
1.8-oz. stalk 2.3
diced, 1 cup 5.5
Rhubarb, canned, in extra heavy syrup *(Oregon)*, ½ cup..........44.0
Rhubarb, frozen:
uncooked, diced, 1 cup 7.0
cooked with sugar, 1 cup 74.9
Rice, ¼ cup dry, except as noted:
Arborio, see "white," below
blend:
   (Lundberg Christmas) 37.0
   black japonica *(Lundberg/Lundberg* Organic) 38.0
   brown *(Lundberg* Countrywild/Wild Blend) 35.0
   brown *(Lundberg* Jubilee) 39.0
   brown *(Lundberg* Organic Wild Blend)................35.0
   brown and wild *(Lundberg* Organic California)................34.0
brown:
   (Fantastic Foods) 36.0
   (Lundberg Royal) 38.0
   (Success), ½ cup 33.0
   basmati *(Arrowhead Mills)* 33.0
   basmati *(Lundberg* Organic California).................34.0
   basmati *(Lundberg Nutra-Farmed* California) 38.0
   wehani *(Lundberg/Lundberg* Organic)....................38.0
brown, long-grain:
   (Arrowhead Mills)..33.0
   (Carolina)..32.0
   (Lundberg Organic) 38.0
   (Lundberg Nutra-Farmed)....................................37.0
   (Mahatma/River)..32.0
   1 cup* 44.8
brown, medium-grain *(Lundberg* Organic Golden Rose) 34.0
brown, medium-grain, 1 cup*................................45.8
brown, short-grain:
   (Arrowhead Mills)..36.0
   (Lundberg Organic) 40.0
   (Lundberg Nutra-Farmed)....................................40.0

brown, whole-grain, instant *(Minute)*, about ⅔ cup* 34.0
jasmine:
    (Fantastic Foods) 38.0
    (Mahatma Thai Fragrant) 36.0
    soft *(A Taste of Thai)* 36.0
sushi *(Lundberg* Organic) 36.0
white:
    (River) 37.0
    (Success), ½ cup 44.0
    Arborio *(Fantastic Foods)* 45.0
    Arborio *(Lundberg Nutra-Farmed* California) 35.0
    basmati *(Fantastic Foods)* 38.0
    basmati *(Lundberg* Organic California) 38.0
    basmati *(Lundberg Nutra-Farmed* California) 41.0
    jasmine *(Lundberg* Organic California) 36.0
    jasmine *(Lundberg Nutra-Farmed* California) 36.0
white, long-grain:
    (Carolina) 35.0
    (Mahatma) 35.0
    (Minute), about 1 cup* 36.0
    1 cup* 44.5
    basmati *(Arrowhead Mills)* 34.0
    instant *(Carolina)* 36.0
    instant *(Mahatma)* 36.0
    instant *(Minute)*, about ¾ cup* 36.0
    instant, 1 cup* 35.1
    parboiled *(Carolina* Gold) 37.0
    precooked *(Minute* Boil-in-Bag), about 1 cup* 42.0
white, medium-grain: 38.7
white, medium-grain, 1 cup* 53.2
white, short-grain:
    (Mahatma Valencia) 36.0
    ¼ cup 39.6
    1 cup* 53.4
white, glutenous or sweet 37.8
white, glutenous or sweet, 1 cup* 36.7
yellow or saffron, see "Rice dish, mix"
Rice, wild, see "Wild rice"
Rice bar, see "Granola and cereal bar"
Rice beverage, 8 fl. oz., except as noted:
(Hain Rice Supreme Original) 16.0

Rice beverage *(cont.)*

(Westbrae Natural)...18.0
(Westbrae Natural Natural Singles), 6.3 fl. oz. 14.0
cinnamon flavor *(Hain* Rice Supreme) 22.0
vanilla *(Westbrae Natural)*...22.0
vanilla *(Westbrae Natural* Natural Singles), 6.3 fl. oz. 17.0
Rice bran, crude, 1 cup...58.6
Rice cake (see also "Popcorn cake"), 1 cake, except as noted:
plain *(Quaker/Mother's)*..7.0
apple, Granny smith *(Estee)*, 5 cakes.................................13.0
apple cinnamon *(Lundberg Nutra-Farmed)*.........................18.0
banana *(Quaker)*..11.0
banana-nut *(Estee)*, 5 cakes...14.0
berry, mixed *(Estee)*, 5 cakes...14.0
brown rice:
    (Lundberg Nutra-Farmed/Lundberg Organic) 15.0
    (Lundberg Nutra-Farmed/Lundberg Organic No Salt) 16.0
    apple cinnamon or honey nut *(Hain)*..............................11.0
    apple cinnamon or honey nut, mini *(Hain)*, 6 cakes.......13.0
    barbecue or mild cheddar flavor *(Hain* Ringers),
       37 pieces 21.0
    corn or sesame seed, .3-oz. cake 7.3
    devil's food flavor, mini *(Hain)*, 5 cakes........................12.0
    mini *(Hain)*, 8 cakes 13.0
    multigrain, buckwheat, or rye, .3-oz. cake........................7.2
    peanut butter crunch, mini *(Hain)*, 5 cakes 11.0
    ranch flavor, mini *(Hain)*, 6 cakes...................................9.0
    strawberry cheesecake flavor, mini *(Hain)*, 5 cakes......12.0
buttery caramel *(Lundberg Nutra-Farmed)* 18.0
chocolate crunch *(Quaker)*..12.0
cinnamon spice *(Estee)*, 5 cakes...14.0
cinnamon streusel *(Quaker)*..12.0
honey nut *(Lundberg Nutra-Farmed)* 18.0
koku sesame or seaweed *(Lundberg* Organic)......................17.0
mochi sweet *(Lundberg Nutra-Farmed/Lundberg* Organic)......15.0
multigrain, with seeds *(Lundberg* Organic)..........................16.0
peanut butter *(Quaker)*...12.0
peanut butter crunch *(Estee)*, 5 cakes 13.0
sesame, toasted *(Lundberg Nutra-Farmed)* 15.0
sesame tamari *(Lundberg Nutra-Farmed/Lundberg* Organic) 16.0
tamari seaweed *(Lundberg* Organic)......................................15.0

wild rice *(Lundberg Nutra-Farmed/Lundberg* Organic) 15.0
Rice dish, canned:
with chicken and vegetables *(Chef Boyardee* Microwave),
    1 bowl 32.0
fried *(La Choy)*, 1 cup 64.0
Rice dish, dried (see also "Rice dish, mix"):
black beans, Santa Fe *(AlpineAire)*, 1 cup.......................69.0
Mexican, with cheese *(AlpineAire)*, 1 cup 39.0
wild rice pilaf *(AlpineAire)*, 1 cup 53.0
Rice dish, frozen, 1 pkg., except as noted:
and beans, Santa Fe *(Lean Cuisine Everyday Favorites)*,
    10⅜ oz. 54.0
and broccoli au gratin *(Freezer Queen* Family Side Dish),
    1 cup 38.0
and broccoli in cheese sauce *(Birds Eye)*, 10-oz. pkg..............44.0
cheesy, with broccoli *(Green Giant)*, 3.5 oz., approx. ½ cup 20.0
cheesy, with chicken and broccoli *(Marie Callender's* Meals),
    12 oz. 44.0
fried:
    chicken *(Michelina's Yu Sing)*, 8 oz.................................58.0
    with chicken and egg rolls *(Banquet)*, 8.5 oz. 51.0
    pork *(Michelina's Yu Sing)*, 8.5 oz....................................69.0
    pork and shrimp *(Michelina's Yu Sing)*, 8 oz....................64.0
    shrimp *(Michelina's Yu Sing)*, 8 oz...................................63.0
with peas and mushrooms *(Green Giant* Medley), 3.5 oz.,
    approx. ½ cup...18.0
pilaf *(Green Giant)*, 3.5 oz., approx. ½ cup......................15.0
risotto Parmigiana *(Michelina's)*, 8 oz.............................50.0
teriyaki stir-fry *(Amy's)*, 1 cup...64.0
Thai stir-fry *(Amy's)*, 9.5 oz...36.0
white and wild rice:
    (Birds Eye), 1 cup...31.0
    with broccoli in cheese sauce *(Marie Callender's* Skillet
      Meals), 1 cup..35.0
    with green beans *(Green Giant)*, 3.5 oz., approx. ½ cup.......18.0
Rice dish, mix, dry, except as noted:
Alfredo broccoli *(Lipton* Rice & Sauce), ½ cup 43.0
beans and rice:
    black beans *(Carolina)*, 1 cup*...39.0
    black beans *(Goya)*, ¼ cup...34.0
    black beans *(Mahatma)*, 1 cup*.......................................39.0

Rice dish, mix, beans and rice *(cont.)*

black beans, spicy Jamaican *(Fantastic Foods
Jamaican Cup)*, 2.4 oz. 52.0
black beans and brown rice, Jamaican *(Fantastic Foods
Healthy Complements)*, ⅓ cup 30.0
pinto beans *(Mahatma)*, 1 cup* 41.0
pinto beans, Tex-Mex *(Fantastic Foods Cup)*, 2.3 oz. 48.0
red beans *(Carolina)*, 1 cup* 40.0
red beans *(Goya)*, ¼ cup 35.0
red beans *(Mahatma)*, 1 cup* 40.0
red beans *(Rice-A-Roni)*, about 1 cup* 51.0
red beans *(Nile Spice)*, 1 cont. 35.0
red beans *(Success)*, ½ cup 51.0
red beans and brown rice *(Fantastic Foods Healthy
Complements New Orleans)*, ⅓ cup 28.0
spicy *(Near East)*, 1 cont. 49.0
beef/beef flavor:
   (Lipton Rice & Sauce), ½ cup, 1 cup* 47.0
   (Rice-A-Roni), about 1 cup* 51.0
   (Rice-A-Roni ⅓ Less Salt), about 1 cup* 53.0
   (Success), ½ cup 43.0
   and mushroom *(Rice-A-Roni)*, about 1 cup* 50.0
broccoli:
   (Rice-A-Roni), about 1 cup* 41.0
   au gratin *(Rice-A-Roni)*, about 1 cup* 46.0
   au gratin *(Rice-A-Roni ⅓ Less Salt)*, about 1 cup* 49.0
   au gratin risotto *(Knorr Italian Rices)*, ⅓ cup.......................54.0
   and cheese *(Mahatma)*, 1 cup* 41.0
   and cheese *(Success)*, ½ cup 40.0
brown, hearty harvest *(Lundberg Organic)*, ½ pkg., 1 cup*.......30.0
brown and wild *(Success)*, ½ cup 41.0
Cajun style:
   (Lipton Rice & Sauce), ½ cup, 1 cup* 46.0
   with beans *(Lipton Rice & Sauce)*, ½ cup, 1 cup* 52.0
   with red beans *(Fantastic Foods Cup)*, 2.3 oz. 46.0
Cantonese style *(Health Valley)*, ½ cup.....................................27.0
cheddar:
   broccoli *(Bowl Appétit!)*, 1 bowl..52.0
   broccoli *(Lipton Rice & Sauce)*, ½ cup, 1 cup* 46.0
   white, and herbs *(Rice-A-Roni)*, about 1 cup* 49.0
cheese, nacho *(Mahatma)*, 1 cup* 49.0

cheese, three, risotto *(Marrakesh Express)*, ¼ cup, 1 cup*........44.0
chicken/chicken flavor:
    (Carolina), 1 cup*..42.0
    (Health Valley), ½ cup..26.0
    (Lipton Rice & Sauce), ½ cup, 1 cup*......................46.0
    (Mahatma), 1 cup*..42.0
    (Rice-A-Roni), about 1 cup*..................................52.0
    (Rice-A-Roni ⅓ Less Salt), about 1 cup*...................53.0
    (Rice-A-Roni Low Fat), about 1 cup*........................41.0
    (Success Classic), ½ cup......................................32.0
    broccoli *(Lipton* Rice & Sauce), ½ cup, 1 cup*.............46.0
    and broccoli *(Rice-A-Roni)*, about 1 cup*.................41.0
    creamy *(Lipton* Rice & Sauce), ½ cup, 1 cup*.............45.0
    and garlic *(Rice-A-Roni)*, about 1 cup*...................42.0
    grilled *(Success)*, ½ cup......................................42.0
    herb-roasted *(Rice-A-Roni)*, about 1 cup*................41.0
    with mushrooms *(Rice-A-Roni)*, about 1 cup*.............52.0
    and Parmesan risotto *(Lipton* Rice & Sauce), ½ cup,
      1 cup*..43.0
    pilaf *(Knorr* Pilaf Rices), ⅓ cup............................45.0
    vegetable, herb *(Bowl Appétit!)*, 1 bowl...................50.0
    vegetable, savory *(Rice-A-Roni* Low Fat), about 1 cup*....41.0
    and vegetables *(Rice-A-Roni)*, about 1 cup*..............52.0
coconut-ginger *(A Taste of Thai)*, ¾ cup*....................42.0
curried basmati rice with lentils *(Fantastic Foods* Healthy
    Complements), ¼ cup..30.0
curry, Bombay, with lentils *(Fantastic Foods* Cup), 2.4 oz. 53.0
eggplant risotto *(Real Torino* Risotto Dinner), ¼ cup 51.0
fried rice:
    (Rice-A-Roni), about 1 cup*..................................51.0
    (Rice-A-Roni ⅓ Less Salt), about 1 cup*...................52.0
    chicken *(Lipton* Rice & Sauce), ½ cup, 1 cup*.............49.0
garlic, roasted, pesto *(Lundberg* Organic), ½ pkg., 1 cup* 52.0
garlic basil *(A Taste of Thai)*, ¾ cup*.......................35.0
garlic primavera risotto *(Lundberg)*, ¼ box...................29.0
golden *(A Taste of Thai)*, ¾ cup*.............................38.0
gumbo *(Mahatma)*, 1 cup*.....................................31.0
herb, Italian, risotto *(Lundberg)*, ¼ box.....................28.0
herb and butter *(Lipton* Rice & Sauce), ½ cup, 1 cup*............43.0
herb and butter *(Rice-A-Roni)*, about 1 cup*.................53.0
jambalaya *(Mahatma)*, 1 cup*.................................42.0

Rice dish, mix *(cont.)*

lemon herb with jasmine pilaf *(Knorr Pilaf Rices)*, ⅓ cup 55.0

and lentil:

    chili *(Lundberg One Step Entree)*, 1 cup* 42.0

    curry *(Lundberg One Step Entree)*, 1 cup* 38.0

    garlic basil *(Lundberg One Step Entree)*, 1 cup*.................37.0

long-grain and wild rice:

    (Mahatma), 1 cup* 41.0

    (Near East), 2 oz. 43.0

    (Rice-A-Roni Original), about 1 cup* 43.0

    (Success), ½ cup 42.0

    chicken-almond *(Rice-A-Roni)*, about 1 cup* 51.0

    with herbs *(Minute)*, about 1 cup* 50.0

    pilaf *(Rice-A-Roni)*, about 1 cup*...43.0

medley *(Lipton Rice & Sauce)*, ½ cup, 1 cup* 44.0

Mexican style *(Goya)*, ¼ cup 37.0

Mexican style *(Rice-A-Roni)*, about 1 cup* 41.0

mushroom:

    flavor *(Lipton Rice & Sauce)*, ½ cup, 1 cup* 45.0

    and herb *(Lipton Rice & Sauce)*, ½ cup, 1 cup*.................49.0

    risotto *(Knorr Italian Rices)*, ⅓ cup......................................62.0

    risotto *(Marrakesh Express)*, ¼ cup, 1 cup* 46.0

    risotto, porcini *(Alessi)*, ⅓ cup..44.0

    wild *(Lundberg Organic)*, ½ pkg., 1 cup* 53.0

onion herb risotto *(Knorr Italian Rices)*, ⅓ cup.........................66.0

Oriental stir-fry *(Rice-A-Roni)*, about 1 cup*..............................54.0

Parmesan, creamy, risotto *(Lundberg)* ¼ box 27.0

pilaf (see also specific listings):

    (Carolina Classic), 1 cup* 43.0

    (Knorr Pilaf Rices Original), ⅓ cup 46.0

    (Lipton Rice & Sauce), ½ cup, 1 cup* 44.0

    (Mahatma Classic), 1 cup* 43.0

    (Rice-A-Roni), about 1 cup* 52.0

    (Success), ½ cup 44.0

    with orzo *(Casbah)*, ¾ cup 38.0

    primavera *(Nile Spice* Chef Express), 2.2-oz. cont. 50.0

primavera *(Goya)*, ¼ cup 35.0

primavera *(Health Valley)*, ½ cup..26.0

risotto (see also specific listings):

    (Fantastic Foods Healthy Complements Classico), ¼ cup.....31.0

    Milanese *(Alessi)*, ⅓ cup...42.0

Milanese *(Knorr* Italian Rices), ⅓ cup 59.0
Milanese *(Marrakesh Express),* ¼ cup, 1 cup* 50.0
primavera *(Marrakesh Express),* ¼ cup, 1 cup* 46.0
saffron, see "yellow," below
scampi style *(Lipton* Rice & Sauce), ½ cup, 1 cup*................44.0
Southwestern *(Bowl Appétit!),* 1 bowl 52.0
Spanish (see also "yellow," below):
  (Carolina Authenic), 1 cup* 42.0
  (Fantastic Foods Healthy Complements Hacienda),
    ⅜ cup 36.0
  (Lipton Rice & Sauce), ½ cup, 1 cup* 47.0
  (Mahatma), 1 cup* 42.0
  (Rice-A-Roni), about 1 cup* 46.0
  (Success), ½ cup 43.0
  picante, fiesta *(Lundberg* Organic), ½ pkg., 1 cup*.............53.0
  pilaf *(Casbah),* ¾ cup 40.0
Stroganoff *(Rice-A-Roni),* about 1 cup* 49.0
sun-dried tomato risotto *(Alessi),* ⅓ cup 42.0
sweet red pepper risotto *(Real Torino* Risotto Dinner), ¼ cup ...54.0
teriyaki *(Lipton* Rice & Sauce), ½ cup, 1 cup* 45.0
Thai style *(Health Valley),* ½ cup 27.0
tomato-basil risotto *(Lundberg),* ¼ box 30.0
tomato and peas risotto *(Marrakesh Express),* ¼ cup, 1 cup* ...45.0
tomato and rice *(Near East),* 1 cont. 27.0
vegetable:
  mixed, risotto *(Real Torino* Risotto Dinner), ¼ cup...............54.0
  pilaf *(Near East),* 1 cont. 50.0
  primavera risotto *(Knorr* Italian Rices), ⅓ cup.....................61.0
  shiitake *(Health Valley),* ½ cup......................................26.0
vegetarian, chicken, savory *(Lundberg* Organic), ½ pkg.,
  1 cup* 53.0
yellow, 1 cup*:
  (Goya), 2 oz. 40.0
  (Goya Spanish Style), ¼ cup 37.0
  saffron *(Carolina)* 43.0
  saffron *(Mahatma)*...43.0
  saffron jasmine *(Casbah),* ¾ cup 38.0
  spicy *(Mahatma)*...41.0
zucchini and leeks risotto *(Real Torino* Risotto Dinner),
  ¼ cup 54.0
Rice entree, see "Rice dish"

Rice flour:

brown:

(Arrowhead Mills), ¼ cup 27.0

(Hodgson Mill), scant ¼ cup 23.0

(Lundberg Organic), ¼ cup 22.0

(Lundberg Nutra-Farmed), ¼ cup 26.0

1 cup 120.8

white (Arrowhead Mills), ¼ cup 28.0

white, 1 cup 126.6

Rice pasta, see "Pasta"

Rice pudding, ready-to-serve, 5-oz. can 31.2

Rice pudding mix:

whole milk, ½ cup* 30.1

2% milk (Jell-O Americana), ½ cup* 29.0

2% milk, ½ cup* 30.2

cinnamon (Lundberg Elegant), ½ cup 16.0

coconut (Lundberg Elegant), ½ cup 13.0

honey almond (Lundberg Elegant), ½ cup 15.0

Rice seasoning mix, Mexican:

(Bearitos), 1 tsp. 1.0

(Lawry's Spices & Seasonings), 1½ tsp. 9.0

Rice snack:

brown, chips (Eden), 50 chips, 1.1 oz. 19.0

puffs, five-flavor, arare (Eden), 30 puffs, 1.1 oz. 24.0

Rice syrup, brown (Lundberg Sweet Dreams Nutra-Farmed/

Organic), ¼ cup 42.0

Rice wafer, see "Cracker"

Rigatoni, plain, see "Pasta"

Rigatoni dish, mix, white cheddar and broccoli sauce (Pasta

Roni), about 1 cup* 48.0

Rigatoni entree, frozen, 1 pkg., except as noted:

cheese, stuffed (Michelina's), 8.5 oz. 41.0

jumbo, with meatballs (Lean Cuisine Hearty Portion Meals),

15⅜ oz. 64.0

with meat sauce (Freezer Queen Family Entree), 1 cup 38.0

pomodoro (Michelina's), 8 oz. 40.0

pomodoro, with broccoli and olives (Michelina's), 9 oz. 43.0

with vegetables in cheese sauce (Marie Callender's Skillet

Meals), 1 cup 32.0

Risotto, see "Rice dish, mix" and "Rice dish, frozen"

Rock candy syrup (Trader Vic's), 2 tbsp. 23.0

Rockfish, without added ingredients 0
Roe (see also "Caviar" and "Taramosalata"), raw:
1 oz. 4
1 tbsp. 2
Roll (see also "Biscuit," "Croissant," and "Focaccia"), 1 roll:
brown-and-serve or dinner 21.7
dinner, all varieties *(Awrey's)*, .9 oz. 22.0
egg 18.2
French 19.1
hamburger:
    (Arnold), 1.76 oz. 25.0
    (Pepperidge Farm), 1.5 oz. 21.0
    mixed-grain 19.2
    reduced-calorie..18.1
    whole-wheat 22.0
    white...21.7
hamburger or hot dog *(Sunbeam)*, 1.4 oz. 20.0
Kaiser:
    (Awrey's), 2½ oz. 37.0
    (Francisco International), 2.15 oz. 33.0
    or hard..30.0
hoagie *(Awrey's)*, 3¼ oz. 46.0
hoagie 17.9
hot dog/frankfurter:
    (Arnold), 1.5 oz. 21.0
    (Pepperidge Farm), 1.8 oz. 24.0
    foot-long...43.3
    mixed-grain 19.2
    reduced-calorie..18.1
    white..21.7
    whole-wheat 22.0
oat bran...13.3
onion 21.7
rye, large...22.8
rye, medium...19.1
sandwich bun:
    potato sesame *(Arnold)*, 1.76 oz. 29.0
    sesame *(Arnold)*, 1.76 oz. 23.0
    sesame *(Pepperidge Farm)*, 1.6 oz. 22.0
wheat 13.0

Roll, refrigerated, 1 roll:
crescent *(Pillsbury)*, 1 oz. 11.0
crescent *(Pillsbury* Reduced Fat), 1 oz. 12.0
dinner *(Pillsbury)*, 1.4 oz. 18.0
Roll, sweet, see "Bun, sweet"
Roll mix, hot *(Pillsbury)*, 1 roll* 21.0
Roseapple, raw, 1 oz. 1.6
Roselle, fresh, raw, trimmed, 1 cup 6.4
Rosemary, fresh:
1 tbsp..4
1 tsp..1
Rosemary, dried:
1 tbsp..2.1
1 tsp..8
Rotini dish, mix:
cheese:
    with broccoli *(Kraft Velveeta* Dinner), about 1 cup* ...47.0
    four-cheese sauce *(Knorr)*, ⅓ cup 21.0
    four-cheese sauce *(Near East)*, 1 cont. 21.0
    three *(Bowl Appétit!)*, 1 bowl 53.0
    three *(Lipton* Pasta & Sauce), ¾ cup 41.0
chicken and broccoli *(Near East)*, 1 cont. 34.0
chicken and broccoli *(Nile Spice* Chef Express), 1 cont. ...33.0
with mushroom sauce, delicate *(Knorr)*, ⅔ cup 50.0
primavera *(Lipton* Pasta & Sauce), ¾ cup 42.0
Roughy, orange, fresh, without added ingredients 0
Rum sauce, butter *(Sable & Rosenfeld)*, 2 tbsp. 27.0
Rutabaga, fresh:
raw, 1 large, 1.7 lbs. 62.8
raw, cubed, 1 cup 11.4
boiled, drained, cubed, 1 cup 14.9
boiled, drained, mashed, 1 cup 21.0
Rutabaga, canned, diced *(Sunshine)*, ½ cup 7.0
Rye, whole-grain:
(Arrowhead Mills), ¼ cup 34.0
1 cup...117.9
Rye flakes, rolled *(Arrowhead Mills)*, ⅓ cup 24.0
Rye flour:
(Arrowhead Mills), ¼ cup 20.0
(Hodgson Mill Organic), ¼ cup 22.0
(Robin Hood Best for Bread), ¼ cup 24.9

1 cup..88.0
medium, 1 cup...79.0
light, 1 cup...81.8
whole-grain *(Hodgson Mill)*, scant ¼ cup......................22.0
Rye malt syrup, see "Malt syrup"

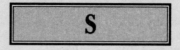

FOOD AND MEASURE　　　　　　**CARBOHYDRATE GRAMS**

Sablefish, without added ingredients 0
Safflower seed kernels, dried, 1 oz. 9.7
Safflower seed meal, partially defatted, 1 oz. 13.8
Saffron:
1 tbsp. 1.4
1 tsp. 5
Sage, ground:
1 tbsp. 1.2
1 tsp. 4
Salad, fresh, with dressing, 3.5 oz., except as noted:
all-American toss *(Dole* Great Restaurant) 7.0
Caesar:
　　(Dole Complete) 7.0
　　(Dole Complete Family) 8.0
　　(Dole Complete Low Fat) 8.0
　　(Dole Lunch for One), 5.75 oz. 17.0
　　creamy garlic *(Dole* Complete) 8.0
　　roasted garlic *(Dole* Complete Light Dressing) 8.0
cheese toss, triple *(Dole* Great Restaurant) 4.0
Greek marinade, classic *(Dole* Great Restaurant) 5.0
Italian, low-fat *(Dole Lunch for One),* 7 oz. 25.0
Italian, zesty *(Dole* Complete Light Dressing) 11.0
Mediterranean marinade *(Dole* Great Restaurant) 5.0
Oriental *(Dole* Complete) 12.0
ranch, classic *(Dole Lunch for One),* 7 oz. 20.0
Romano *(Dole* Complete) 8.0
sunflower ranch *(Dole* Complete) 5.0
tomato and mozzarella medley *(Dole* Great Restaurant) 7.0
Salad blend, fresh, 3 oz.:
(Dole Classic Greener Selection) 3.0
American blend *(Dole Special Blends)* 3.0
coleslaw *(Dole* Classic) 5.0
European blend *(Dole Special Blends)* 3.0
French blend *(Dole Special Blends)* 4.0

iceberg (Dole Classic) 4.0
Italian blend (Dole Special Blends) 3.0
Mediterranean blend (Dole Special Blends) 3.0
Romaine blend (Dole Special Blends)...........................3.0
Tuscan blend (Dole Special Blends).............................4.0
Verona blend (Dole Special Blends)..............................2.0
Salad dressing, 2 tbsp., except as noted:
bacon and tomato (Henri's)...10.0
bacon and tomato (Kraft)..2.0
balsamic vinaigrette:
   (Henri's Fat Free) 4.0
   (Wish-Bone)..3.0
   honey and tarragon (Hellmann's/Best Foods).........6.0
   roasted tomato (Hellmann's/Best Foods) 3.0
   roasted tomato and garlic (Hellmann's/Best Foods
     Fat Free)..4.0
berry vinaigrette (Wish-Bone)..2.0
blue cheese:
   (Just 2 Good!)...6.0
   (Kraft Roka)..2.0
   chunky (Hellmann's/Best Foods)............................1.0
   chunky (Hellmann's/Best Foods Refrigerated)........2.0
   chunky (Seven Seas)..2.0
   chunky (Wish-Bone)...2.0
   chunky (Wish-Bone Fat Free) 7.0
   flavored (Kraft Free) 11.0
buttermilk ranch (Hellmann's/Best Foods Refrigerated)................3.0
buttermilk ranch (Kraft)..1.0
Caesar:
   (Hellmann's/Best Foods Fat Free) 8.0
   (Just 2 Good! Classic)...5.0
   (Kraft Classic)..1.0
   (Kraft Free Classic)..11.0
   (Seven Seas Classic) 2.0
   (Weight Watchers)..7.0
   (Wish-Bone Classic) 2.0
cilantro pepita (El Torito)..2.0
creamy (Hellmann's/Best Foods)....................................2.0
creamy (Hellmann's/Best Foods Refrigerated) 1.0
creamy (Henri's Fat Free 8 oz.)...................................11.0
creamy (Henri's Fat Free 16 oz.)..................................12.0

Salad dressing, Caesar *(cont.)*

creamy *(Just 2 Good!)* 7.0
creamy *(Wish-Bone)* 1.0
Italian *(Kraft)* 2.0
Italian *(Kraft Free)* 4.0
oil and vinegar *(Hellmann's/Best Foods)* 6.0
ranch *(Henri's)* 2.0
ranch *(Kraft)* 1.0
carrot ginger *(Cary Randall's)* 1.0
Chardonnay vinaigrette *(Hellmann's/Best Foods)* 5.0
cheese, two, Italian *(Seven Seas)* 3.0
coleslaw *(Henri's* Fat Free) 13.0
coleslaw *(Kraft)* 7.0
cucumber *(Henri's* Fat Free) 14.0
cucumber ranch *(Kraft/Kraft* Reduced Fat) 2.0
Dijon vinaigrette, creamy *(Hain)* 3.0
dill, creamy *(Nasoya)* 3.0
French:
(*Hellmann's/Best Foods* Fat Free) 11.0
(Henri's Fat Free) 11.0
(Henri's Light) 13.0
(Henri's Original) 6.0
(Kraft Catalina) 7.0
(Kraft Catalina Reduced Fat) 9.0
(Kraft Catalina Free) 8.0
(Trader Vic's San Francisco Style) 0
(Wish-Bone Deluxe) 5.0
creamy *(Estee)* 2.0
creamy *(Hellmann's/Best Foods)* 4.0
creamy *(Kraft)* 5.0
with honey *(Kraft Catalina)* 7.0
style *(Just 2 Good!* Deluxe) 7.0
style *(Kraft Free)* 11.0
style *(Weight Watchers)* 9.0
garlic:
creamy *(Kraft)* 2.0
ranch *(Hellmann's/Best Foods)* 2.0
ranch *(Kraft)* 1.0
ranch *(Kraft Free)* 11.0
roasted, vinaigrette *(Cary Randall's)* 1.0
roasted, vinaigrette *(Wish-Bone)* 2.0

green goddess *(Seven Seas)*...1.0
(Henri's Renaissance) 2.0
(Henri's Tas-Tee) 8.0
(Henri's Tas-Tee Light) 11.0
herb, garden *(Nasoya)*...3.0
herb, Italian, ranch *(Hellmann's/Best Foods)* 1.0
herb vinaigrette *(Seven Seas)*..<1.0
herbs and spices *(Seven Seas)*..1.0
honey Dijon:
    (Hellmann's/Best Foods Fat Free) 12.0
    (Just 2 Good!) 8.0
    (Kraft)...6.0
    (Kraft Free) 10.0
    (Weight Watchers)..11.0
    ranch *(Hellmann's)*, 2-oz. pkt. 12.0
honey mustard:
    (Cary Randall's)..8.0
    (Henri's)...10.0
    (Henri's Fat Free) 12.0
    (Seven Seas) 6.0
    spicy *(Cary Randall's)*...7.0
Italian:
    (Estee)...1.0
    (Hellmann's/Best Foods)..3.0
    (Hellmann's/Best Foods Fat Free) 4.0
    (Henri's Fat Free) 4.0
    (Henri's Traditional) 2.0
    (Just 2 Good!)...5.0
    (Just 2 Good! Country) 3.0
    (Kraft Presto)..2.0
    (Kraft Reduced Fat) 3.0
    (Kraft Zesty) 2.0
    (Kraft Free) 4.0
    (Seven Seas Viva)...2.0
    *(Seven Seas Viva Free/*Reduced Fat) 2.0
    (Trader Vic's San Francisco Style) ....<1.0
    (Weight Watchers)..2.0
    (Wish-Bone) 3.0
    (Wish-Bone Classic House/Fat Free) 2.0
    (Wish-Bone Robusto)..4.0
    creamy *(Hain)*..8.0

Salad dressing, Italian *(cont.)*
creamy *(Hellmann's/Best Foods)*..3.0
creamy *(Henri's* Fat Free) 12.0
creamy *(Kraft)* 2.0
creamy *(Kraft Free)*...12.0
creamy *(Nasoya)* 3.0
creamy *(Seven Seas)*..1.0
creamy *(Seven Seas* Reduced Fat) 2.0
creamy *(Seven Seas Free)*...12.0
creamy *(Weight Watchers)* 7.0
creamy *(Wish-Bone)*..4.0
creamy garlic flavor *(Henri's)*...6.0
golden *(Hellmann's/Best Foods)*...3.0
with olive oil blend *(Kraft* House) 2.0
with olive oil blend *(Seven Seas* Reduced Fat) 2.0
Javanese *(Trader Vic's* South Pacific Style) 1.0
lemongrass herb *(Annie Chun's* Marinade & Dressing) 6.0
mango lime vinaigrette *(Chi-Chi's)*...7.0
mayonnaise type, see "Mayonnaise dressing"
mustard vinaigrette *(Henri's)*...5.0
olive oil vinaigrette *(Wish-Bone)*...4.0
onion, spring, ranch *(Hellmann's/Best Foods)* 2.0
orange Oriental *(Hellmann's/Best Foods Citrus Splash)*..............7.0
orange vinaigrette *(Hellmann's/Best Foods Citrus Splash)* 6.0
Oriental *(Wish-Bone)* 7.0
Parmesan:
basil Italian *(Just 2 Good!)*..6.0
onion *(Wish-Bone)* 5.0
peppercorn *(Hellmann's/Best Foods)*, 2-oz. pkt....................4.0
ranch *(Henri's* Fat Free) 10.0
pepper, roasted, vinaigrette *(Cary Randall's)*..............................2.0
peppercorn ranch:
(Henri's)...3.0
(Kraft) 1.0
(Kraft Free) 11.0
pesto, hemp, vinaigrette *(Cary Randall's)* 1.0
poppyseed rancher's *(Hain)* 3.0
ranch (see also specific listings):
(Chi-Chi's Serrano) 2.0
(Hellmann's/Best Foods Fat Free) 11.0
(Hellmann's/Best Foods Refrigerated Light) 4.0

(Henri's Chef's Recipe) 3.0
(Henri's Chef's Recipe Light) 12.0
(Henri's Fat Free) 11.0
(Just 2 Good!) 5.0
(Kraft/Kraft Reduced Fat) 1.0
(Kraft Free) 11.0
(Seven Seas) 2.0
(Seven Seas Reduced Fat) 5.0
(Seven Seas Free) 11.0
(Weight Watchers) 1.0
(Wish-Bone) 1.0
(Wish-Bone Fat Free) 9.0
creamy *(Hellmann's/Best Foods)* 1.0
Southwest *(Henri's)* 5.0
raspberry vinaigrette:
   (Hellmann's/Best Foods Fat Free) 9.0
   (Henri's Fat Free) 10.0
   (Seven Seas Free) 7.0
red wine vinaigrette:
   (Henri's Fat Free) 3.0
   (Wish-Bone) 9.0
   (Wish-Bone Fat Free) 7.0
red wine vinegar:
   (Kraft Free) 3.0
   (Seven Seas Free) 3.0
   and oil *(Seven Seas)* 2.0
   and oil *(Seven Seas* Reduced Fat) 3.0
Roquefort 2.3
ruby red ginger *(Hellmann's/Best Foods Citrus Splash)* 8.0
Russian:
   (Kraft) 10.0
   (Seven Seas Viva) 3.0
   (Wish-Bone) 15.0
salsa vinaigrette *(Chi-Chi's)* 4.0
serrano grape vinaigrette *(El Torito)* 7.0
serrano ranch *(El Torito)* 2.0
sesame:
   cilantro *(Annie Chun's* Noodle & Salad Dressing) 4.0
   garlic *(Nasoya)* 3.0
   with soy *(Trader Vic's* South Pacific Style) 3.0
sour cream and onion ranch *(Kraft)* 1.0

Salad dressing *(cont.)*

sour cream and onion ranch *(Kraft Free)* 11.0
sweet and sour *(Henri's)* 8.0
sweet and spicy *(Wish-Bone)* 6.0
sweet and spicy French *(Just 2 Good!)* 9.0

tamari:
    mustard *(San-J)* 5.0
    peanut *(San-J)* 9.0
    sesame *(San-J)* 8.0
    vinaigrette *(San-J)* 7.0

tangerine, tangy *(Hellmann's/Best Foods Citrus Splash)* 6.0
tangerine balsamic *(Hellmann's/Best Foods Citrus Splash)* 7.0
teriyaki ginger *(Henri's)* 4.0

Thousand Island:
    (Hain) 6.0
    (Hellmann's/Best Foods Refrigerated) 5.0
    (Henri's) 5.0
    (Henri's Fat Free) 9.0
    (Henri's Light) 8.0
    (Just 2 Good!) 9.0
    (Kraft) 5.0
    (Kraft Reduced Fat) 7.0
    (Kraft Free) 9.0
    (Nasoya) 6.0
    with bacon *(Kraft)* 5.0
    creamy *(Hellmann's/Best Foods)* 4.0

tomato:
    and herb Italian *(Kraft)* 3.0
    roasted, vinaigrette *(Henri's)* 3.0
    sun-dried, basil *(Cary Randall's)* 2.0
    sun-dried, vinaigrette *(Wish-Bone)* 2.0

vinaigrette, see specific listings
white wine vinaigrette *(Wish-Bone)* 4.0

Salad dressing mix, 2 tbsp.*:

Caesar *(Good Seasons Gourmet)* 3.0
cheese garlic *(Good Seasons)* 1.0
garlic, roasted *(Good Seasons)* 2.0
garlic and herbs *(Good Seasons)* 1.0
herb, zesty *(Good Seasons Fat Free)* 2.0
honey French *(Good Seasons/Good Seasons Fat Free)* 5.0
honey mustard *(Good Seasons)* 3.0

honey mustard *(Good Seasons* Fat Free) 5.0
Italian:
    (Good Seasons Fat Free) 3.0
    mild *(Good Seasons)*..2.0
    regular or zesty *(Good Seasons)*............................1.0
    regular or zesty *(Good Seasons* Reduced Calorie) 2.0
Mexican spice *(Good Seasons)*....................................2.0
Oriental sesame *(Good Seasons)*..................................3.0
Parmesan Italian *(Good Seasons* Gourmet) 2.0
peanut *(A Taste of Thai)*..7.0
Salami, 2 oz., except as noted:
beef:
    (Boar's Head)..0
    (Hebrew National Presliced), 3 slices, 2 oz. 0
    (Hebrew National Presliced Lean), 4 slices, 2 oz. 1.0
    (Sara Lee Deli), 3 slices, 1.6 oz...............................0
    .8-oz. slice 4
cooked:
    (Boar's Head)..0
    (Russer) 3.0
    (Russer Light) 4.0
    beef, .8-oz. slice 6
    beef and pork, .8-oz. slice 5
Genoa:
    (Boar's Head)..1.0
    (Di Lusso)..0
    (Fiorucci), 1 oz. 1.0
    (Russer) 0
    (Sara Lee), 4 slices, 1.1 oz....................................0
hard or dry:
    (Boar's Head), 1 oz. ....<1.0
    (Homeland) 0
    (Oscar Mayer), 3 slices, 1 oz..................................1.0
    (Russer) 0
    (Sara Lee), 4 slices, 1.1 oz....................................0
    pork, 4-oz. pkg. 1.8
    pork, .3-oz. slice 2
    pork and beef, 4-oz. pkg..2.9
    pork and beef, .3-oz. slice 3
pork, .8-oz. slice 5

"Salami," vegetarian, frozen *(Worthington* Meatless),
  3 slices, 2 oz. 2.0
Salisbury steak, see "Beef dinner" and "Beef entree"
Salmon, fresh, canned, or frozen, without added ingredients 0
Salmon, smoked, 2 oz., except as noted:
(Ocean Beauty)...<1.0
Chinook, regular or lox, 4 oz.......................................0
lox or Nova *(Vita)*..<1.0
Nova *(Nathan's Famous)*..2.0
roasted or Atlantic *(Ducktrap River)* 0
Salmon burger, frozen *(Ocean Beauty)*, 3.2-oz. burger................1.0
"Salmon" burger, vegetarian *(Dr. Praeger's* Veggie),
  2.8-oz. piece 3.0
Salmon croquette, frozen *(Dr. Praeger's)*, 2.2-oz. piece 12.0
Salmon entree, frozen, grilled:
creamy dill *(Mrs. Paul's)*, 1 fillet 1.0
honey mustard *(Mrs. Paul's)*, 1 fillet...........................3.0
Salmon nuggets, frozen, 4 oz.:
unheated 13.4
heated 15.8
Salmon paté, smoked *(Ducktrap River)*, ¼ cup, 2 oz. 1.0
Salsa, tomato (see also "Picante sauce"), 2 tbsp., except
  as noted:
(Buckaroo Greenhorn Salsa & Dip)..............................1.0
(D.L. Jardine's Bobos)...4.0
(Featherweight)..3.0
(Kraft Free Dip)..3.0
(La Victoria Salsa Verde)...1.0
(Sonoma) 3.0
(Tostitos Restaurant Style), 4 tbsp..............................6.0
all varieties *(La Victoria* Thick 'n' Chunky) 2.0
all varieties *(Pace* Thick & Chunky)..............................3.0
black bean:
  (Buckaroo Whistle-Berries) 2.0
  medium *(Buckaroo* Buckshot).................................3.0
  medium *(D.L. Jardine's* Buckshot) 3.0
  and corn *(Buckaroo)*..4.0
  and corn, medium *(Muir Glen* Organic)......................3.0
cherry *(Buckaroo* Wild & Woolly)..................................5.0
chili, green *(Buckaroo)*..1.0
chili, green *(La Victoria)*..2.0

chipotle medium *(Muir Glen* Organic)..2.0
con queso or cheese, see "Cheese dip"
creamy *(Breakstone's Free* Dip) 3.0
creamy *(Knudsen Free* Dip)...3.0
garden *(Chi-Chi's)* 3.0
garden style, medium or mild *(Ortega)*.....................................2.0
garlic *(Christopher Ranch* California Style) 2.0
garlic, roasted:
    (Buckaroo)..2.0
    (Tostitos), 4 tbsp. 6.0
    hot or mild *(Muir Glen* Organic) 3.0
    medium *(Muir Glen* Organic) 2.0
garlic cilantro, medium *(Muir Glen* Organic)..............................2.0
green or red *(La Victoria* Jalapeña)...2.0
hot:
    (D.L. Jardine's Habañero XXX) 2.0
    (Shotgun Willie's Jalapeño/Habañero Hotter'n Hell)................2.0
    habañero *(Muir Glen* Organic)......................................2.0
hot or medium *(Taco Bell Home Originals)*..............................2.0
hot, medium, or mild:
    (Chi-Chi's) 2.0
    (El Torito Original Restaurant) 2.0
    (Muir Glen Organic)...2.0
    (Tostitos), 4 tbsp. 6.0
mango-pineapple *(Sonoma* Coasteña) 5.0
medium *(D.L. Jardine's* Texacante) 2.0
medium *(La Victoria* Suprema) 1.0
medium or mild *(El Torito* Fire-Roasted)...................................2.0
medium or mild *(Ortega* Thick and Chunky) 2.0
mild *(La Victoria* Suprema) 2.0
mild *(Taco Bell Home Originals)* 3.0
peach *(Buckaroo* Twenty-Four Kick) 3.0
peach or raspberry *(D.L. Jardine's)* 4.0
pepper, garden, medley, medium *(Muir Glen* Organic) 2.0
pepper, roasted, and onion, medium *(Muir Glen* Organic)............2.0
picante, medium or mild *(La Victoria)* 1.0
pinto bean, spicy *(Buckaroo* Cowboy) 3.0
roasted tomato *(Chi-Chi's)*..2.0
roasted tomato, fire, medium *(Muir Glen* Organic) 2.0
tomatillo, green *(D.L. Jardine's* Salsa Verde Dip)......................2.0

Salsa seasoning mix, ½ tsp.:
(Bearitos) 1.0
(Lawry's Spices & Seasonings) 1.0
Salsify, fresh:
raw *(Frieda's),* ¾ cup, 3 oz. 16.0
raw, sliced, 1 cup...24.7
boiled, drained, sliced, 1 cup 20.7
Salt, 1 tbsp. 0
Salt, seasoned (see also specific listings) *(Lawry's),* ¼ tsp. 0
Salt, substitute, 1 tsp. 0
Salt pork, raw..0
Sandwich, see specific listings
Sandwich sauce, see "Sloppy Joe sauce"
Sandwich spread:
(Hellmann's/Best Foods), 1 tbsp. 3.0
(Kraft/Kraft Reduced Fat), 1 tbsp. 3.0
(Loma Linda), ¼ cup 7.0
1 tbsp. 3.4
2 tbsp. 6.9
Sapodilla, fresh, raw:
(Frieda's), 3-oz. fruit...17.0
6-oz. fruit..33.9
pulp, 1 cup 48.1
Sapote, fresh, raw:
(Frieda's), 5 oz. 47.0
trimmed, 7.9-oz. sapote 76.0
Sardine, fresh see "Herring"
Sardine, canned:
in mustard sauce *(Underwood),* 3.75-oz. can............2.0
in oil, 4 oz. 0
in olive oil, lemon or spice *(Goya),* ¼ cup..................0
in olive oil, skinless, boneless *(Granadaisa),* ¼ cup 0
smoked lightly, in lemon, tomato, or hot sauce *(Bela),* ¼ cup.........0
in tomato sauce *(Goya),* ¼ cup.................................1.0
Satay sauce, see "Peanut sauce"
Sauce, see specific listings
Sauerkraut:
(Boar's Head), 2 tbsp. 1.0
(Claussen), ¼ cup...1.0
(Del Monte), 2 tbsp. ....<1.0
(Del Monte Bavarian Style), 2 tbsp. 4.0

(Eden Organic), ½ cup...4.0
(Hebrew National), 2 tbsp. 1.0
(Seneca), 2 tbsp. 1.0
(Seneca Bavarian), 2 tbsp. 3.0
undrained, 1 cup...10.1
Sausage (see also specific listings), cooked, except as noted:
(Jones Dairy Farm Light), 2 links...............................1.0
(Jones Dairy Farm Patties), 1 patty..............................0
(Little Sizzlers), 3 links or 2 patties.............................0
andouille, Cajun *(Aidells)*, 3.5-oz. link.......................1.0
breakfast:
    (Healthy Choice), 2 links or 1 patty 3.0
    all varieties, except brown sugar and honey
        (Johnsonville), 3 links 1.0
    brown sugar and honey *(Johnsonville)*, 3 links.........5.0
    pork *(Perri)*, 3 links 1.0
    turkey *(Butterball)*, 2 links, 2 oz. 0
brown-and-serve, precooked:
    (Little Sizzlers), 3 links or 2 patties 1.0
    all varieties, except apple cinnamon *(Jones Dairy Farm*
        Golden Brown), 2 links or 1 patty....................1.0
    apple cinnamon *(Jones Dairy Farm Golden Brown)*,
        2 links..2.0
    breakfast *(Swift Premium Brown 'N Serve* Original),
        2 patties or 2 links....................................2.0
chicken, teriyaki, fresh, raw *(Aidells)*, 3.5-oz. link.......6.0
chicken:
    and apple, fresh, raw *(Aidells)*, 1.9-oz. link 1.0
    and apple, smoked *(Aidells)*, 3.5-oz. link 1.0
    and apple, smoked, mini *(Aidells)*, 6 links, 2 oz. 1.0
    lemon, smoked *(Aidells)*, 3.5-oz. link......................1.0
    Romano, roasted garlic and parsley, raw *(Perdue)*, 2 oz.......1.0
chicken and turkey, see "turkey and chicken," below
chorizo, see "Chorizo"
dinner *(Jones Dairy Farm)*, 1.4-oz. link.......................1.0
duck and turkey, smoked *(Aidells)*, 3.5-oz. link 1.0
Italian:
    all varieties *(Johnsonville)*, 3-oz. link 1.0
    all varieties *(Perri)*, 2.7-oz. link or 4-oz. patty 1.0
    chicken, raw, sweet *(Perdue)*, 1 link.......................1.0
    pork, 4-oz. link 1.2

Sausage, Italian *(cont.)*

pork, 2.4-oz. link 1.0
pork, raw *(Aidells)*, 3.5-oz. link 0
pork, raw, 4-oz. link 7
pork, raw, 3.2-oz. link 6
precooked, mild *(Johnsonville)*, 2.7-oz. link 2.0
turkey, hot *(Butterball)*, 4 oz. 0
turkey, hot or sweet *(Perdue)*, 1 link 1.0
turkey, hot or sweet, raw *(Aidells)*, 3.5-oz. link ..1.0
turkey, sweet *(Butterball)*, 3.8-oz. link 0
lamb and beef with rosemary, raw *(Aidells)*, 3.5-oz. link 2.0
pork, link:
   (Jones Dairy Farm Little), 3 links 1.0
   (Oscar Mayer Little Friers), 2 links, 1.8 oz. ..1.0
   raw, 1 oz. 3
   whiskey fennel, smoked *(Aidells)*, 3.5-oz. link 1.0
pork, patty, raw, 2 oz. 6
pork roll, regular or spicy *(Jones Dairy Farm* Original), 2 oz. 1.0
pork and beef, link, .5 oz. 4
pork and beef, patty, .8 oz. 7
pork and veal, smoked *(Aidells* Bier), 3.5-oz. link 0
smoked:
   (Johnsonville Light), 2.3-oz. link 3.0
   (Johnsonville Swisswurst), 2.7-oz. link 2.0
   beef *(Healthy Choice)*, 2 oz. 6.0
   beef, 1.5-oz. sausage 1.0
   cheddar *(Johnsonville* Beddar with Cheddar), 2.7-oz. link 2.0
   cheddar *(Johnsonville* Beddar with Cheddar Light),
      2.3-oz. link 3.0
   cocktail *(Johnsonville* Little Smokies), 6 links, 2 oz. 1.0
   hot *(Boar's Head)*, 3.2-oz. link 1.0
   hot, regular or beef *(Johnsonville* Hot Links), 2.7-oz. link 2.0
   pork, 2.4-oz. link 1.4
   pork, .6-oz. link 3
   pork and beef, 2.4-oz. link 1.0
   pork and beef, .6-oz. link 2
   pork and beef, with flour and nonfat dry milk, 2.4-oz. link 2.7
   pork and beef, with nonfat dry milk, 2.4-oz. link 3
   turkey, pork, and beef *(Healthy Choice)*, 2 oz. 6.0
summer, see "Sausage sticks" and "Summer sausage"
tomato basil, turkey, pork, beef *(Healthy Choice)*, 2 oz. 6.0

turkey, cranberry, smoked *(Aidells)*, 3.5-oz. link............................1.0
turkey, with scallions and herbs, fresh *(Aidells)*, raw,
   3.5-oz. link..1.0
turkey and chicken:
   artichoke, smoked *(Aidells)*, 3.5-oz. link 2.0
   Burmese, curry, smoked *(Aidells)*, 3.5-oz. link....................3.0
   habañero and green chili, smoked *(Aidells)*, 3.2-oz. link.........2.0
   New Mexico, smoked *(Aidells)*, 3.5-oz. link 2.0
   pesto, smoked *(Aidells)*, 3.5-oz. link 1.0
   sun-dried tomato and basil, raw *(Aidells)*, 3.5-oz. link...........1.0
   sun-dried tomato and basil, smoked *(Aidells)*, 3.5-oz. link 0
   Thai, fresh, raw *(Aidells)*, 3.5-oz. link...................................1.0
   Thai, smoked, cooked *(Aidells)*, 3.5-oz. link............................0
Sausage, canned, Vienna (see also "Sausage hash"):
pickled, regular or hot *(Hormel)*, 6 links, 2 oz. 1.0
Vienna:
   (Armour), 3 links...5.0
   (Goya), 3 links..1.0
   (Hormel), 2 oz. 0
   (Libby's), 3 links, 1.7 oz. ....<1.0
   7 sausages, 4 oz. 2.3
   1 sausage, approx. .6 oz. 3
   chicken *(Hormel)*, 2 oz. 1.0
"Sausage," vegetarian:
.9-oz. link...2.5
1.3-oz. patty...3.7
canned *(Worthington Saucettes)*, 1.3-oz. link..............................1.0
frozen:
   (Morningstar Farms Breakfast Links), 2 links, 1.6 oz..............2.0
   (Morningstar Farms Breakfast Patties), 1.3-oz. patty 3.0
   (Worthington Prosage), 2 links, 1.6 oz.................................2.0
   (Worthington Prosage), 1.3-oz. patty 3.0
   crumbles *(Morningstar Farms* Sausage Style Recipe),
      ⅔ cup 5.0
   roll *(Worthington Prosage)*, ⅝" slice...................................2.0
Sausage hash, canned *(Mary Kitchen)*, 1 cup 23.0
Sausage sandwich, 4.5-oz. piece:
and egg, biscuit *(Hormel Quick Meal)*.......................................31.0
and egg and cheese, muffin *(Hormel Quick Meal)*......................29.0
Sausage sticks:
all varieties *(Rustlers Roundup)*, 1 piece 1.0

Sausage sticks *(cont.)*
beef and cheese *(Pemmican)*, 1.5-oz. pkg. 3.0
beef steak, kippered, tender, original, peppered, or teriyaki
    (Pemmican), 1.4-oz. piece...3.0
pepperoni and cheese *(Pemmican)*, 1.5-oz. pkg. 2.0
smoked *(Big Mama)*, 2-oz. pkg. 2.0
summer sausage, beef, cheddar, or spicy *(Johnsonville* Stix),
    1-oz. piece...0
Savory, ground:
1 tbsp. 3.0
1 tsp. 1.0
Scallion, see "Onion, green"
Scallops, meat only:
raw, 2 large or 5 small, 1.1 oz. 7
raw, 4 oz. 2.7
breaded, fried, 2 large, 1.1 oz. 3.1
"Scallops," imitation, from surimi, 4 oz. 12.0
Scallops, smoked *(Ducktrap River)*, ¼ cup, 2 oz. 3.0
"Scallops," vegetarian, canned *(Worthington Skallops)*,
    ½ cup 3.0
Scallop entree, frozen, fried *(Mrs. Paul's)*, 13 pieces 27.0
Scallop squash, fresh:
raw, sliced, 1 cup 5.0
boiled, drained:
    sliced, 1 cup 5.9
    sliced, ½ cup 3.0
    mashed, 1 cup 7.9
    mashed, ½ cup 4.0
Scone, all varieties *(Healthy Valley* Fat Free), 1 piece 43.0
Scorpion drink mix *(Trader Vic's)*, 4 fl. oz. 29.0
Scrapple *(Jones Dairy Farm* Country Style), 2 oz. 7.0
Scrod, fresh, see "Cod"
Scungilli, canned, sliced *(La Monica* Conch), ⅓ cup 1.0
Scup, without added ingredients 0
Sea bass, without added ingredients 0
Sea breeze drink mixer *(Mr & Mrs T)*, 4 fl. oz. 19.0
Sea trout, without added ingredients 0
Seafood, see specific listings
Seafood sauce (see also specific listings), cocktail, ¼ cup:
(Crosse & Blackwell Cocktail) 23.0
(Crosse & Blackwell Shrimp) 25.0

(Del Monte Cocktail) 24.0
(Kraft Cocktail) 13.0
Seafood seasoning, see "Fish seasoning and coating mix"
Seasoning and coating mix (see also specific listings):
(Don's Chuck Wagon Bake and Fry Mix), ¼ cup....................21.0
country mild recipe *(Shake 'n Bake)*, ⅛ pkt................................5.0
Seasonings, see specific listings
Seaweed:
agar *(Eden* Bar/Flakes), 1 tbsp...2.0
agar, raw, 2 tbsp. 7
arame *(Eden)*, ½ cup 7.0
hiziki *(Eden)*, ½ cup 6.0
Irish moss, raw, 2 tbsp. 1.2
kelp, raw, 2 tbsp. 1.0
kombu *(Eden)*, ½ of 7" piece 2.0
laver, 10 sheets 1.3
laver, 2 tbsp. 5
nori *(Eden)*, 1 sheet 1.0
nori, toasted *(Eden)*, 1 sheet 1.0
spirulina, dried, 1 cup 3.6
wakame:
   (Eden), ½ cup 4.0
   flakes *(Eden)*, 1 tsp. 0
   raw, 2 tbsp. 9
Semolina, whole-grain:
1 oz. 20.6
1 cup 121.6
Semolina flour:
(Arrowhead Mills), ½ cup 50.0
pasta *(Hodgson Mill)*, scant ¼ cup 22.0
Serrano chili, see "Pepper, chili"
Sesame butter, see "Tahini"
Sesame flour, 1 oz.:
high-fat...7.5
partially defatted..10.0
low-fat..10.1
Sesame meal, partially defatted, 1 oz. 7.4
Sesame paste (see also "Tahini"), from whole sesame
   seeds, 1 tbsp. 4.1
Sesame seasoning, plain, garlic, or seaweed *(Eden* Organic
   Sesame Shake), ½ tsp. 0

Sesame seeds:
whole, brown *(Arrowhead Mills)*, ¼ cup......................................8.0
whole, dried, 1 cup...33.8
whole, dried, 1 tbsp..2.1
whole, roasted and toasted, 1 oz..7.3
kernels *(Arrowhead Mills)*, ¼ cup......................................5.0
kernels, decorticated:
   whole, 1 oz...2.7
   whole, 1 cup..14.1
   whole, 1 tbsp..8
   toasted, 1 oz..7.4
   toasted, salted or unsalted, 1 cup...........................33.3
Sesbania flower, steamed, 1 cup......................................5.4
Shad, without added ingredients..0
Shaddock, see "Pummelo"
Shallot, fresh, raw:
(Frieda's), 1.1 oz...5.0
peeled, 1 oz..4.8
chopped, 1 tbsp...1.7
Shallot, freeze-dried:
¼ cup..2.9
1 tbsp...7
Shark, without added ingredients..0
Sheepshead, without added ingredients...............................0
Shellie beans, canned, 1 cup..15.2
Shells, pasta, plain, see "Pasta"
Shells, pasta, dinner, frozen, stuffed *(Healthy Choice* Meal),
   10.35-oz. pkg..60.0
Shells, pasta, dish, mix, about 1 cup*:
(Kraft Velveeta Original Dinner)....................................44.0
and cheddar, white *(Pasta Roni)*....................................40.0
and cheese:
   bacon *(Kraft Velveeta* Dinner)...............................43.0
   creamy *(Land O Lakes)*, 3.5 oz., 1 cup*..............40.0
   salsa *(Kraft Velveeta* Dinner), about 1 cup*.........47.0
Shells, pasta, entree, frozen, 1 pkg.:
and cheese, American *(Stouffer's)*, 1 cup....................36.0
and cheese, with jalapeños *(Michelina's)*, 8 oz............45.0
and cheese sauce *(Freezer Queen* Meal), 8.5 oz.........43.0
Sherbet, ½ cup:
berry rainbow *(Dreyer's/Edy's)*.....................................29.0

orange:
    (Breyers All Natural) 27.0
    (Turkey Hill)...20.0
    Swiss *(Dreyer's/Edy's)*...30.0
    with vanilla ice cream *(Breyers* Take Two All Natural) 20.0
    and vanilla ice cream *(Turkey Hill* Premium Orange
      Swirl) 19.0
    vanilla swirl *(Dreyer's/Edy's)*................................23.0
rainbow *(Breyers* All Natural) 27.0
rainbow *(Turkey Hill)* 26.0
raspberry *(Breyers* All Natural) 28.0
raspberry-chocolate swirl *(Dreyer's/Edy's)*.................28.0
tropical rainbow *(Dreyer's/Edy's)* 29.0
Sherbet bar, 1 bar:
(Popsicle Cyclone 8 Pack), 1.8 fl. oz...11.0
chocolate:
    (Fudgsicle 8 Pack), 2.5 fl. oz. 17.0
    (Fudgsicle Fat Free 10 Pack), 1.75 fl. oz. 13.0
    (Fudgsicle No Sugar 12 Pack), 1.75 fl. oz. 9.0
    (Fudgsicle Pop 12 Pack), 1.75 fl. oz....................12.0
    (Fudgsicle Variety 18 Pack), 1.75 fl. oz. 24.0
chocolate-vanilla swirl *(Fudgsicle* Variety 18 Pack), 1.75 fl. oz. ...23.0
orange-lemon *(Popsicle* Smile! 6 Pack)......................20.0
vanilla *(Fudgsicle* Variety 18 Pack), 1.75 fl. oz............22.0
and vanilla ice cream:
    orange-raspberry sherbet *(Creamsicle* 8 Pack), 2.5 fl. oz. 19.0
    orange-raspberry sherbet *(Creamsicle* 12 Pack),
      1.75 fl. oz..14.0
Shortening, 1 tbsp..0
Shrimp, meat only:
raw:
    4 oz. 1.0
    1 medium...2
    1 small...0
breaded, fried, 4 large, 1.1 oz.....................................3.4
Shrimp, canned, drained, 1 cup 1.3
Shrimp, freeze-dried, whole *(AlpineAire),* ½ cup.........2
"Shrimp," imitation, from surimi, 1 oz. 2.6
Shrimp, smoked, Maine *(Ducktrap River),* ¼ cup, 2 oz. ...0
Shrimp dinner, frozen, and vegetables *(Healthy
    Choice* Meal), 11.8-oz. pkg.....................................39.0

Shrimp entree, dried:
Alfredo *(AlpineAire)*, 1¼ cups 44.0
Newburg *(AlpineAire)*, 1¼ cups 49.0
Shrimp entree, frozen, 1 pkg., except as noted:
Alfredo, with fettuccine *(Michelina's)*, 8 oz. 31.0
and angel-hair pasta *(Lean Cuisine Cafe Classics)*, 10 oz. 35.0
Buffalo *(Mrs. Paul's/Van de Kamp's)*, 20 pieces.......................35.0
butterfly *(Mrs. Paul's)*, 7 pieces 27.0
butterfly *(Van de Kamp's)*, 7 pieces 30.0
fried rice, see "Rice dish, frozen"
linguine *(Mrs. Paul's/Van de Kamp's)*, 1½ cups 30.0
lo mein *(Michelina's Yu Sing)*, 8 oz...38.0
popcorn *(Mrs. Paul's)*, 20 pieces 31.0
popcorn *(Van de Kamp's)*, 20 pieces 30.0
stir-fry *(Mrs. Paul's/Van de Kamp's)*, 1⅔ cups 54.0
stuffed *(Van de Kamp's)*, 3 pieces...32.0
Shrimp entree mix, frozen *(Birds Eye Shrimp Voila!)*,
    2 cups 27.0
Shrimp sauce, see "Seafood sauce"
Sisymbrium seeds, whole, dried:
1 oz. 16.5
1 cup 43.1
Sloppy Joe dip:
(Fritos), 6 oz. 19.0
with corn chips, see "Corn chips and dip"
Sloppy Joe sauce, ¼ cup, except as noted:
(Del Monte Original Recipe)..16.0
(Heinz), ½ cup 14.0
(Hormel Not-So-Sloppy-Joe)..13.0
(Hunt's Manwich Bold)...13.0
(Hunt's Manwich Original)..7.0
(Hunt's Manwich Thick & Chunky)...9.0
barbecue *(Hunt's Manwich)* 14.0
hickory flavor *(Del Monte)* 18.0
Sloppy Joe seasoning mix *(Bearitos)*, 2 tsp. 6.0
Smelt, rainbow, without added ingredients 0
Snack bar, see "Granola and cereal bar"
Snack mix (see also "Trail mix" and specific listings),
    ½ cup, except as noted:
(Act II Original/Cheese/Honey BBQ), ¾ cup..............................20.0
(Boston's)...20.0

(Cheez-It Party Mix) 19.0
(Cheez-It Party Mix Reduced Fat) 21.0
(Chex Bold Party Mix) 20.0
(Chex Traditional),* ⅔ cup 22.0
(Doo Dads)...20.0
(Gardetto's Snak•ens Original Recipe) 18.0
(Gardetto's Snak•ens Original Recipe Reduced Fat)....19.0
(Kellogg's Snack 'Ums Big Boomin' Pops), 1 cup 27.0
(Kellogg's Snack 'Ums Big Rollin' Froot Loops!), 1 cup 28.0
(Kellogg's Snack 'Ums Rice Krispies Treats Krunch), 1 cup 26.0
(Planters Carribean Crunch), ¼ cup...................14.0
(Ritz Traditional) 21.0
(Rold Gold), ¾ cup, 1.2 oz. 18.0
baked *(Cheez-It* Get Nutty) 16.0
cheddar cheese *(Chex)*.......................................21.0
cheddar flavor *(Ritz),* 1.5-oz. pkg. 27.0
cheddar flavor *(Ritz)* 20.0
honey nut *(Chex)* 22.0
hot and spicy *(Chex),* ⅔ cup 21.0
Italian cheese blend or special recipe *(Gardetto's)*....20.0
nacho *(Cheez-It* Party Mix) 20.0
nacho fiesta *(Chex),* ⅔ cup................................22.0
peanut butter *(Wheatables* Snack Mix) 21.0
peanut lovers *(Chex)* 19.0
pretzel, deli-style mustard *(Gardetto's)* 24.0
sour cream and onion *(Gardetto's)* 21.0
toasted honey *(Wheatables* Snack Mix) 20.0
Snail, sea, see "Whelk"
Snap beans (see also "Green beans"), all varieties
    (Frieda's), ⅔ cup, 3 oz. 6.0
Snapper, without added ingredients 0
Snow peas, see "Peas, edible-podded"
Snow pea sprouts *(Jonathan's),* 1 cup 8.0
Soft drink, carbonated:
apple cider *(R.W. Knudsen* Sparkling), 8 fl. oz...........28.0
berry *(After the Fall Berrymeister Spritzer),* 12 fl. oz. 42.0
birch beer, brown or clear *(Canada Dry),* 8 fl. oz. 27.0
blueberry *(Minute Maid),* 8 fl. oz. 29.0
boysenberry *(R.W. Knudsen Spritzer),* 12 fl. oz. 40.0
boysenberry *(R.W. Knudsen Spritzer Light),* 12 fl. oz...28.0
cherries and cream *(Stewart's* Old Fashioned), 12 fl. oz...48.0

Soft drink *(cont.)*
cherry:
    (Crush), 8 fl. oz. 34.0
    (7Up), 8 fl. oz. 26.0
    black *(After the Fall Spritzer)*, 12 fl. oz. 45.0
    black *(Canada Dry)*, 8 fl. oz. 33.0
    black *(Koala)*, 11 fl. oz. 32.0
    black *(Koala)*, 8 fl. oz. 23.0
    black *(Minute Maid)*, 8 fl. oz. 29.0
    black *(R.W. Knudsen Sparkling)*, 8 fl. oz. 28.0
    black *(R.W. Knudsen Spritzer)*, 12 fl. oz. 42.0
    black *(R.W. Knudsen Spritzer)*, 10 fl. oz. 35.0
    lime *(Slice)*, 12 fl. oz. 43.0
    spice *(Slice)*, 12 fl. oz. 40.0
    wild *(Canada Dry)*, 8 fl. oz. 28.0
citrus *(Citra)*, 8 fl. oz. 25.0
citrus *(Orangina)*, 8 fl. oz. 23.0
club soda *(Canada Dry/Schweppes)*, 8 fl. oz. 0
cola:
    (Canada Dry Jamaica)*, 8 fl. oz. 27.0
    (Coca-Cola Classic/*Coca-Cola* Classic Caffeine Free)*,
        8 fl. oz. 27.0
    (Pepsi Regular/Caffeine Free)*, 12 fl. oz. 41.0
    (Santa Cruz Organic Gold)*, 12 fl. oz. 36.0
    (Slice), 12 fl. oz. 43.0
    cherry *(Cherry Coke)*, 8 fl. oz. 28.0
    cherry *(R.W. Knudsen Spritzer)*, 12 fl. oz. 42.0
    cherry, wild *(Pepsi)*, 12 fl. oz. 43.0
    cherry type, 16 fl. oz. 51.0
    ginseng *(Natural Brew)*, 12 fl. oz. 42.0
Collins mixer *(Canada Dry/Schweppes)*, 8 fl. oz. 21.0
cranberry:
    (R.W. Knudsen Spritzer), 12 fl. oz. 45.0
    (R.W. Knudsen Spritzer), 10 fl. oz. 38.0
    cider *(R.W. Knudsen* Sparkling)*, 8 fl. oz. 45.0
cranberry-raspberry *(Koala)*, 11 fl. oz. 29.0
cranberry-raspberry *(Koala)*, 8 fl. oz. 21.0
cream/creme:
    (A&W), 8 fl. oz. 28.0
    (After the Fall Creamie Vanilla Spritzer), 12 fl. oz. 42.0
    (Barq's French Vanilla)*, 8 fl. oz. 30.0

    (Barq's Red), 8 fl. oz..31.0
    (Canada Dry Vanilla Cream), 8 fl. oz......................30.0
    (Hires), 8 fl. oz. 32.0
    (Mug), 12 fl. oz. 48.0
    (R.W. Knudsen Spritzer Vanilla Creme), 12 fl. oz. 35.0
    (Stewart's), 12 fl. oz. 45.0
(Dr Pepper), 8 fl. oz. 27.0
(Dr. Slice), 12 fl. oz..39.0
fruit punch *(Minute Maid),* 8 fl. oz. 32.0
fruit punch *(Slice),* 12 fl. oz. 50.0
ginger ale:
    (After the Fall Nantucket Spritzer), 12 fl. oz. 40.0
    (Canada Dry Golden), 8 fl. oz. 24.0
    (Canada Dry/Schweppes), 8 fl. oz. 22.0
    (R.W. Knudsen Spritzer), 12 fl. oz. 40.0
    cherry *(Canada Dry),* 8 fl. oz. 27.0
    cranberry *(After the Fall Spritzer),* 12 fl. oz. 37.0
    cranberry *(Canada Dry),* 8 fl. oz. 25.0
    lemon *(Canada Dry),* 8 fl. oz. 25.0
    raspberry *(After the Fall Spritzer),* 12 fl. oz. 35.0
    raspberry *(Schweppes),* 8 fl. oz. 26.0
    strawberry *(After the Fall Spritzer),* 12 fl. oz. 37.0
ginger beer *(Schweppes),* 8 fl. oz. 25.0
grape:
    (After the Fall Concord Grape Spritzer), 12 fl. oz. 43.0
    (Canada Dry Concord), 8 fl. oz. 29.0
    (Crush), 8 fl. oz. 35.0
    (Minute Maid), 8 fl. oz. 34.0
    (R.W. Knudsen Spritzer), 12 fl. oz. 41.0
    (Schweppes), 8 fl. oz...33.0
    (Slice), 12 fl. oz. 51.0
    (Stewart's Classic), 12 fl. oz. 48.0
    sparkling, red or white *(R.W. Knudsen),* 8 fl. oz..............31.0
grapefruit *(Schweppes),* 8 fl. oz..................................27.0
grapefruit-kiwi-lime *(Koala),* 12 fl. oz..........................32.0
grapefruit-kiwi-lime *(Koala),* 8 fl. oz. 22.0
kiwi-lime *(R.W. Knudsen Spritzer),* 10 fl. oz. 32.0
kiwi-strawberry *(After the Fall Spritzer),* 12 fl. oz. 38.0
lemon:
    (Stewart's Meringue), 12 fl. oz. 50.0
    bitter *(Canada Dry),* 8 fl. oz. 26.0

Soft drink, lemon *(cont.)*
- bitter *(Schweppes)*, 8 fl. oz. 28.0
- sour *(Canada Dry)*, 8 fl. oz. 21.0
- sour *(Schweppes)*, 8 fl. oz. 26.0

lemonade (see also "Lemonade"):
- Jamaican *(R.W. Knudsen Spritzer)*, 12 fl. oz. 41.0
- Jamaican *(R.W. Knudsen Spritzer)*, 10 fl. oz. 34.0

lemon-lime:
- *(R.W. Knudsen Spritzer)*, 12 fl. oz. 42.0
- *(Schweppes)*, 8 fl. oz. 25.0
- *(Slice)*, 12 fl. oz. 40.0
- *(Slice* Diet)*, 12 fl. oz. 1.0

lime:
- *(After the Fall Caribbean Lime Spritzer)*, 12 fl. oz. 41.0
- *(Canada Dry* Island)*, 8 fl. oz. 33.0
- Key *(Stewart's)*, 12 fl. oz. 46.0
- mandarin *(R.W. Knudsen Spritzer)*, 12 fl. oz. 42.0

mango:
- *(After the Fall Hawaiian Mango Spritzer)*, 12 fl. oz. 45.0
- *(R.W. Knudsen Mango Fandango Spritzer)*, 12 fl. oz. 45.0
- *(R.W. Knudsen Spritzer Light)*, 12 fl. oz. 28.0

mango-ginger *(After the Fall Spritzer)*, 12 fl. oz. 36.0

(Mello Yello), 8 fl. oz. 32.0

(Mountain Dew Regular/Caffeine Free)*, 12 fl. oz. 46.0

(Mr. Pibb), 8 fl. oz. 26.0

orange:
- *(After the Fall Mimosa Orange Spritzer)*, 12 fl. oz. 39.0
- *(Canada Dry* Sunripe)*, 8 fl. oz. 29.0
- *(Crush)*, 8 fl. oz. 34.0
- *(Fanta)*, 8 fl. oz. 32.0
- *(Minute Maid)*, 8 fl. oz. 32.0
- *(Slice)*, 12 fl. oz. 46.0
- *(Slice* Caffeine Free)*, 12 fl. oz. 51.0
- *(Slice* Diet)*, 12 fl. oz. 1.0
- and cream *(Stewart's* Country)*, 12 fl. oz. 48.0
- and cream *(Stewart's* Country Diet)*, 12 fl. oz. 3.0

orange-mango:
- *(Koala)*, 12 fl. oz. 30.0
- *(Koala)*, 11 fl. oz. 25.0
- *(Koala)*, 8 fl. oz. 20.0

orange–passion fruit:
(Koala), 8 fl. oz. 25.0
(R.W. Knudsen Spritzer), 12 fl. oz. 40.0
(R.W. Knudsen Spritzer), 10 fl. oz. 33.0
peach:
(After the Fall Georgia Peach Spritzer), 12 fl. oz. 37.0
(Canada Dry), 8 fl. oz. 30.0
(Crush), 8 fl. oz. 33.0
(Minute Maid), 8 fl. oz. 29.0
(R.W. Knudsen Spritzer), 10 fl. oz. 31.0
(R.W. Knudsen Spritzer), 12 fl. oz. 37.0
pineapple:
(After the Fall Mandarin Spritzer), 12 fl. oz. 38.0
(Canada Dry), 8 fl. oz. 26.0
(Crush), 8 fl. oz. 34.0
(Minute Maid), 8 fl. oz. 30.0
(Slice), 12 fl. oz. 51.0
pineapple–passion fruit *(After the Fall Tropical Passion*
Spritzer), 12 fl. oz. 42.0
raspberry:
(After the Fall Spritzer), 12 fl. oz. 42.0
red *(R.W. Knudsen Spritzer)*, 12 fl. oz. 38.0
red *(R.W. Knudsen Spritzer)*, 10 fl. oz. 35.0
red *(R.W. Knudsen Spritzer Light)*, 12 fl. oz. 28.0
raspberry-guava:
(Koala), 12 fl. oz. 35.0
(Koala), 11 fl. oz. 30.0
(Koala), 8 fl. oz. 21.0
(Red Flash), 8 fl. oz. 28.0
root beer:
(A&W), 8 fl. oz. 31.0
(Barq's), 8 fl. oz. 30.0
(Barrelhead), 8 fl. oz. 27.0
(Hires), 8 fl. oz. 31.0
(Mug), 12 fl. oz. 43.0
(Santa Cruz Organic), 12 fl. oz. 36.0
(Stewart's), 12 fl. oz. 40.0
seltzer, plain or flavored *(Canada Dry/Schweppes)*, 8 fl. oz. 0
(7Up), 8 fl. oz. 26.0
(Slice Red), 12 fl. oz. 51.0
sour mixer *(Canada Dry)*, 8 fl. oz. 22.0

Soft drink *(cont.)*
(Sprite), 8 fl. oz. 26.0
(Storm), 12 fl. oz. 39.0
(Surge), 8 fl. oz. 31.0
strawberry:
    (Canada Dry California), 8 fl. oz. 27.0
    (Crush), 8 fl. oz. 30.0
    (Minute Maid), 8 fl. oz. 33.0
    (R.W. Knudsen Spritzer), 12 fl. oz. 42.0
    (R.W. Knudsen Spritzer), 10 fl. oz. 35.0
    (Slice), 12 fl. oz. 47.0
    cider *(R.W. Knudsen* Sparkling), 8 fl. oz. 28.0
strawberry-kiwi *(R.W. Knudsen Spritzer Light)*, 12 fl. oz. 28.0
strawberry-kiwi-peach *(Koala)*, 8 fl. oz. 25.0
tangerine:
    (After the Fall Spritzer), 12 fl. oz. 44.0
    (R.W. Knudsen Spritzer), 12 fl. oz. 40.0
    (R.W. Knudsen Spritzer), 10 fl. oz. 33.0
    (R.W. Knudsen Spritzer Light), 12 fl. oz. 28.0
tonic water, 8 fl. oz.:
    (Canada Dry) 24.0
    (Schweppes) 23.0
    cranberry *(Schweppes)* 21.0
vanilla, see "cream/creme," above
Sole, fresh, without added ingredients.............................0
Sole entree, frozen, ½ of 10-oz. pkg.:
au gratin *(Oven Poppers)*...4.0
crab-stuffed *(Oven Poppers)*..15.0
stuffed:
    with broccoli and cheese *(Oven Poppers)*.............4.0
    with garlic, shrimp, and almonds *(Oven Poppers)*...........15.0
    with shrimp and lobster *(Oven Poppers)* 7.0
Sopressata sausage:
hot *(Beretta)*, 2 oz. ....<1.0
hot *(Boar's Head Cinghiale)*, 1 oz....................................<1.0
with wine *(Fiorucci)*, 1 oz. 0
Sorbet, ½ cup:
(Ben & Jerry's Doonesberry) 33.0
berries, wild, chunky *(Real Fruit)* 27.0
boysenberry *(Dreyer's/Edy's Whole Fruit)*.....................37.0

cherry *(Mama Tish's Fruttuoso Sorbetto Premium*
   Italian Ices)...22.0
chocolate:
   (Dreyer's/Edy's Whole Fruit).................................40.0
   (Häagen-Dazs)...28.0
   (Mama Tish's Fruttuoso Sorbetto Premium Italian Ices).......25.0
   devil's food *(Ben & Jerry's)*...............................36.0
   Dutch *(Sharon's Sorbet)*......................................22.0
coconut *(Sharon's Sorbet)*...22.0
lemon:
   (Dreyer's/Edy's Whole Fruit).................................35.0
   (Häagen-Dazs Zesty)..31.0
   (Mama Tish's Fruttuoso Sorbetto Premium Italian Ices).......21.0
   (Sharon's Sorbet)..19.0
   peel, chunky *(Real Fruit)*......................................25.0
   swirl *(Ben & Jerry's)*...30.0
lemon-strawberry *(Mama Tish's Fruttuoso Sorbetto*
   Premium Italian Ices)..19.0
mango:
   (Dreyer's/Edy's Whole Fruit).................................33.0
   (Häagen-Dazs)...31.0
   (Sharon's Sorbet)..20.0
orange *(Häagen-Dazs)*...30.0
orange and vanilla ice cream *(Dreyer's/Edy's* 50/50 Bar
   Grand Light)...18.0
passion fruit, purple *(Ben & Jerry's)*.......................22.0
peach:
   (Dreyer's/Edy's Whole Fruit).................................32.0
   (Häagen-Dazs Orchard)......................................35.0
   chunky *(Real Fruit* Georgia).................................28.0
raspberry:
   (Dreyer's/Edy's Whole Fruit).................................33.0
   (Häagen-Dazs)...30.0
   (Mama Tish's Fruttuoso Sorbetto Premium Italian Ices).......24.0
   (Sharon's Sorbet)..20.0
   chunky, red *(Real Fruit)*.......................................27.0
strawberry:
   (Dreyer's/Edy's Whole Fruit).................................31.0
   (Häagen-Dazs)...32.0
   (Mama Tish's Fruttuoso Sorbetto Premium Italian Ices).......20.0
   chunky *(Real Fruit* Mountain)...............................26.0

Sorbet *(cont.)*
tropical blend, chunky *(Real Fruit)*....................................29.0
vanilla *(Häagen-Dazs)*...30.0
vanilla, dark *(Sharon's Sorbet)*...15.0
Sorbet bar, 1 bar:
orange and vanilla ice cream *(Häagen-Dazs)*.......................16.0
with marshmallow swirl *(Cool Cotton Candy)*.......................20.0
strawberry and vanilla ice cream *(Häagen-Dazs)*...................15.0
Sorghum, whole-grain, 1 cup...143.3
Sorghum syrup:
(Arrowhead Mills), 1 tbsp. 16.0
1 cup...247.2
1 tbsp..15.7
Sorrel, see "Dock"
Soup, canned, ready-to-serve, 1 cup, except as noted:
asparagus, cream of *(Baxters)*..13.0
bean:
    (Dominique's U.S. Senate) 29.0
    black *(Greene's Farm),* ½ of 15-oz. can 32.0
    black *(Hain)*...18.0
    black *(Health Valley* Organic)......................................25.0
    black *(Progresso* Hearty)...30.0
    black, Indian, with rice *(Shari Ann's* Organic) 30.0
    black, vegetable *(Amy's)*..22.0
    five, with barley *(Coco Pazzo* Tuscan) 31.0
    and ham *(Campbell's* Chunky)....................................29.0
    and ham *(Campbell's Home Cookin')*..............................32.0
    and ham *(Healthy Choice)*...28.0
    Mexican, spicy *(Shari Ann's* Organic)...........................38.0
    and pasta *(Baxters* Healthy Reward Italian).....................19.0
    and pasta, Mediterranean *(Healthy Choice)*.....................26.0
    three, with sage *(Coco Pazzo* Tuscan) 35.0
    white, with escarole *(Coco Pazzo* Tuscan).......................31.0
    white, Italian *(Shari Ann's* Organic) 32.0
beef:
    barley *(Progresso* 99% Fat Free)................................20.0
    and mushroom *(Progresso)*..12.0
    pasta *(Campbell's* Chunky) 18.0
    and potato *(Healthy Choice)*.....................................21.0
    and potato, baked *(Progresso)*...................................18.0
    and vegetable *(Progresso)* 12.0

vegetable, chunky *(Campbell's* Low Sodium),
    10¾-oz. can...11.0
with vegetables, country *(Campbell's* Chunky).....................14.0
with vegetables, country *(Campbell's* Chunky),
    10¾-oz. can...22.0
beef broth:
    (College Inn/College Inn Fat Free) 0
    (Health Valley) 0
    (Health Valley Quart) 2.0
    clear *(Swanson)* 1.0
broccoli-carotene *(Health Valley* Fat Free)....................16.0
broccoli-cheddar *(Healthy Choice)*.............................19.0
chicken:
    Alfredo *(Healthy Choice)*...20.0
    barley *(Progresso)*...16.0
    broccoli, cheese, and potato *(Campbell's* Chunky)......14.0
    broccoli, cheese, and potato *(Campbell's* Chunky),
       10¾-oz. can...17.0
    chunky..16.5
    hearty *(Healthy Choice)* 23.0
    with meatballs *(Progresso* Chickarina)......................12.0
    mushroom chowder *(Campbell's* Chunky) 18.0
    noodle *(Campbell's* Low Sodium), 10¾-oz. can.......18.0
    noodle *(Campbell's Simply Home)* 12.0
    noodle *(Hain)*...24.0
    noodle *(Hain* No Salt) 13.0
    noodle *(Health Valley* 99% Fat Free) 20.0
    noodle *(Healthy Choice)* 18.0
    noodle *(Progresso)*...9.0
    noodle *(Progresso* 99% Fat Free)..............................13.0
    noodle, chunky 17.5
    noodle, chunky, 19-oz. can..38.3
    noodle, classic *(Campbell's* Chunky) 16.0
    noodle, classic *(Campbell's* Chunky), 10¾-oz. can 20.0
    noodle, egg *(Wolfgang Puck's)* 16.0
    noodle, hearty *(Campbell's Healthy Request)*.............16.0
    noodle, with meatballs, chunky 8.4
    noodle, with meatballs, chunky, 20-oz. can...............19.1
    with noodles, egg *(Campbell's Home Cookin')*............13.0
    with noodles, egg *(Campbell's Home Cookin')*,
       10¾-oz. can...16.0

Soup, canned, ready-to-serve, chicken *(cont.)*

and pasta *(Campbell's Simply Home)* 14.0
and pasta, with roasted garlic *(Campbell's Home
  Cookin')* 17.0
with pasta *(Healthy Choice)* 19.0
with pasta and mushrooms *(Campbell's Chunky)* 16.0
roasted, garden herb *(Progresso)* 7.0
roasted, with long-grain and wild rice *(Campbell's Select)* ...17.0
rice *(Campbell's Home Cookin')* 19.0
rice *(Campbell's Home Cookin')*, 10¾-oz. can 22.0
rice *(Health Valley 99% Fat Free)* 21.0
rice *(Healthy Choice)* 16.0
rice, chunky 13.0
rice, chunky, 19-oz. can 29.2
rice, hearty *(Campbell's Healthy Request)* 14.0
rice, wild *(Progresso)* 15.0
rice, wild *(Progresso 99% Fat Free)* 12.0
with rice *(Rienzi)* 17.0
with rice, white and wild *(Campbell's Simply Home)* 19.0
and rotini *(Progresso Hearty)* 11.0
savory, with white/wild rice *(Campbell's Chunky)* 18.0
spicy, with vegetables *(Campbell's Chunky)* 13.0
vegetable *(Campbell's Healthy Request)* 18.0
vegetable *(Campbell's Home Cookin')* 18.0
vegetable *(Progresso)* 13.0
vegetable, chunky 18.9
vegetable, chunky, 19-oz. can 42.4
vegetable, with pasta *(Progresso Homestyle)* 11.0
vegetable, roast *(Wolfgang Puck's)* 17.0
with vegetables, hearty *(Campbell's Chunky)* 12.0
with vegetables, Indian style *(Campbell's Home Cookin')* 20.0
chicken broth:
  (Campbell's Low Sodium), 10½-oz. can 2.0
  (Campbell's Healthy Request) 1.0
  (College Inn/College Inn No Fat/Low Salt) 1.0
  (Hain/Hain No Salt) 3.0
  (Health Valley) 0
  (Health Valley Quart) 2.0
  (Swanson/Swanson Fat Free) 1.0
  clear *(Swanson)* ....<1.0
  with Italian herbs or roasted garlic *(Swanson)* 3.0

with onion *(Swanson)* 5.0
chicken corn chowder:
   (Campbell's Chunky) 18.0
   (Campbell's Chunky), 10¾-oz. can 22.0
   (Campbell's Healthy Request) 24.0
   (Healthy Choice) 28.0
chili beef *(Healthy Choice)* 34.0
chili beef with beans *(Campbell's* Chunky) 38.0
chili pepper *(A Taste of Thai)* 5.0
clam chowder, Manhattan:
   (Campbell's Chunky) 20.0
   (Campbell's Chunky), 10¾-oz. can 25.0
   (Progresso) 11.0
   chunky 18.8
clam chowder, New England:
   (Campbell's Chunky) 21.0
   (Campbell's Chunky), 10¾-oz. can 26.0
   (Campbell's Healthy Request) 17.0
   (Campbell's Home Cookin') 14.0
   (Campbell's Home Cookin'), 10¾-oz. can 17.0
   (Campbell's Home Cookin' 98% Fat Free) 17.0
   (Dominique's) 13.0
   (Healthy Choice) 24.0
   (Snow's) 14.0
coconut-ginger *(A Taste of Thai)* 11.0
consommé, clear *(Dominique's* Madrilène) ....<1.0
consommé, red *(Dominique's* Madrilène) 2.0
corn chowder *(Greene's Farm)*, ½ of 15-oz. can 26.0
corn tortilla *(Buckaroo)* 22.0
corn and vegetable *(Health Valley* Fat Free) 17.0
crab, cream of *(Chincoteague* Chesapeake Bay) 23.0
crab, vegetable *(Chincoteague* Red Crab) 12.0
escarole *(Progresso)* 3.0
gazpacho *(Dominique's)* 12.0
gumbo, zesty *(Healthy Choice)* 15.0
leek *(Baxter's* Scotch) 8.0
lemongrass *(A Taste of Thai)* 6.0
lentil:
   (Amy's) 19.0
   (Health Valley Organic) 18.0
   (Health Valley Organic No Salt) 21.0

Soup, canned, ready-to-serve, lentil *(cont.)*

    (Progresso Classics) 22.0

    (Progresso 99% Fat Free) 20.0

    (Rienzi) 22.0

    green, French, spicy *(Shari Ann's* Organic) 22.0

    with ham 20.2

    with ham, 20-oz. can 46.3

    sausage *(Dominique's)* 25.0

    savory *(Campbell's Home Cookin')* 23.0

    vegetarian *(Hain)* 30.0

lobster bisque *(Baxters)* 12.0

macaroni and bean *(Progresso* Classics) 23.0

macaroni and bean *(Rienzi)* 26.0

minestrone:

    (Amy's) 17.0

    (Baxters Healthy Reward Homestyle) 21.0

    (Campbell's Simply Home) 21.0

    (Hain) 20.0

    (Health Valley Fat Free) 21.0

    (Health Valley Organic) 17.0

    (Healthy Choice) 26.0

    (Progresso 99% Fat Free) 19.0

    (Rienzi) 21.0

    (Shari Ann's Organic) 20.0

    chunky 20.7

    chunky, 19-oz. can 46.6

    hearty *(Campbell's* Plus!) 26.0

    hearty *(Campbell's Healthy Request)* 22.0

    old world *(Campbell's Home Cookin')* 25.0

    Tuscany style *(Campbell's Home Cookin')* 21.0

mulligatawny, see "vegetable," below

mushroom:

    barley *(Hain)* 26.0

    barley *(Health Valley* Organic) 17.0

    cream of *(Amy's)*, ¾ cup 10.0

    cream of *(Campbell's* Low Sodium), 10½-oz. can 18.0

    cream of *(Campbell's Home Cookin'* 98% Fat Free) 15.0

    cream of *(Hain)* 28.0

    rice, country *(Campbell's Home Cookin')* 16.0

    mushroom broth *(Health Valley)* 2.0

noodle *(Amy's* No Chicken) 12.0

noodles, Oriental, with vegetables *(Campbell's Home Cookin')* 18.0
onion, French:
    (Progresso Distinctive Recipe) 9.0
    (Wolfgang Puck's Country) 16.0
    vegetarian *(Shari Ann's* Organic) 9.0
pasta:
    Bolognese *(Health Valley* Fat Free) 20.0
    cacciatore *(Health Valley* Fat Free) 20.0
    fagioli *(Health Valley* Fat Free) 25.0
    Romano *(Health Valley* Fat Free) 20.0
    rotini *(Health Valley* Fat Free) 20.0
    and vegetables, hearty *(Campbell's* Plus!) 20.0
pea, split:
    (Amy's) 19.0
    (Campbell's Low Sodium), 10½-oz. can 38.0
    (Health Valley Organic) 23.0
    (Shari Ann's Organic Great Plains) 26.0
    and carrot *(Health Valley* Fat Free) 25.0
    green *(Progresso* Classics) 25.0
    and ham *(Campbell's* Chunky) 27.0
    with ham *(Campbell's* Healthy Request) 29.0
    with ham *(Campbell's* Home Cookin') 30.0
    with ham *(Healthy Choice)* 28.0
    with ham *(Progresso* Distinctive Recipe) 20.0
    with ham, chunky 26.8
    with ham, chunky, 19-oz. can 60.2
    vegetarian *(Hain)* 20.0
penne *(Progresso* Hearty) 14.0
pepper steak *(Campbell's* Chunky) 18.0
potato:
    baked, with bacon bits and chives *(Campbell's* Chunky) 20.0
    baked, with cheddar and bacon bits *(Campbell's* Chunky) 23.0
    baked, with steak and cheese *(Campbell's* Chunky) 21.0
    baked style *(Healthy Choice)* 26.0
    with broccoli and cheese chowder *(Progresso)* 21.0
    and cheddar *(Shari Ann's* Organic) 15.0
    creamy, with roasted garlic *(Campbell's* Healthy Request) 22.0
    creamy, with roasted garlic *(Campbell's* Home Cookin') 21.0
    ham, creamy *(Healthy Choice)* 25.0
    ham chowder, old-fashioned *(Campbell's* Chunky) 16.0

Soup, canned, ready-to-serve *(cont.)*

    leek *(Baxter's* Healthy Reward)...............................16.0
    leek *(Health Valley* Organic)..................................15.0
  rotini, tomato-basil *(Progresso)*.................................22.0
  sirloin burger with vegetables *(Campbell's* Chunky) 18.0
  sirloin burger with vegetables *(Campbell's* Chunky),
    10¾-oz. can 22.0
  steak and potato *(Campbell's* Chunky)........................19.0
  steak and potato *(Campbell's* Chunky), 10¾-oz. can 24.0
  tomato:
    (Campbell's) 22.0
    (Muir Glen Organic Fresh Pack) 12.0
    (Health Valley Organic)......................................18.0
    chunky *(Hain)* 27.0
    cream of *(Amy's)* 17.0
    cream of *(Shari Ann's* Organic) 17.0
    creamy *(Campbell's)* 26.0
    garden *(Campbell's* Home Cookin')..........................22.0
    garden *(Healthy Choice)*......................................20.0
    ravioli, cheese, with vegetables *(Campbell's* Chunky) 26.0
    ravioli with vegetables, hearty *(Campbell's* Healthy
      Request) 26.0
    with red bell pepper *(Shari Ann's* Organic)..................19.0
    with roasted garlic *(Shari Ann's* Organic)..................12.0
    with tomato pieces *(Campbell's* Low Sodium),
      10½-oz. can...28.0
    vegetable *(Health Valley* Fat Free)..........................17.0
    with vegetables *(Wolfgang Puck's* Country) 18.0
  tortellini, cheese, with chicken and vegetables *(Campbell's*
    Chunky) 18.0
  tortellini, cheese and herb *(Progresso)*.......................23.0
  turkey:
    chunky..14.1
    chunky, with wild rice *(Greene's Farm)*, ½ of 15-oz. can 19.0
    chunky, with wild rice *(Healthy Choice)*.....................17.0
    noodle *(Progresso)*..11.0
    rice, with vegetables *(Progresso)* 18.0
  vegetable:
    (Campbell's Chunky)...22.0
    (Campbell's Chunky), 10¾-oz. can..........................28.0
    (Health Valley Organic).......................................18.0

(Progresso Classics) 17.0
barley *(Health Valley* Fat Free) 19.0
barley *(Shari Ann's* Organic)..........................18.0
bean, black *(Health Valley* Fat Free)..............24.0
bean, five *(Health Valley* Fat Free) 32.0
country *(Campbell's Home Cookin')*................21.0
country *(Campbell's Home Cookin')*, 10¾-oz. can ...27.0
country *(Healthy Choice)*.................................22.0
fiesta *(Campbell's Home Cookin')*...................24.0
garden *(Campbell's Simply Home)*..................21.0
garden *(Healthy Choice)*.................................25.0
garden, 14 vegetables *(Health Valley* Fat Free)....17.0
hearty *(Campbell's Healthy Request)*..............20.0
Indian, hot *(Patak's* Sabzi Mulligatawny)........20.0
Indian, mild, tomato and lentil *(Patak's)*..........20.0
with pasta *(Rienzi)*..20.0
with pasta, hearty *(Campbell's* Chunky) 24.0
roasted, with barley and wild rice *(Campbell's* Plus!) ...25.0
Southwestern, with black beans *(Campbell's Healthy*
  Request)...28.0
thick *(Wolfgang Puck's* Country)....................25.0
vegetable beef:
  (Campbell's Home Cookin')...........................15.0
  (Healthy Choice)...20.0
  hearty *(Campbell's Healthy Request)*..............20.0
  old-fashioned *(Campbell's* Chunky)................17.0
  old-fashioned *(Campbell's* Chunky), 10¾-oz. can ...20.0
  with pasta *(Campbell's Simply Home)*.............19.0
vegetable broth:
  (College Inn Fat Free) 5.0
  (Hain/Hain No Salt)......................................8.0
  (Health Valley) 5.0
  (Health Valley Quart) 3.0
  clear *(Swanson)* 3.0
vichyssoise *(Dominique's)*..............................17.0
wild rice *(Hain)*...15.0
Soup, canned, condensed, ½ cup undiluted, except as noted:
asparagus, cream of:
  (Campbell's) 11.0
  diluted with equal volume water, 1 cup.............10.7
  diluted with equal volume whole milk, 1 cup.........16.4

Soup, canned, condensed *(cont.)*

bean:

with bacon *(Campbell's)* 25.0

black *(Campbell's)* 19.0

black, diluted with equal volume water, 1 cup 19.8

with frankfurters, diluted with equal volume water, 1 cup 22.8

with ham and bacon *(Campbell's Healthy Request)* 26.0

with pork, diluted with equal volume water, 1 cup 22.8

beef:

broth, double rich, double strength *(Campbell's)* 1.0

consommé *(Campbell's)* 2.0

consommé, diluted with equal volume water, 1 cup 1.8

mushroom, diluted with equal volume water, 1 cup 6.3

noodle *(Campbell's)* 8.0

noodle, diluted with equal volume water, 1 cup 9.0

with vegetables and barley *(Campbell's)* 11.0

broccoli, cream of:

(Campbell's) 9.0

(Campbell's 98% Fat Free) 12.0

(Campbell's Healthy Request) 9.0

cheese *(Campbell's)* 9.0

cheese, cream of *(Campbell's 98% Fat Free)* 11.0

celery, cream of:

(Campbell's) 9.0

(Campbell's 98% Fat Free) 11.0

(Campbell's Healthy Request) 11.0

diluted with equal volume water, 1 cup 8.8

diluted with equal volume whole milk, 1 cup 14.5

cheese:

diluted with equal volume water, 1 cup 10.5

diluted with equal volume whole milk, 1 cup 16.2

cheddar *(Campbell's)* 10.0

nacho, fiesta *(Campbell's)* 11.0

chicken:

alphabet, with vegetables *(Campbell's)* 11.0

and broccoli, cream of *(Campbell's)* 9.0

broth *(Campbell's)* 2.0

broth, diluted with equal volume water, 1 cup 9

cream of *(Campbell's)* 11.0

cream of *(Campbell's 98% Fat Free)* 9.0

cream of *(Campbell's Healthy Request)* 12.0

cream of, diluted with equal volume water, 1 cup 9.3
cream of, diluted equal volume whole milk, 1 cup 15.0
cream of, and broccoli *(Campbell's Healthy Request)* 10.0
cream of, with herbs *(Campbell's)* 9.0
with dumplings *(Campbell's)* 10.0
with dumplings, diluted with equal volume water, 1 cup 6.0
gumbo *(Campbell's)* 9.0
gumbo, diluted with equal volume water, 1 cup 8.3
mushroom, diluted with equal volume water, 1 cup 9.3
mushroom, cream of *(Campbell's)* 9.0
noodle *(Campbell's)* 9.0
noodle *(Campbell's Healthy Request)* 9.0
noodle, diluted with equal volume water, 1 cup 9.4
noodle, creamy or curly *(Campbell's)* 12.0
noodle, double, in chicken broth *(Campbell's)* 15.0
noodle, home style *(Campbell's)* 9.0
noodle O's *(Campbell's)* 10.0
rice *(Campbell's)* 9.0
with rice *(Campbell's Healthy Request)* 10.0
with rice, diluted with equal volume water, 1 cup 7.2
with rice, white and wild *(Campbell's)* 9.0
and stars *(Campbell's)* 9.0
vegetable *(Campbell's/Campbell's Healthy Request)* 12.0
vegetable, Southwestern style *(Campbell's)* 18.0
chili beef, diluted with equal volume water, 1 cup 21.5
chili beef with beans, fiesta *(Campbell's)* 24.0
clam bisque *(Chincoteague)*, ½ cup 13.0
clam chowder, Manhattan:
   (Campbell's) 12.0
   (Chincoteague) 13.0
   diluted with equal volume water, 1 cup 12.2
clam chowder, New England:
   (Campbell's) 13.0
   (Campbell's 98% Fat Free) 14.0
   (Chincoteague) 10.0
   (Jake's), ⅔ cup undiluted 20.0
   (Olde Cape Cod All Natural) 11.0
   diluted with equal volume water, 1 cup 12.4
   diluted equal volume whole milk, 1 cup 16.6
corn chowder *(Chincoteague)* 16.0
corn chowder *(Olde Cape Cod All Natural Old Fashioned)* 18.0

Soup, canned, condensed *(cont.)*
crab and cheddar *(Chincoteague* Chesapeake Bay).....................10.0
lobster bisque *(Chincoteague)* 10.0
lobster bisque *(Old Cape Cod* All Natural Gourmet)....................8.0
minestrone:
   (Campbell's) 15.0
   (Campbell's Healthy Request)..17.0
   diluted with equal volume water, 1 cup 11.2
mushroom:
   barley, diluted with equal volume water, 1 cup....................11.7
   with beef stock, diluted with equal volume water, 1 cup.......11.7
   beefy *(Campbell's)* 6.0
   cream of *(Campbell's/Campbell's* 98% Fat Free) 9.0
   cream of *(Campbell's Healthy Request)* 10.0
   cream of, diluted with equal volume water, 1 cup..................9.3
   cream of, diluted with equal volume whole milk, 1 cup 15.0
   cream of, with roasted garlic *(Campbell's)*...........................10.0
   golden *(Campbell's)*...10.0
noodle, souper stars *(Campbell's)* 7.0
noodles and ground beef *(Campbell's)* 11.0
onion:
   diluted with equal volume water, 1 cup 8.4
   cream of *(Campbell's)* 13.0
   cream of, diluted with equal volume water, 1 cup.................12.7
   cream of, diluted with equal volume whole milk, 1 cup 18.4
   French *(Campbell's)*...10.0
oyster chowder *(Olde Cape Cod)* 11.0
oyster stew:
   (Campbell's) 6.0
   diluted with equal volume water, 1 cup 4.1
   diluted with equal volume whole milk, 1 cup 9.8
pasta, with chicken in chicken broth *(Campbell's Rugrats)* 9.0
pea:
   green *(Campbell's)* 29.0
   green, diluted with equal volume water, 1 cup 26.5
   green, diluted with equal volume whole milk, 1 cup 32.2
   split, with ham *(Campbell's)* 28.0
   split, with ham, diluted with equal volume water, 1 cup........28.0
pepperpot *(Campbell's)*..9.0
pepperpot, diluted with equal volume water, 1 cup......................9.4

potato, cream of:
    (Campbell's) 14.0
    diluted with equal volume water, 1 cup 11.5
    diluted with equal volume whole milk, 1 cup 17.2
Scotch broth *(Campbell's)* 9.0
Scotch broth, diluted with equal volume water, 1 cup 9.5
shrimp, cream of:
    (Campbell's) 8.0
    diluted with equal volume water, 1 cup 8.2
    diluted with equal volume whole milk, 1 cup 13.9
shrimp bisque *(Chincoteague)* 10.0
shrimp and tomato bisque *(Olde Cape Cod)* 8.0
stockpot, diluted with equal volume water, 1 cup 11.5
tomato:
    (Campbell's) 19.0
    (Campbell's Healthy Request) 18.0
    diluted with equal volume water, 1 cup 16.6
    diluted with equal volume whole milk, 1 cup 22.9
    beef with noodle, diluted with equal volume water, 1 cup 21.2
    bisque *(Campbell's)* 24.0
    bisque, diluted with equal volume water, 1 cup 23.7
    bisque, diluted with equal volume whole milk, 1 cup 29.4
    Italian, with basil and oregano *(Campbell's)* 23.0
    rice, diluted with equal volume water, 1 cup 21.9
    rice, old-fashioned *(Campbell's)* 23.0
turkey:
    noodle *(Campbell's)* 10.0
    noodle, diluted with equal volume water, 1 cup 8.6
    vegetable *(Campbell's)* 11.0
    vegetable, diluted with equal volume water, 1 cup 8.6
vegetable:
    (Campbell's) 17.0
    (Campbell's Old Fashioned) 10.0
    (Campbell's Healthy Request) 16.0
    beef *(Campbell's)* 14.0
    beef *(Campbell's Healthy Request)* 11.0
    beef diluted with equal volume water, 1 cup 10.2
    with beef broth, diluted with equal volume water, 1 cup 13.0
    California style *(Campbell's)* 10.0
    pasta, hearty *(Campbell's)* 18.0
    pasta, hearty *(Campbell's Healthy Request)* 16.0

Soup, canned, condensed, vegetable *(cont.)*
    vegetarian *(Campbell's)* 18.0
    vegetarian, diluted with equal volume water, 1 cup 12.0
won ton *(Campbell's)* 5.0
Soup, canned, semicondensed, ⅔ cup undiluted, except
    as noted:
black bean *(Pepperidge Farm)* 19.0
chicken curry *(Pepperidge Farm)* 16.0
chicken with wild rice *(Pepperidge Farm)* 8.0
clam chowder, Manhattan *(Bookbinder's)*, ½ cup undiluted 12.0
clam chowder, New England *(Pepperidge Farm)* 13.0
consommé *(Pepperidge Farm* Madrilène) 6.0
corn chowder *(Pepperidge Farm)* 14.0
crab bisque *(Bookbinder's)*, ½ cup undiluted 10.0
gazpacho *(Pepperidge Farm)* 12.0
lobster bisque *(Bookbinder's)*, ½ cup undiluted 10.0
lobster bisque *(Pepperidge Farm)* 12.0
mushroom, shiitake *(Pepperidge Farm)* 10.0
onion, French *(Pepperidge Farm)* 7.0
pepperpot *(Bookbinder's)*, ½ cup undiluted 16.0
vichyssoise or watercress *(Pepperidge Farm)* 11.0
Soup, dried (see also "Soup, mix"):
bean, multi *(AlpineAire)*, 1½ cups 28.0
broccoli, cream of *(AlpineAire)*, 1 cup 21.0
corn chowder *(AlpineAire Kernel's)*, ⅞ cup 35.0
minestrone *(AlpineAire Alpine)*, 1½ cups 33.0
potato with cheddar, creamy *(AlpineAire)*, 1½ cups 36.0
split pea *(AlpineAire Soup-er)*, 1 cup 34.0
Soup, frozen, 7.5 oz.:
barley mushroom *(Tabatchnick)* 13.0
bean, Yankee *(Tabatchnick)* 27.0
broccoli, cream of *(Tabatchnick)* 12.0
cabbage *(Tabatchnick)* 14.0
chicken, New York *(Tabatchnick)* 6.0
chicken with dumplings *(Tabatchnick)* 13.0
corn chowder *(Tabatchnick)* 22.0
lentil *(Tabatchnick)* 25.0
minestrone *(Tabatchnick)* 27.0
mushroom *(Tabatchnick No Salt)* 13.0
mushroom, cream of *(Tabatchnick)* 12.0
onion *(Tabatchnick)* 11.0

pea *(Tabatchnick/Tabatchnick* No Salt)..31.0
potato, New England *(Tabatchnick)*...................................21.0
potato, old-fashioned *(Tabatchnick)*..................................16.0
spinach, cream of *(Tabatchnick)*..11.0
tomato-rice *(Tabatchnick)*...11.0
vegetable *(Tabatchnick/Tabatchnick* No Salt) 20.0
wild rice *(Tabatchnick)*...24.0
Soup, mix (see also "Soup, dried," and "Soup base mix"),
   dry, except as noted:
asparagus, creamy *(Fantastic Foods* Cup), 1.2 oz. 22.0
bean:
   (Hodgson Mill Choice), ¼ cup...27.0
   black *(Fantastic Foods* Hearty Cup Jumpin'), 2.2 oz. 39.0
   black *(Knorr* TasteBreaks), 1 cont. 36.0
   black *(Near East)*, 1 cont. 40.0
   black *(Nile Spice)*, 1 cont. 35.0
   black, spicy, with couscous *(Health Valley)*, ⅓ cup..............29.0
   black, zesty, with rice *(Health Valley)*, ⅓ cup 22.0
   five *(Fantastic Foods* Hearty Cup), 2.3 oz. 43.0
   navy *(Knorr* TasteBreaks), 1 cont. 25.0
   navy *(Nile Spice* Home Style), 1 cont. 37.0
   red, and rice *(Near East)*, 1 cont. 40.0
bean and barley, 7 beans *(Arrowhead Mills)*, ⅓ cup..................35.0
bean and ham *(Hormel* Micro Cup), 1 cup................................29.0
bean and pasta, see "pasta and bean," below
beef noodle *(House of Tsang)*, 1 cont. 23.0
beef vegetable *(Hormel* Micro Cup), 1 cup 15.0
beefy mushroom *(Lipton Recipe Secrets)*, 1½ tbsp. 7.0
beefy onion *(Lipton Recipe Secrets)*, 1 tbsp. 5.0
broccoli, cream of *(Knorr Recipe Classics* Soup/Recipe),
   2 tbsp. 10.0
broccoli-cheddar, creamy *(Fantastic Foods* Cup), 1.4 oz. 26.0
broccoli and cheese *(Lipton Cup-a-Soup)*, 1 pkt. 9.0
broccoli-cheese with ham *(Hormel* Micro Cup), 1 cup 10.0
cheddar-broccoli *(Nile Spice* Home Style), 1 cont. 19.0
chicken:
   cream of *(Lipton Cup-a-Soup)*, 1 pkt. 12.0
   noodle *(Herb-ox)*, 1 cont. 19.0
   noodle *(Hormel* Micro Cup), 1 cup.......................................13.0
   noodle *(House of Tsang)*, 1 cont. 25.0
   noodle *(Knorr* Savory), 3 tbsp..11.0

Soup, mix, chicken *(cont.)*
    noodle *(Lipton Cup-a-Soup)*, 1 pkt...................................8.0
    noodle *(Nile Spice* Home Style), 1 cont....................16.0
    noodle, hearty *(Knorr* TasteBreaks), 1 cont. 20.0
    and rice *(Hormel* Micro Cup), 1 cup........................17.0
    with rice *(Knorr* Savory), 3 tbsp............................14.0
    with rice *(Wyler's Mrs. Grass)*, ¼ pkg....................15.0
    vegetable *(Nile Spice* Home Style), 1 cont. 21.0
chili:
    (Fantastic Foods Hearty Cha-Cha Cup), 2.4 oz. 37.0
    (Herb-ox), 1 cont. 37.0
    without beans *(Herb-ox)*, 1 cont. 17.0
clam chowder, New England *(Hormel* Micro Cup), 1 cup 17.0
coconut-ginger *(A Taste of Thai)*, 2 tsp.............................2.0
corn:
    (House of Tsang Velvet), 1 cont. 34.0
    chowder *(Knorr* TasteBreaks), 1 cont. 26.0
    chowder, roasted *(Near East)*, 1 cont. 28.0
    chowder, with tomatoes *(Health Valley)*, ½ cup 21.0
    sweet *(Nile Spice* Home Style), 1 cont. 22.0
corn and potato chowder, creamy *(Fantastic Foods* Cup),
    1.6 oz. 34.0
couscous:
    black bean salsa *(Fantastic Foods* Cup), 2.4 oz................46.0
    corn, sweet *(Fantastic Foods* Cup), 1.8 oz. 36.0
    eggplant, mushroom, tomato *(Marrakesh Express*
        Zuppa Cup), 1.5 oz. 33.0
    with lentils *(Fantastic Foods* Hearty Cup), 2.3 oz. 44.0
    nacho cheddar *(Fantastic Foods* Cup), 1.9 oz. 36.0
    onion, toasted *(Marrakesh Express* Zuppa Cup), 1.5 oz........35.0
    vegetable Creole *(Fantastic Foods* Cup), 2.1 oz. 41.0
garlic herb *(Knorr Recipe Classics* Soup/Recipe), 3 tbsp. 13.0
garlic-mushroom *(Lipton Recipe Secrets)*, 1⅓ tbsp.................4.0
garlic-mushroom, creamy *(Fantastic Foods* Cup), 1.5 oz. 28.0
gazpacho *(Nile Spice)*, 1 cont. 23.0
herb, savory, with garlic *(Lipton Recipe Secrets)*, 1 tbsp. 6.0
herb with red pepper *(Lipton Recipe Secrets* Fiesta), 1⅓ tbsp.....6.0
hot and sour *(Knorr Recipe Classics* Soup/Recipe), 2 tbsp. 8.0
leek *(Knorr Recipe Classics* Soup/Recipe), 2 tbsp. 9.0
lentil:
    (Fantastic Foods Hearty Country Cup), 2.3 oz.....................41.0

(Herb-ox), 1 cont..35.0
(Nile Spice Home Style), 1 cont. 34.0
with couscous *(Health Valley)*, ⅓ cup.................28.0
hearty *(Knorr* TasteBreaks), 1 cont....................38.0
minestrone:
   (Fantastic Foods Hearty Cup), 1.5 oz. 29.0
   (Near East), 1 cont. 27.0
   (Nile Spice Home Style), 1 cont. 30.0
   Mediterranean style *(Knorr Savory)*, 3 tbsp. 18.0
miso, dark *(San-J)*, 1 cont. 4.0
miso, mild *(San-J)*, 1 cont. 6.0
mushroom, country *(Nile Spice* Home Style), 1 cont. 26.0
mushroom and noodle *(House of Tsang)*, 1 cont. 23.0
noodle (see also specific soup listings and "wonton," below):
   (Fantastic Foods Chicken Free Ramen Cup), 1.5 oz. 26.0
   all varieties *(Westbrae Natural)*, ½ pkg. 30.0
   all varieties, except chicken mushroom, creamy chicken,
      picante chicken, or tomato *(Maruchan* Ramen), 1.5 oz.....26.0
   beef:
      (Maruchan Instant Lunch), 2.25 oz. 38.0
      picante *(Maruchan* Instant Lunch), 2.25 oz.........37.0
      picante *(Maruchan* Picante Style), 2.25 oz. 36.0
      vegetable *(Herb-ox)*, 1 cont. 23.0
   chicken (see also "chicken," above):
      (Maruchan Instant Lunch), 2.25 oz. 37.0
      broth, real *(Wyler's Mrs. Grass)*, ¼ pkg. 10.0
      creamy *(Maruchan* Instant Lunch), 2.25 oz..........38.0
      creamy or picante *(Maruchan* Ramen), 1.5 oz. 27.0
      curry *(Maruchan* Instant Lunch), 2.25 oz............39.0
      flavored *(Wyler's Mrs. Grass* Homestyle), ¼ pkg. ...10.0
      flavored, with vegetables *(Health Valley)*, ½ cup.....24.0
      mushroom *(Maruchan* Instant Lunch), 2.25 oz..........35.0
      mushroom *(Maruchan* Ramen), 1.5 oz...................25.0
      picante *(Maruchan* Instant Lunch/Picante Style),
         2.25 oz..36.0
   chili with beans *(Maruchan* Instant Lunch), 2.25 oz. 39.0
   Italian *(Maruchan* Instant Lunch), 2.25 oz. 34.0
   pork *(Maruchan* Instant Lunch), 2.25 oz................36.0
   shrimp:
      (Maruchan Instant Lunch), 2.25 oz. 38.0
      picante *(Maruchan* Instant Lunch), 2.25 oz.........36.0

Soup, mix, noodle, shrimp *(cont.)*

    picante *(Maruchan* Picante Style), 2.25 oz. 35.0
   tomato *(Maruchan* Ramen), 1.5 oz. 28.0
   tomato-vegetable *(Maruchan* Instant Lunch), 2.25 oz. 39.0
   vegetable:
      (Maruchan Instant Lunch), 2.25 oz. 35.0
      curry *(Fantastic Foods* Ramen Cup), 1.5 oz. 28.0
      miso *(Fantastic Foods* Ramen Cup), 1.3 oz. 25.0
      picante *(Maruchan* Instant Lunch/Picante Style),
        2.25 oz. 34.0
      tomato *(Fantastic Foods* Ramen Cup), 1.5 oz. 31.0
onion:
   (Lipton Recipe Secrets), 1 tbsp. 4.0
   (Wyler's Mrs. Grass), ¼ pkt. 6.0
   (Wyler's Mrs. Grass Reduced Sodium), ¼ pkt. 7.0
   French *(Knorr Recipe Classics* Soup & Recipe), 2 tbsp. 6.0
   golden *(Lipton Recipe Secrets),* 1⅔ tbsp. 10.0
onion-mushroom *(Lipton Recipe Secrets),* 2 tbsp. 6.0
onion-mushroom *(Mrs. Grass),* ¼ pkt. 10.0
oxtail, see "tomato-beef flavor," below
pasta Italiano *(Health Valley),* ⅓ cup 31.0
pasta marinara, Mediterranean, or Parmesan *(Health Valley),*
   ½ cup 20.0
pasta and beans:
   (Marrakesh Express Zuppa Pasta Fagioli), 1.4-oz. cup 29.0
   black beans *(Marrakesh Express* Zuppa), 1.5-oz. cup...........32.0
   white beans, Tuscan *(Marrakesh Express* Zuppa), 1.3-oz. cup ..27.0
pea, green *(Lipton Cup-a-Soup),* 1 pkt. 12.0
pea, split:
   (Fantastic Foods Hearty Cup), 2 oz. 35.0
   (Knorr TasteBreaks), 1 cont. 28.0
   (Near East), 1 cont. 35.0
   (Nile Spice Home Style), 1 cont. 35.0
   garden, with carrots *(Health Valley),* ⅓ cup 22.0
potato, creamy, with broccoli *(Health Valley),* ⅓ cup 17.0
potato-cheese with ham *(Hormel* Micro Cup), 1 cup 15.0
potato-leek:
   (Herb-ox), 1 cont. 24.0
   (Knorr TasteBreaks), 1 cont. 22.0
   (Nile Spice Home Style), 1 cont. 19.0
   creamy *(Fantastic Foods* Cup), 1.1 oz. 21.0

red pepper, roasted and rice *(Marrakesh Express)*,
    1.4-oz. cup 30.0
rice, Spanish *(Herb-ox)*, 1 cont. 54.0
rotini, roasted chicken *(Near East)*, 1 cont. 21.0
spinach, cream of *(Knorr Recipe Classics* Soup/Recipe),
    2 tbsp. 10.0
tomato:
    (Lipton Cup-a-Soup), 1 pkt. 20.0
    with basil *(Knorr Recipe Classics* Soup/Recipe), 3 tbsp. 13.0
    beef flavor *(Knorr Recipe Classics* Soup/Recipe), 2 tbsp. 9.0
    herb *(Nile Spice* Home Style), 1 cont. 20.0
vegetable:
    (Knorr Recipe Classics Soup/Recipe), 2 tbsp. 10.0
    (Lipton Recipe Secrets), 1⅔ tbsp. 7.0
    (Wyler's Mrs. Grass Homestyle), ¼ pkt. 7.0
    barley *(Fantastic Foods* Hearty Cup), 1.5 oz. 29.0
    chicken flavor *(Knorr* TasteBreaks), 1 cont. 21.0
    chicken flavor *(Lipton Cup-a-Soup)*, 1 pkt. 10.0
    cream of *(Knorr* Savory), 3 tbsp. 12.0
    herb *(Arrowhead Mills)*, ⅓ cup 30.0
    and noodle *(House of Tsang)*, 1 cont. 25.0
    spring *(Knorr Recipe Classics* Soup/Recipe), 2 tbsp. 5.0
    spring *(Lipton Cup-a-Soup)*, 1 pkt. 8.0
    vegetarian *(Knorr* TasteBreaks), 1 cont. 32.0
vichyssoise *(Nile Spice)*, 1 cont. 18.0
wild rice *(Herb-Ox)*, 1 cont. 33.0
wild rice and herb *(Arrowhead Mills)*, ⅓ cup 28.0
wonton:
    all varieties, except hot and sour and wonton skins
        (Maruchan Instant Wonton), 1.49 oz. 19.0
    hot and sour *(Maruchan* Instant Wonton), 1.49 oz. 21.0
    wonton skins *(Maruchan* Instant Wonton), 1.49 oz. 14.0
Soup base mix, ⅛ pkg.:
bean, three, chili *(Wyler's Soup Starter)* 28.0
beef stew, hearty *(Wyler's Soup Starter)* 16.0
beef vegetable *(Wyler's Soup Starter)* 21.0
chicken, with white and wild rice *(Wyler's Soup Starter*
    Quick Cook) 15.0
chicken noodle *(Wyler's Soup Starter)* 15.0
chicken vegetable, hearty *(Wyler's Soup Starter* Quick Cook) 14.0
potato-garlic and chives *(Wyler's Soup Starter)* 23.0

Sour cream, see "Cream, sour"
Sour cream sauce mix, dry, except as noted:
1¼-oz. pkt. 17.0
8 fl. oz.* 34.0
Soursop, fresh, raw:
7" x 5¼"-diam. soursop, 1.4 lb. 105.3
pulp, 1 cup 37.9
Soy beverage, 8 fl. oz., except as noted:
(Edensoy Light Original) 14.0
(Edensoy/Edensoy Extra Original) 13.0
(Edensoy/Edensoy Extra Original), 8.45 fl. oz. 14.0
(Hain Soy Supreme Original) 9.0
(Health Valley Soy Moo Fat Free/Low Fat) 13.0
(NutraBlend Original) 9.0
(WestSoy Drink) 14.0
(WestSoy Drink Nonfat ½ Gallon) 16.0
(WestSoy Drink Nonfat 32 oz.) 15.0
(WestSoy Drink Nonfat Singles), 6.3 fl. oz. 12.0
(WestSoy Lite) 15.0
(WestSoy Lite Lunch Box), 8.45 fl. oz. 16.0
(WestSoy Original/Plus) 18.0
(WestSoy Plus Lunch Box), 8.45 fl. oz. 19.0
(WestSoy Plus Singles), 6.3 fl. oz. 14.0
(WestSoy Unsweetened) 5.0
apple *(NutraBlend)* 25.0
apple juice *(WestSoy* Singles Blast), 6.3 fl. oz. 18.0
berry juice *(WestSoy* Singles Blast), 6.3 fl. oz. 19.0
blend *(EdenBlend* Original) 18.0
chai soy *(WestSoy* Singles), 6.3 fl. oz. 20.0
chocolate, creamy *(WestSoy* VigorAid) 38.0
cocoa *(WestSoy* Lite) 28.0
cocoa *(WestSoy* Plus) 29.0
coffee:
    (Café Westbrae) 25.0
    French vanilla *(Café Westbrae)* 23.0
    French vanilla or mocha *(WestSoy* Lite Café Singles),
      6.3 fl. oz. 18.0
    mocha *(Café Westbrae)* 24.0
malted:
    almond *(WestSoy),* 1 pkg. 27.0
    almond *(WestSoy* Lite), 1 pkg. 26.0

carob *(WestSoy)*, 1 pkg..33.0
cocoa-mint *(WestSoy)*, 1 pkg......................................32.0
cocoa-mint *(WestSoy* Lite), 1 pkg...........................26.0
vanilla *(WestSoy)*, 1 pkg. 28.0
vanilla royale *(WestSoy)*, 1 pkg.............................26.0
"milk," nondairy *(WestSoy* Plus)...............................18.0
"milk," nondairy, vanilla *(WestSoy* Plus)................19.0
orange *(NutraBlend)*..24.0
orange juice *(WestSoy* Singles Twist), 6.3 fl. oz. 16.0
vanilla:
   (Edensoy Light) 21.0
   (Edensoy/Edensoy Extra)..............................23.0
   (Edensoy/Edensoy Extra), 8.45 fl. oz.........24.0
   (Hain Soy Supreme) 12.0
   (NutraBlend) 15.0
   (WestSoy Drink)..22.0
   (WestSoy Drink Nonfat) 17.0
   (WestSoy Drink Nonfat Singles), 6.3 fl. oz. 13.0
   (WestSoy Lite)...21.0
   (WestSoy Lite Lunch Box), 8.45 fl. oz........22.0
   (WestSoy Lite Singles), 6.3 fl. oz.................16.0
   (WestSoy Plus)...19.0
   (WestSoy Plus Lunch Box), 8.45 fl. oz.......20.0
   (WestSoy Plus Singles), 6.3 fl. oz................15.0
   French *(WestSoy VigorAid)* 44.0

Soy beverage mix, dry, ¼ cup:
(Loma Linda Soyagen All Purpose/No Sucrose).....................12.0
carob *(Loma Linda Soyagen)*..13.0
Soy creamer, see "Creamer, nondairy"
Soy flour:
(Arrowhead Mills), ½ cup 16.0
(Hodgson Mill Organic), scant ¼ cup 9.0
stirred, 1 cup:
   full-fat, raw 29.6
   full-fat, roasted 28.6
   defatted 38.4
   low-fat 33.4
Soy meal, defatted, raw, 1 cup................................49.0
Soy milk, see "Soy beverage"
Soy nuts, roasted:
(Frieda's), ⅓ cup..9.0

Soy nuts *(cont.)*
all varieties *(Tofutti* Totally Nuts), 1 oz. 8.0
toasted *(AlpineAire)*, 2.5 oz. 19.0
Soy protein:
(Tofutti Ultra Soy Protein Power), 2 rounded tbsp. 0
concentrate, 1 oz. 8.8
isolate, 1 oz. 2.1
Soy sauce, 1 tbsp.:
(Chun King) 1.0
(Chun King Light) 2.0
(House of Tsang Light/Low Sodium) 0
(Kikkoman) 0
(Kikkoman Lite) 1.0
(La Choy) 2.0
(La Choy Light) 3.0
all varieties, except tamari *(Westbrae)* 2.0
dark *(House of Tsang)* 1.0
ginger-flavored *(House of Tsang)* 4.0
ginger-flavored *(House of Tsang* Low Sodium) 2.0
Polynesian style *(Trader Vic's)* 1.0
shoyu *(San-J* Organic) 1.0
shoyu, all varieties *(Eden)* 2.0
tamari:
    (Eden Organic) 2.0
    (San-J Reduced Sodium) 2.0
    all varieties, except reduced-sodium *(San-J)* 1.0
    wheat-free *(Westbrae Natural)* ....<1.0
Soybeans, green (see also "Edamame"):
raw, 1 cup 28.3
boiled, drained, 1 cup 19.9
Soybeans, fermented, see "Miso" and "Natto"
Soybeans, mature:
dry *(Arrowhead Mills)*, ¼ cup 14.0
dry, raw, 1 cup 56.1
boiled, 1 cup 17.1
boiled, 1 tbsp. 1.1
dry-roasted, 1 cup 56.3
roasted, salted or unsalted, 1 cup 57.7
Soybeans, mature, canned, ½ cup:
(Westbrae Natural) 11.0
black *(Eden* Organic) 8.0

Soybeans, mature, sprouted:
raw *(Jonathan's)*, 3 oz......8.0
raw, ½ cup......3.3
raw, 10 sprouts......1.0
steamed, 1 cup......6.1
Soybean cake or curd, see "Tofu"
Soybean kernels, roasted, toasted:
1 oz. or 95 kernels......8.7
whole, 1 cup......33.0
Soybean sprouts, see "Soybeans, mature, sprouted"
Spaghetti, plain, see "Pasta"
Spaghetti dish, mix, about 1 cup*, except as noted:
cheese, zesty *(Kraft Spaghetti Classics)*......46.0
Italian, mild or tangy *(Kraft Spaghetti Classics)*......46.0
with meat sauce *(Kraft Spaghetti Classics)*......47.0
with tomato sauce, beef-flavored or traditional *(Classico It's Pasta Anytime)*, 15.25-oz. cont. 93.0
Spaghetti entree, canned or packaged:
with franks *(Franco-American* Spaghettios), 1 cup......32.0
with franks, rings *(Kid's Kitchen)*, 1 cup......32.0
and meatballs:
   (Chef Boyardee), 1 cup......32.0
   (Dinty Moore American Classics), 1 bowl......44.0
   (Franco-American Spaghettios), 1 cup......31.0
   (Kid's Kitchen), 1 cup......31.0
   in tomato sauce *(Chef Boyardee* Microwave), 1 bowl......25.0
   in tomato sauce *(Franco-American* Superiore), 1 cup......39.0
tomato and cheese sauce *(Franco-American* Spaghettios),
   1 cup......36.0
Spaghetti entree, dried:
marinara, with mushrooms *(AlpineAire)*, 1 cup......53.0
and meatballs *(AlpineAire)*, 12 oz. 37.0
Spaghetti entree, frozen, 1 pkg., except as noted:
Bolognese *(Michelina's)*, 8.5 oz. 47.0
cheesy bake *(Stouffer's)*, 12 oz.......47.0
cheesy bake *(Stouffer's* 40 oz.), 1 cup......37.0
marinara *(Michelina's)*, 8 oz.......46.0
with meat sauce:
   (Lean Cuisine Everyday Favorites), 11½ oz.......50.0
   (Morton), 8.5 oz. 30.0
   (Stouffer's), 12 oz.......56.0

Spaghetti entree, frozen, with meat sauce *(cont.)*
    and garlic bread *(Marie Callender's Meals)*, 17 oz.................85.0
and meatballs:
    (Lean Cuisine Everyday Favorites), 9½ oz.....................37.0
    with sauce *(Michelina's)*, 9 oz. 43.0
    in sauce *(Stouffer's)*, 12⅝ oz.......................................49.0
with onions, green peppers, and mushrooms
    (Michelina's), 9 oz. 45.0
and sauce, with seasoned beef *(Healthy Choice* Entree),
    10 oz. 43.0
with tomato and basil sauce *(Michelina's)*, 8 oz. 46.0
Spaghetti sauce, see "Pasta sauce"
Spaghetti squash, fresh:
raw *(Frieda's)*, ¾ cup, 3 oz. 6.0
raw, cubed, 1 cup...7.0
baked or boiled, drained, 1 cup..10.0
Spareribs, without added ingredients....................................0
Spearmint:
fresh, 2 tbsp...1.0
dried, 1 tbsp... .8
dried, 1 tsp... .3
Spelt, see "Cereal, ready-to-eat"
Spelt flour, ¼ cup:
(Arrowhead Mills) 24.0
(Hodgson Mill Organic)...22.0
Spinach, fresh:
raw, untrimmed, 1 lb...11.4
raw, trimmed:
    (Andy Boy), 3 oz. 10.0
    chopped *(Dole)*, 1 cup, 2 oz. 2.0
    chopped, 1 cup...2.0
    salad *(Mann's)*, 3 oz. 10.0
boiled, drained, 1 cup 6.8
Spinach, canned:
(S&W), ½ cup...4.0
1 cup...6.8
drained, 1 cup..7.3
leaf or chopped *(Del Monte)*, ½ cup.................................4.0
leaf or chopped *(Popeye/Sunshine)*, ½ cup......................4.0
Spinach, frozen (see also "Spinach dish, frozen"):
(Green Giant), ½ cup...5.0

leaf *(Birds Eye* Southern), 1 cup 2.0
leaf, cut *(Freshlike)*, 1 cup..2.0
leaf or chopped:
    (Birds Eye), ⅓ cup 3.0
    unprepared, 10-oz. pkg. 11.4
    unprepared, 1 cup 6.2
    boiled, drained, 10-oz. pkg. 11.7
    boiled, drained, ½ cup 5.1
chopped *(Freshlike)*, ⅓ cup 2.0
chopped *(Seabrook Farms)*, 1 cup..2.0
in butter sauce, cut leaf *(Green Giant)*, ½ cup 4.0
Spinach, malabar, fresh, cooked:
1 bunch...5
1 cup 1.2
Spinach, mustard:
raw, untrimmed, 1 lb...16.5
raw, chopped, 1 cup 5.9
boiled, drained, chopped, 1 cup 5.0
Spinach, New Zealand:
raw, untrimmed, 1 lb...8.2
raw, chopped, 1 cup 1.4
boiled, drained, chopped, 1 cup 4.0
Spinach, vine, see "Vine spinach"
Spinach dish, frozen, ½ cup, except as noted:
creamed:
    (Birds Eye)..7.0
    (Green Giant)..9.0
    (Seabrook Farms)..10.0
    (Stouffer's) 12.0
    (Tabatchnick), 7.5 oz. 8.0
pancake *(Dr. Praeger's)*, 1.3-oz. cake...8.5
soufflé *(Stouffer's)* 9.0
Spinach salad, see "Salad blend"
Spinach-feta pocket, frozen *(Amy's)*, 4.5 oz. 34.0
Spinach-feta snack, frozen *(Amy's)*, ½ pkg., 5–6 pieces...........24.0
Spiny lobster, meat only:
raw, 1 lobster, 7.4 oz...5.1
raw, 4 oz. 2.8
boiled, poached, or steamed, 2-lb. lobster in shell 5.1
boiled or steamed, 4 oz..3.5
Spiral pasta, plain, see "Pasta"

Spiral pasta entree, frozen, spicy tomato sauce with
   (*Michelina's*), 8-oz. pkg. 41.0
Split peas, mature:
dry:
   1 cup 118.9
   green (*Arrowhead Mills*), ¼ cup........................31.0
   green (*Goya*), ¼ cup 27.0
   yellow (*Goya*), ¼ cup 28.0
boiled, 1 cup 41.1
boiled, 1 tbsp. 2.6
Sports drink, 8 fl. oz.:
all flavors:
   (*All Sport*)..20.0
   (*Gatorade*) 14.0
   (*R.W. Knudsen Recharge*) 18.0
lemon-lime (*AriZona Total Sport*)............................16.0
Spot, without added ingredients..............................0
Spread, see specific listings
Spring onion, see "Onion, green"
Sprouts (see also specific listings):
hot and spicy (*Jonathan's*), 1 cup................................4.0
mixed:
   (*Jonathan's*) 3 oz. 21.0
   (*Jonathan's* Gourmet), 1 cup.............................3.0
   (*Jonathan's* Salad Sprouts), 1 cup 10.0
Squab, without added ingredients............................0
Squash (see also specific squash listings), winter, frozen
   (*Birds Eye*), ½ cup 12.0
Squid, meat only:
raw, 4 oz. 3.5
fried, 4 oz. 8.8
Starfruit, see "Carambola"
Steak sandwich, see "Beef sandwich/pocket"
Steak sauce, 1 tbsp.:
(*A.1.*)..3.0
(*A.1.* Bold & Spicy) 5.0
(*A.1.* Sweet & Tangy) 8.0
(*A.1.* Thick & Hearty) 6.0
(*Crosse & Blackwell*)..7.0
(*Heinz 57*) 4.0
(*HP*)..3.0

(Peter Luger Steak House)...7.0
peppercorn *(Lawry's* Weekday Gourmet).....................3.0
Stir-fry sauce, 1 tbsp., except as noted:
(House of Tsang Classic)..4.0
(House of Tsang Bangkok Padang)............................4.0
(House of Tsang Saigon Sizzle).................................8.0
(Kikkoman)..4.0
sweet and sour *(House of Tsang)*...............................8.0
Szechuan *(House of Tsang)*.......................................4.0
Szechuan *(San-J* Cooking Sauce), 2 tbsp....................1.0
teriyaki *(House of Tsang Korean)*...............................6.0
Stir-fry seasoning, 1 tbsp.:
herb and roasted garlic *(Lawry's)*.............................1.0
lemon-basil *(Lawry's)*..3.0
sesame-ginger *(Lawry's)*..3.0
sweet and spicy *(Lawry's)*..4.0
Stomach, pork, without added ingredients...................0
Straightneck squash, fresh:
raw, sliced, 1 cup...5.3
boiled, drained, sliced, 1 cup......................................7.8
boiled, drained, sliced, ½ cup.....................................3.9
Straightneck squash, canned, 1 cup:
drained, diced..6.2
mashed, 1 cup..7.1
Straightneck squash, frozen, 1 cup:
unprepared, sliced..6.2
boiled, drained, sliced...10.6
Strawberries, fresh:
(Dole), 8 medium, 5.3 oz..12.0
halves, 1 cup...10.7
puree, 1 cup..16.3
Strawberries, canned:
in light syrup *(Oregon),* ½ cup.................................23.0
in heavy syrup, 1 cup..59.8
Strawberries, dried:
(Frieda's), ½ cup, 1.4 oz..34.0
freeze-dried *(AlpineAire),* ½ oz................................12.0
Strawberries, frozen:
unsweetened, unthawed, 1 cup..................................13.6
unsweetened, thawed, 1 cup......................................20.2

Strawberries, frozen *(cont.)*
whole, sweetened:
(Birds Eye), ½ cup 25.0
10-oz. pkg. 59.6
thawed, 1 cup..53.6
halves, sweetened *(Birds Eye)*, ½ cup 31.0
halves, sweetened *(Birds Eye Lite)*, ½ cup 17.0
sliced, sweetened:
10-oz. pkg. 73.6
thawed, 1 cup..66.1
Strawberry drink blend, 8 fl. oz., except as noted:
banana *(WhipperSnapper)*, 10 fl. oz. 40.0
banana nectar *(Libby's)*, 11.5-fl.-oz. can.................52.0
guava nectar *(Santa Cruz Organic)* 24.0
kiwi:
(Kool-Aid Bursts Slammin' Strawberry-Kiwi), 1 bottle 24.0
(Tropicana Twister), 10 fl. oz. 42.0
lemonade *(Turkey Hill)* 29.0
nectar *(Libby's)*, 11.5-fl.-oz. can.........................49.0
lemonade *(Santa Cruz Organic)* 24.0
melon *(Fruitworks)*, 12 fl. oz...............................44.0
pineapple colada cocktail *(AriZona)* 34.0
punch *(Hawaiian Punch Strawberry Surfin')*.................31.0
smoothie *(Rocket Juice Strawberry Shield)*, 16 fl. oz. 48.0
mix*:
kiwi *(Kool-Aid Slammin' Strawberry-Kiwi)*.................25.0
kiwi *(Kool-Aid Slammin' Strawberry-Kiwi* Sugar
Sweetened)..17.0
lemonade *(Country Time Lem'n Berry Sippers)* 0
lemonade *(Kool-Aid Soarin' Strawberry Lemonade)* 25.0
lemonade *(Kool-Aid Soarin' Strawberry Lemonade* Sugar
Sweetened)..17.0
raspberry *(Kool-Aid)*.......................................25.0
raspberry *(Kool-Aid* Sugar Sweetened) 16.0
Strawberry drink mix, 8 fl. oz.*:
(Kool-Aid)..25.0
(Kool-Aid Sugar Sweetened) 18.0
Strawberry filling, see "Pastry filling" and "Pie filling"
Strawberry juice:
(Juicy Juice), 8 fl. oz.......................................29.0
(Juicy Juice), 8.45-fl.-oz. box 31.0

(Juicy Juice), 4.23-fl.-oz. box 15.0
Strawberry milk drink:
(Hershey's), 1 box 33.0
(Hershey's Reduced Fat), 1 cup 31.0
(Nesquik), 1 cup 33.0
mix:
    (Nesquik), 2 tbsp..22.0
    dry, 2–3 heaping tsp. or ¾-oz. pkt. 21.8
    prepared with milk, 8 fl. oz. 32.7
Strawberry pie glaze *(Smucker's)*, 2 oz. 21.0
Strawberry syrup:
(Hershey's), 2 tbsp. 26.0
(Knott's Berry Farm), ¼ cup 52.0
(Maple Grove Farms), ¼ cup 57.0
(Nesquik), 2 tbsp. 27.0
(R.W. Knudsen), ¼ cup 38.0
(Smucker's), ¼ cup 52.0
(Smucker's Sundae), 2 tbsp. 25.0
Strawberry topping, 2 tbsp.:
(Kraft)..29.0
(Mrs. Richardson's Fat Free) 18.0
(Smucker's)..26.0
String beans, see "Green beans"
Stroganoff sauce mix, dry, except as noted:
(Natural Touch), 4 tbsp. 10.0
1.6-oz. pkt. 26.5
Strudel (see also "Toaster pastry"), apple, 2.5-oz. piece............29.2
Stuffing:
corn bread or seasoned *(Arnold)*, ¾ cup 28.0
corn bread or seasoned *(Pepperidge Farm)*, ¾ cup 33.0
Stuffing mix, ½ cup*, except as noted:
(Croutettes), 1 cup 25.0
all varieties *(Stove Top* Flexible Serving)....................19.0
all varieties *(Stove Top* Microwave), ...20.0
for beef *(Stove Top)* 22.0
chicken *(Pepperidge Farm One Step)* 24.0
chicken flavor *(Stove Top)* 20.0
chicken flavor *(Stove Top* Lower Sodium) 21.0
corn bread *(Stove Top)* 21.0
herbs, savory *(Stove Top)* 20.0
long-grain and wild rice *(Stove Top)* 22.0

Stuffing mix *(cont.)*

mushroom and onion *(Stove Top)*	20.0
for pork or turkey *(Stove Top)*	20.0
sage flavor *(Stove Top* Traditional)	21.0
San Francisco style *(Stove Top)*	20.0
turkey *(Pepperidge Farm One Step)*	22.0
Sturgeon, without added ingredients	0

Subway, 1 serving:

7 under 6 subs, without cheese or mayo:

chicken breast, roasted	40.0
ham	39.0
roast beef	39.0
Subway Club	40.0
turkey breast	39.0
turkey breast and ham	40.0
Veggie Delite	37.0

7 under 6 deli sandwiches, without cheese or mayo:

ham	30.0
roast beef, tuna, or turkey breast	31.0

7 under 6 salads:

all varieties, except roasted chicken and *Veggie Delight*	11.0
roasted chicken	12.0
Veggie Delite	9.0

Subway Classic Subs, 6":

Cold Cut Trio or *Italian B.M.T.*	40.0
meatball	46.0
steak and cheese or *Subway Melt*	41.0
Subway Seafood & Crab, with light mayo	46.0
tuna, with light mayo	39.0

Subway Classic deli style sandwich, tuna | 34.0

Subway Classic Salads, without dressing:

Cold Cut Trio or *Italian B.M.T.*	11.0
meatball	18.0
steak and cheese or *Subway Melt*	12.0
Subway Seafood & Crab, with light mayo	17.0
tuna, with light mayo	11.0

Subway Select Subs, 6":

asiago Caesar chicken	46.0
honey mustard melt	47.0
horseradish roast beef or Southwest steak and cheese	42.0

wraps:
    select, asiago chicken...52.0
    steak and cheese...53.0
    turkey breast and bacon...52.0
breads:
    deli-style roll...27.0
    6" harvest wheat..39.0
    6" hearty Italian...36.0
    6" Italian 33.0
    6" Parmesan oregano 34.0
    6" sesame Italian 34.0
    6" whole-wheat 36.0
    wrap 45.0
condiments:
    bacon or cheese, 2 strips or triangles........................0
    mayonnaise, regular or light, 1 tbsp..........................0
    mustard, 2 tsp...1.0
    vinegar or olive oil blend, 1 tsp................................0
select sauces, 1 tbsp.:
    asiago Caesar or Southwest....................................1.0
    honey mustard 5.0
    horseradish 2.0
salad dressing, 2-oz. pkt.:
    French, fat-free 17.0
    Italian, fat-free 4.0
    ranch, fat-free 14.0
cookies, 1 piece:
    chocolate chip or oatmeal raisin..............................29.0
    chocolate chunk 30.0
    peanut butter 26.0
    M&M's..29.0
    sugar 28.0
    white macadamia nut 27.0
Succotash, fresh, boiled, drained, 1 cup 46.8
Succotash, canned:
cream-style corn, 1 cup 46.8
whole-kernel *(Seneca),* ½ cup 18.0
whole-kernel corn, 1 cup 35.6
Succotash, frozen:
unprepared, 10-oz. pkg..56.6

Succotash, frozen *(cont.)*
unprepared, 1 cup...31.1
boiled, drained, 1 cup 33.9
Sucker, without added ingredients 0
Sugar, beet or cane:
brown:
   1 oz. 27.6
   1 cup, not packed 141.0
   1 cup, packed 221.0
granulated:
   1 oz. 28.3
   1 cup 199.8
   1 tbsp. 12.0
   1 tsp. 4.0
powdered or confectioner's:
   1 oz. 28.2
   1 cup, sifted..99.5
   1 tbsp., unsifted 8.0
Sugar, maple:
1 oz. 25.5
1 tsp. 2.7
"Sugar," substitute, see "Sweetener"
Sugar, turbinado *(Hain),* 1 tsp..............................4.0
Sugar apple, fresh, raw:
2⅞"-diam. apple...36.6
pulp, 1 cup..59.1
Sugar loaf squash *(Frieda's),* ¾ cup, 3 oz...................7.0
Sugar snap peas, see "Peas, edible-podded"
Summer sausage (see also "Sausage sticks"):
(Johnsonville Original/Old World), 2 oz. 1.0
beef or garlic *(Johnsonville),* 2 oz.............................1.0
beef and pork, .8-oz. slice 1
smoked *(Old Smokehouse),* 2 oz. 2.0
Sunburst squash *(Frieda's),* ⅔ cup, 3 oz.....................3.0
Sunchoke, see "Jerusalem artichoke"
Sunfish, pumpkin-seed, without added ingredients..............0
Sunflower seeds, shelled, except as noted:
(Arrowhead Mills Hulled), ¼ cup 6.0
(Frito-Lay), 3 tbsp., 1 oz. 5.0
(Planters), ¼ cup 8.0
(Planters In Shell), 3.25 oz. 8.0

candy-coated *(AlpineAire)*, 2.5 oz. 33.0
dried:
    kernels, 1 oz. 5.3
    kernels, 1 cup 27.0
    in shell, 1 cup (edible yield 1.6 oz.)..............................8.6
dry-roasted:
    (River Queen Salted), ¼ cup, 1.1 oz. 7.0
    (River Queen Unsalted), ¼ cup, 1.2 oz. 8.0
    kernels, 1 oz. 6.8
    kernels, 1 cup 30.8
oil-roasted, kernels, 1 oz...4.2
oil-roasted, kernels, 1 cup..19.9
roasted and salted, in shell *(Planters)*, 3-oz. pkg..........8.0
roasted and salted, in shell *(Planters)*, ¾ cup 5.0
toasted, kernels, 1 oz. 5.8
toasted, kernels, 1 cup...27.6
Sunflower seed butter, 1 tbsp..4.4
Sunflower seed flour, partially defatted:
1 cup..22.9
1 tbsp...1.4
Sunflower sprouts *(Jonathan's)*, 1 cup...........................2.0
Surimi[1], 4 oz. 7.8
Swamp cabbage, fresh:
raw, .5-oz. shoot.. .4
raw, chopped, 1 cup...1.8
boiled, drained, chopped, 1 cup.......................................3.6
Sweet dumpling squash *(Frieda's)*, ¾ cup, 3 oz. 7.0
Sweet peas, see "Peas, green"
Sweet potato, fresh (see also "Yam"):
raw, 1 sweet potato, 5" long, 4.7 oz.............................31.5
raw, cubed, 1 cup..32.3
baked in skin:
    1 large, 6.3 oz...43.7
    1 medium, 4 oz. 24.3
    mashed, 1 cup...48.5
    mashed, ½ cup 27.7
boiled without skin, 1 medium, 5.3 oz. 36.7
boiled without skin, mashed, 1 cup 79.6

[1]*Processed from walleye (Alaska) pollock.*

Sweet potato, canned:

whole *(Royal Prince* 9 oz.), 3 pieces, 6.1 oz. 48.0
whole *(Royal Prince/Trappey's)*, 4 pieces, 6 oz. 48.0
cut *(Allens/Princella/Sugary Sam)*, ⅔ cup 39.0
cut, vacuum pack, 1 cup 42.3
mashed:
   (Princella/Sugary Sam), ⅔ cup 28.0
   1 cup 59.2
   vacuum pack, 1 cup 53.9
candied *(Royal Prince)*, ½ cup 50.0
orange-pineapple *(Royal Prince)*, ½ cup 50.0
in syrup, 1 cup 47.7
in syrup, drained, 1 cup 49.7

Sweet potato, frozen:

cubed, unprepared, 1 cup 39.1
cubed, baked, 1 cup 41.2
candied *(Mrs. Paul's)*, 5 oz. 73.0
candied, with apple *(Mrs. Paul's)*, 1¼ cups 66.0

Sweet potato chips, see "Potato chips and crisps"

Sweet potato leaf:

raw, 1 leaf, 12¼" long 1.0
raw, chopped, 1 cup 2.2
steamed, 1 cup 4.7

Sweet and sour drink mixer *(Mr & Mrs T)*, 4 fl. oz. 34.0

Sweet and sour sauce (see also "Stir-fry sauce"), 2 tbsp.:

(Chun King) 14.0
(Kikkoman) 9.0
(Kraft) 14.0
(La Choy) 14.0
(San-J Cooking Sauce) 13.0
duck sauce:
   (Gold's) 14.0
   (Ka•Me) 20.0
   (La Choy) 15.0
with pineapple *(Contadina)* 8.0

Sweet and sour sauce mix, dry, except as noted:

2-oz. pkt. 54.5
8 fl. oz.* 72.7

Sweetbreads, see "Pancreas" and "Thymus"

Sweetener, artificial:

(Equal), 1 pkt. ....<1.0

(NutraSweet), 1 tsp...<1.0
(Sweet 'n Low), 1 pkt..1.0
(Weight Watchers), ¼ tsp. 1.0
Swiss chard, fresh:
raw:
    (Frieda's), 1 cup, 3 oz. 3.0
    1 leaf, 1.7 oz. 1.8
    1 cup 1.3
boiled, drained, chopped, 1 cup 7.2
Swordfish, fresh, without added ingredients 0
Syrup, see specific listings
Szechuan sauce, see "Stir-fry sauce"

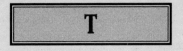

T

FOOD AND MEASURE	CARBOHYDRATE GRAMS

Tabouli salad:
(Cedar's Taboule), 2 tbsp. 3.0
(Cedarlane), ½ cup 17.0
Tabouli salad mix:
(Casbah), 1.25 oz. 24.0
(Fantastic Foods), ¼ cup 26.0
Taco Bell, 1 serving:
breakfast items:
    burrito, country 26.0
    burrito, double bacon and egg 39.0
    burrito, fiesta 25.0
    burrito, grande 43.0
    hash brown nuggets 29.0
    quesadilla, cheese, bacon, or sausage 33.0
burritos:
    bean 54.0
    Big Beef 43.0
    Big Beef Supreme 52.0
    Big Chicken Supreme 50.0
    chili cheese 40.0
    grilled chicken 49.0
    7-layer 65.0
    Supreme 50.0
Chalupa Baja:
    beef 30.0
    chicken 28.0
    steak 27.0
Chalupa Santa Fe:
    beef 31.0
    chicken 30.0
    steak 29.0
Chalupa Supreme:
    beef 29.0
    chicken 28.0

 steak..27.0

Gordita Baja:

 beef 29.0

 chicken 28.0

 steak..27.0

Gordita Santa Fe:

 beef 31.0

 chicken 30.0

 steak..29.0

Gordita Supreme:

 beef or steak..27.0

 chicken 28.0

tacos:

 regular 12.0

 Double Decker..37.0

 Double Decker Supreme.....................................39.0

 soft..20.0

 soft, grilled chicken 20.0

 soft, grilled steak 19.0

 soft, grilled steak *Supreme*.................................21.0

 Soft Taco Supreme..22.0

 Taco Supreme..14.0

specialties:

 Big Beef *MexiMelt*..22.0

 Mexican pizza 42.0

 Mexican pizza, beef 39.0

 Mexican pizza, chicken 41.0

 taco salad, with salsa 69.0

 taco salad, with salsa, without shell.....................36.0

 tostada...27.0

 quesadilla, cheese 31.0

 quesadilla, chicken 33.0

nachos and sides:

 Big Beef nachos supreme.......................................44.0

 nachos..34.0

 nachos *BellGrande*...83.0

 nachos *BellGrande,* chicken.................................82.0

 nachos *BellGrande,* steak 81.0

 pintos 'n cheese 18.0

 rice, Mexican 23.0

Taco Bell, nachos and sides (cont.)

twists, cinnamon 25.0
ice cream dessert, *Choco Taco* 37.0

Taco dinner kit:

(Chi-Chi's), 2 shells and seasonings 30.0
(Ortega), 2 shells, 1 tbsp. sauce, ⅛ envelope 25.0
(Taco Bell Home Originals), 2 tacos* 19.0

soft taco:

(Chi-Chi's), 2 shells and seasonings 54.0
(Ortega), 2 shells, 1 tbsp. sauce, ⅕ envelope 47.0
(Taco Bell Home Originals), 2 tacos* 41.0

Taco John's, 1 serving:

burritos:

bean 54.0
beefy 44.0
chicken fajita 41.0
chicken and potato 56.0
combination 49.0
El Grande 69.0
El Grande, chicken or steak 66.0
meat and potato 58.0
ranch 43.0
steak and potato 56.0
super 51.0

chilito 41.0
quesadilla 41.0
quesadilla, chicken 42.0

tacos:

crispy 13.0
El Grande 30.0
El Grande chicken or steak 24.0
softshell 23.0
softshell chicken or steak 22.0
Taco Bravo 39.0
taco burger 29.0

tostada 13.0
tostada, bean 18.0

platters:

beef and bean chimi 82.0
beef enchilada 80.0
chicken enchilada 72.0

chimichanga	57.0
double enchilada	34.0
smothered burrito	57.0

specialties:

chicken fajita salad	53.0
chicken festiva burrito	56.0
chicken festiva salad	39.0
chicken festiva salad, without dressing	27.0
Mexi Rolls with cheese	53.0
Potato Olés Bravo	55.0
Sierra chicken fillet sandwich	40.0
super nachos	69.0
Super Potato Olés	83.0
taco salad	55.0
taco salad, without dressing	50.0

side orders/extras:

beans, refried	46.0
cheese crisp	10.0
chili, green	19.0
chili, Texas style	23.0
nachos	36.0
Potato Olés	45.0
<Potato Olés, large	59.0
Potato Olés with nacho cheese	51.0
rice, Mexican	44.0
side salad	15.0

desserts:

apple grande	40.0
churro	13.0
cinnamon mint swirl	14.0
choco taco	37.0
Teddy Graham cubs, Kid's Meal	11.0

Taco pocket, frozen *(Michelina's),* 5.5-oz. pkg.	34.0
Taco sauce:	
(Chi-Chi's), 1 tbsp.	1.0
green, medium or mild *(La Victoria),* 1 tbsp.	<1.0
medium or mild *(Taco Bell Home Originals),* 2 tbsp.	3.0
red, medium or mild *(La Victoria),* 1 tbsp.	1.0
Taco seasoning mix:	
(Bearitos), 2¼ tsp.	4.0
(Chi-Chi's), ⅛ pkg.	4.0

Taco seasoning mix *(cont.)*
(El Torito), ⅕ pkg. 5.0
(Hain), 2 tsp. 4.0
(Lawry's Spices & Seasonings), 2 tsp. 3.0
(Natural Touch), 3 tbsp. 5.0
(Ortega), 1 tbsp. 4.0
(Taco Bell Home Originals), about 2 tsp. 3.0
chicken *(Lawry's* Spices & Seasonings), 2 tsp. 5.0
salad *(Lawry's* Spices & Seasonings), 1 tsp. 3.0
Taco shell:
(Ortega), 2 shells 19.0
(Rosarita), 1 shell 7.0
(Rosarita Tostada), 1 shell 9.0
(Taco Bell Home Originals), 3 shells 21.0
corn, white *(Ortega)*, 2 shells 19.0
corn, white or yellow *(Chi-Chi's)*, 2 shells 22.0
Tahini:
(Arrowhead Mills), 2 tbsp. 5.0
(Krinos), 2 tbsp. 5.0
paste, 1 tbsp. 4.1
Tahini sauce mix *(Casbah)*, 1.13 oz., ¼ cup* 10.0
Tamale, canned, 2 pieces, except as noted:
(Gebhardt) 19.0
(Gebhardt Jumbo) 24.0
(Wolf) 23.0
beef:
    (Hormel), 7.5-oz. can 22.0
    (Hormel Jumbo) 21.0
    regular or spicy hot *(Hormel)* 15.0
chicken *(Hormel)* 15.0
Tamale entree, see "Enchilada entree"
Tamale pie, see "Vegetable entree"
Tamale pie, dried, with beef, Western style
    (AlpineAire), 1 cup..50.0
Tamale pocket, frozen, Mexican *(Amy's)*, 4.5 oz. 39.0
Tamari, see "Soy sauce"
Tamarillo *(Frieda's)*, 2 pieces, 4.2 oz. 9.0
Tamarind, fresh, raw:
(Frieda's), 1.1-oz. pod 19.0
1 fruit, 3" x 1", <.1 oz. 1.3
pulp, 1 cup 75.0

Tangerine, fresh:
(Dole), 2 fruits...19.0
1 large, 2½" diam...11.0
sections, 1 cup...21.8
Tangerine, canned:
in juice, 1 cup..23.8
in light syrup:
    (Del Monte Mandarin Orange), ½ cup....................19.0
    (Del Monte Mandarin Orange Snack Cup), 4-oz. cup 17.0
    (Dole Mandarin Orange), ½ cup.............................19.0
    (S&W Mandarin Orange), ½ cup.............................21.0
    1 cup 40.8
Tangerine drink blend:
citrus (Fruit Works), 12 fl. oz................................42.0
ruby red (Tropicana Twister), 10 fl. oz. 40.0
Tangerine juice, 8 fl. oz., except as noted:
fresh, raw...24.9
canned, sweetened..29.9
frozen* (Minute Maid) 30.0
frozen*, sweetened...26.7
Tangerine juice blend, orange (Tropicana Pure Premium),
    8 fl. oz. 25.0
Tapenade, see "Tomato tapenade"
Tapioca, dry:
(Minute), 1½ tsp...5.0
pearl, 1 oz..25.1
pearl, 1 cup 134.8
Tapioca pudding, see "Pudding"
Taramosalata, 1 tbsp.:
(Krinos)...0
(Krinos Lite) 1.0
Taro, fresh:
raw, sliced, 1 cup...27.5
cooked, sliced, 1 cup 45.7
Taro, Tahitian, fresh:
raw, sliced, 1 cup...8.6
cooked, sliced, 1 cup 9.4
Taro chips:
10 chips, .8 oz. 15.7
spiced (Terra Chips), 1 oz.....................................20.0

Taro leaf:
raw, 1 leaf, 11" x 6½", .4 oz. 7
raw, 1 cup 1.9
steamed, 1 cup 5.8
Taro root *(Frieda's)*, ⅔ cup, 3 oz. 22.0
Taro shoots, fresh:
raw, 1 shoot, 2.9 oz. 1.9
raw, sliced, ½ cup 1.0
cooked, sliced, 1 cup 4.5
Tarragon, dried:
ground, 1 tbsp. 2.4
ground, 1 tsp. 8
Tart shell, see "Pastry shell"
Tartar sauce, 2 tbsp.:
(Hellmann's/Best Foods) 3.0
(Hellmann's/Best Foods Low Fat) 7.0
(Kraft) 4.0
(Kraft Fat Free) 5.0
lemon and herb flavor *(Kraft)* .... <1.0
TCBY, all flavors, ½ cup:
ice cream, hand-dipped, low-fat 22.0
ice cream, hand-dipped, low-fat, no sugar added 20.0
sorbet, nonfat and nondairy 24.0
yogurt, frozen, 96% fat free or nonfat 23.0
yogurt, frozen, nonfat, no sugar added 20.0
Tea (see also "Tea, iced"):
(Lipton), 1 bag or 1 tsp. loose 0
brewed, all varieties *(Celestial Seasonings),* 1 cup 0
brewed, herb, all varieties, 1 cup 5
Tea, iced, bottled or canned, 8 fl. oz.:
(AriZona) 25.0
(AriZona Rx Energy) 31.0
(AriZona Rx Health) 19.0
(AriZona Rx Memory) 20.0
(AriZona Rx Stress) 18.0
(Lipton Southern Style No Lemon Extra Sweet) 29.0
(Lipton Southern Style No Lemon Sweetened) 24.0
(Snapple Sun Tea) 23.0
(Snapple Sweet Tea) 31.0
(Snapple Unsweetened) 0
(Turkey Hill) 22.0

(Turkey Hill Decaffeinated) 20.0
(Turkey Hill Diet) 0
all flavors:
    (AriZona Diet) ....<1.0
    (Lipton Brisk Chilled) 20.0
    (Snapple Diet) 1.0
cactus *(Snapple)* 24.0
cherry *(Turkey Hill Cooler)* 24.0
with fruit juices *(R.W. Knudsen Hibiscus Cooler)* 23.0
with fruit juices *(Santa Cruz Organic Hibiscus Cooler)* 23.0
ginseng *(R.W. Knudsen Simply Nutritious Ginseng Boost)* 27.0
ginseng *(Snapple)* 20.0
ginseng extract *(AriZona)* 15.0
green tea:
    with ginseng *(After the Fall Green Tea Express)* 23.0
    with ginseng *(AriZona)* 18.0
    with ginseng *(AriZona Diet)* ....<1.0
    with ginseng and honey *(Turkey Hill Cooler)* 17.0
    lemon *(Snapple)* 25.0
    mandarin orange *(AriZona)* 19.0
    and passion fruit *(Lipton)* 19.0
    plum, Asian *(AriZona)* 18.0
lemon:
    (Snapple) 25.0
    (Turkey Hill Cooler) 24.0
    flavor *(AriZona Thermal)* 23.0
    flavor *(Lipton)* 21.0
    flavor *(Lipton Southern Style)* 25.0
lemon, peach, or raspberry *(AriZona)* 25.0
lemon, peach, or raspberry *(Crystal Light)* 0
and lemonade *(Lipton)* 26.0
lemonade *(Snapple)* 28.0
mint *(Snapple)* 27.0
mint, with spearmint and peppermint *(Turkey Hill Cooler)* 24.0
orange *(Turkey Hill Cooler)* 25.0
orange *(Turkey Hill Cooler Decaffeinated Diet)* 2.0
peach or raspberry:
    (Lipton) 26.0
    (Snapple) 26.0
    (Turkey Hill Cooler) 28.0

Tea, iced, mix:
(Crystal Light), 8 fl. oz.*..0
(Crystal Light Decaffeinated/Sun Tea), 8 fl. oz.*.........<1.0
(Lipton Regular/Decaffeinated), 1½ tsp.............................0
(Nestea/Nestea Decaffeinated), 2 tsp...........................<1.0
(Nestea/Nestea Decaffeinated Sugar Free), 2 tsp....................1.0
all flavors:
    (General Foods International Teas), 8 fl. oz.*.................13.0
    (Lipton), 1⅔ tbsp...22.0
    except tea and lemonade *(Lipton* Diet), 1 tbsp....................1.0
lemon-flavored *(Lipton* Decaffeinated), 8 fl. oz.*...............22.0
and lemonade *(Lipton* Diet), 1 tbsp. 2.0
peach *(Crystal Light),* 8 fl. oz.*...0
unsweetened:
    1 rounded tsp...4
    8 fl. oz.*..5
    herb *(Nestea* Lemon Bliss/Orange Spice), 1 tbsp................3.0
    lemon *(Nestea),* 2 tsp..1.0
    lemon *(Nestea* Ice Teaser), 8 fl. oz. 1.0
    lemon flavor, 1 rounded tsp. 1.1
    lemon flavor, 8 fl. oz.*...1.0
sweetened with sugar:
    lemon or lemonade *(Nestea),* 2 tbsp. 19.0
    lemon flavor, 3 rounded tsp. 22.2
    lemon flavor, 8 fl. oz.*..22.0
Tempeh:
1 oz. 2.7
1 cup 15.6
cooked, 1 oz. 2.6
Tequila sunrise, 6.8-fl.-oz. can 23.8
Teriyaki baste and glaze, 2 tbsp.:
(Kikkoman)..11.0
with honey and pineapple *(Kikkoman)* 18.0
Teriyaki sauce (see also "Grilling sauce," "Marinade," and
    "Stir-fry sauce"), 1 tbsp.:
(Annie Chun's) 5.0
(Chun King/La Choy)..3.0
(San-J Cooking Sauce) 3.0
(Sun Luck Honey Marin) 6.0
1 tbsp. 2.9
hot *(Chun King)* 3.0

hot and spicy *(Annie Chun's)* 5.0
Polynesian style *(Trader Vic's)* 3.0
Teriyaki sauce mix, dry, 1.6-oz. pkt. 27.6
Teriyaki stir-fry entree, frozen *(Lean Cuisine Everyday Favorites)*, 10 oz. 45.0
Thai peanut sauce, see "Peanut sauce"
Thai seasoning sauce *(A Taste of Thai)*, 1 tbsp. 1.0
Thuringer cervelat, see "Summer sausage"
Thyme:
fresh, 1 tsp. 2
dried:
    ground, 1 tbsp. 2.7
    ground, 1 tsp. 9
Thymus, beef or veal, without added ingredients 0
Tikka sauce, see "Curry sauce"
Tilefish, without added ingredients 0
Toaster pastry (see also "Bagel sandwich" and "Breakfast sandwich"), 1 piece:
all varieties *(Weight Watchers)* 38.0
apple *(Pillsbury Toaster Strudel)* 26.0
apple-cinnamon *(Kellogg's Pop•Tarts/Pop•Tarts Pastry Swirls)* 37.0
berry, frosted *(Kellogg's Pop•Tarts Snak-Stix)* 37.0
berry, wild, frosted *(Kellogg's Pop•Tarts)* 39.0
blueberry:
    (Kellogg's Pop•Tarts) 36.0
    (Thomas' Toast-r-Cakes) 15.0
    frosted *(Kellogg's Pop•Tarts)* 37.0
    muffin *(Kellogg's Eggo)* 19.0
brown sugar–cinnamon:
    (Kellogg's Pop•Tarts) 35.0
    (Pillsbury Toaster Strudel) 26.0
    frosted *(Kellogg's Pop•Tarts)* 34.0
    frosted *(Kellogg's Pop•Tarts Low Fat)* 39.0
    frosted *(KoolStuf Toastettes)* 34.0
cheese *(Kellogg's Pop•Tarts Pastry Swirls)* 36.0
cherry:
    (Kellogg's Pop•Tarts) 37.0
    (Pillsbury Toaster Strudel) 26.0
    frosted *(Kellogg's Pop•Tarts)* 38.0
    frosted *(KoolStuf Toastettes Cherry Burst)* 35.0

Toaster pastry *(cont.)*

chocolate chip *(Thomas' Toast-r-Cakes)*......................................17.0
chocolate fudge, frosted *(Kellogg's Pop•Tarts Low Fat)*..............39.0
chocolate fudge or vanilla creme, frosted *(Kellogg's
    Pop•Tarts)*..37.0
cinnamon *(Thomas' Toast-r-Cakes)* 17.0
cinnamon muffin *(Kellogg's Eggo)*..20.0
corn muffin *(Thomas' Toast-r-Cakes)* 17.0
cream cheese and strawberry *(Pillsbury Toaster Strudel)*...........24.0
egg, see "Breakfast sandwich"
fudge, frosted *(KoolStuf Toastettes Super Fudge Blast)* 32.0
grape, frosted *(Kellogg's Pop•Tarts)* 38.0
raisin bran *(Thomas' Toast-r-Cakes)* 15.0
raspberry, frosted *(Kellogg's Pop•Tarts)* 37.0
S'mores, frosted *(Kellogg's Pop•Tarts)*..36.0
S'mores, frosted *(KoolStuf Honey Maid)* 36.0
strawberry:
    (Kellogg's Pop•Tarts/Pop•Tarts Pastry Swirls).....................37.0
    (Pillsbury Toaster Strudel)..26.0
    frosted *(Kellogg's Pop•Tarts)*..38.0
    frosted *(Kellogg's Pop•Tarts Snak-Stix)*..............................37.0
    frosted *(KoolStuf Toastettes Screamin' Strawberry)* 33.0
    muffin *(Kellogg's Eggo)*...20.0
    regular or frosted *(Kellogg's Pop•Tarts Low Fat)*..................39.0
watermelon, wild, frosted *(Kellogg's Pop•Tarts)* 39.0
Wild Magicburst, frosted *(Kellogg's Pop•Tarts)* 37.0
Wild Tropical Blast, frosted *(Kellogg's Pop•Tarts)*.....................39.0
Toffee, see "Candy"
Toffee baking bits *(Skor)*, 1 tbsp..7.0
Toffee dessert topping, see "Chocolate topping"
Tofu:
raw, ¼ block, 4.1 oz...2.2
raw, ½ cup..2.3
dried-frozen (koyadofu), .6-oz. piece 2.5
extra firm *(Nasoya Organic)*, ⅕ block, 3.2 oz. 1.0
firm *(Nasoya Organic)*, ⅕ block, 3.2 oz. 2.0
firm, ½ cup...5.4
5-spice *(Nasoya Organic)*, ¼ block, 3 oz. 0
flavored *(Nasoya Organic French Country)*, ⅕ block, 3.2 oz. 0
fried, ½-oz. piece 1.4

nigari:

    extra firm, ⅕ block, 3.2 oz. 1.8

    firm, ¼ block, 2.9 oz. 2.4

    firm, ½ cup 3.7

    hard, ¼ block, 4.3 oz. 5.4

    soft, 1" cube 3

    soft, ½" cubes, 1 cup 4.5

okara, 1 oz. 3.6

okara, 1 cup 15.3

salted and fermented (fuyu), .4-oz. block 6

silken *(Nasoya* Organic), ⅙ block, 3.2 oz. 2.0

silken, soft *(Mori-Nu),* 3 oz. 2.0

soft *(Nasoya* Organic), ⅕ block, 3.2 oz. 2.0

Tofu, "cheese," see " 'Cheese,' substitute and nondairy"

Tofu dish, mix:

burger *(Fantastic Foods* Tofu Classics), ⅛ cup 12.0

chow mein, Mandarin *(Fantastic Foods* Tofu Classics),

    ⅝ cup 33.0

shells and curry *(Fantastic Foods* Tofu Classics), ½ cup 40.0

Stroganoff, creamy *(Fantastic Foods* Tofu Classics),

    ½ cup 35.0

Tofu salad, ½ cup:

cottage style *(Cedarlane)* 5.0

egg-free or ranchero *(Cedarlane)* 7.0

Tofu sauce *(Westbrae Natural),* 1 tsp. 1.0

Tofu seasoning mix:

breakfast scramble *(Fantastic Foods),* ½ tbsp. 12.0

eggless salad *(Mori-Nu),* ⅓ pkg. 2.0

garden sampler or Italian herb *(Mori-Nu),* ⅓ pkg. 5.0

Shanghai stir-fry *(Mori-Nu),* ⅓ pkg. 6.0

Tom and Jerry drink batter *(Trader Vic's),* 1 tbsp. 23.0

Tomatillo, fresh:

(Frieda's), ⅔ cup, 3 oz. 5.0

1 medium, 1.2 oz. 2.0

chopped or diced, ½ cup 3.8

Tomatillo, in jar:

(La Victoria Entero), 5 pieces, 4.5 oz. 6.0

crushed *(La Victoria),* 4.5 oz. 7.0

Tomato, ripe, fresh:

orange, 3.9-oz. tomato 3.5

orange, chopped, 1 cup 5.0

Tomato *(cont.)*

red, raw:

  (Frieda's Teardrop), ²/₃ cup, 3 oz. 4.0

  untrimmed, 1 lb. 19.2

  1 medium, 2⅗" diam, 4¾ oz. 5.7

  chopped or diced, 1 cup 8.3

  cherry tomato, 1 cup 6.9

  grape *(Frieda's* Baby Roma), ²/₃ cup, 3 oz. 4.0

red, boiled:

  2 medium, 8.7 oz. 14.3

  1 cup 14.0

  ½ cup 7.0

red, stewed, 1 cup 13.2

yellow, raw:

  (Frieda's Teardrop), ²/₃ cup, 3 oz. 4.0

  7.5-oz. tomato 6.3

  chopped, 1 cup 4.1

Tomato, canned (see also "Pasta sauce" and "Tomato sauce"), ½ cup, except as noted:

whole:

  (Contadina) 5.0

  (Del Monte) 6.0

  peeled *(Hunt's)*, 2 pieces 4.0

  peeled *(Muir Glen* Organic) 5.0

  peeled, with basil *(Muir Glen* Organic) 5.0

chunky, chili style *(Del Monte)* 8.0

chunky, pasta style *(Del Monte)* 11.0

crushed:

  (Del Monte Original Recipe) 9.0

  (Eden Organic), ¼ cup 3.0

  (Hunt's) 7.0

  with basil *(Muir Glen* Organic), ¼ cup 4.0

  with garlic *(Del Monte)* 11.0

  Italian recipe *(Del Monte)* 9.0

  with Italian herbs or roasted garlic *(Contadina)*, ¼ cup 3.0

  in tomato purée *(Contadina)*, ¼ cup 4.0

diced:

  (Contadina) 6.0

  (Del Monte/Del Monte No Salt) 6.0

  (Eden Organic) 6.0

  (Hunt's) 6.0

(Muir Glen/Muir Glen No Salt Organic) 4.0
with basil and garlic or garlic and onion (Muir Glen
   Organic) 4.0
with basil, garlic, and oregano (Del Monte) 11.0
with garlic and onion (Del Monte) 8.0
with green chilies (Chi-Chi's), ¼ cup.....................................4.0
with green chilies (Del Monte) 6.0
with green chilies (Eden Organic) 5.0
with green chilies or Italian herbs (Muir Glen Organic)...........4.0
with green pepper and onion (Del Monte).............................9.0
with Italian herbs or roasted garlic (Contadina) 10.0
with jalapeños (Del Monte)..6.0
with sautéed onion (Contadina) 9.0
with green chilies, 1 cup 8.7
ground, peeled (Muir Glen Organic), ¼ cup 2.0
paste, see "Tomato paste"
purée, see "Tomato purée"
stewed:
(Del Monte Original Recipe) 9.0
(Hunt's) 7.0
(Muir Glen Organic) 7.0
1 cup 17.3
Cajun or Mexican recipe (Del Monte).....................................9.0
Italian recipe (Del Monte)...8.0
wedges (Del Monte) 9.0
wedges, in tomato juice, 1 cup 16.5
Tomato, dried:
1 piece, 32 pieces per cup 1.1
chopped or halves (Frieda's), ⅓ cup, 1.1 oz. 19.0
diced, bits (Sonoma), 2 tsp. 3.0
flakes (AlpineAire), ½ cup 10.0
halves (Sonoma), 2 pieces...2.0
marinated:
halves (Sonoma), 2–3 pieces, .35 oz. 3.0
julienne (Sonoma), 8 strips, .35 oz. 3.0
julienne, and roasted garlic (Sonoma), 8 strips, .35 oz...........4.0
in safflower oil (Rienzi), 4 pieces, 1.4 oz. 8.0
seasoning blend:
(Sonoma Toss-Ta), ½ cup..13.0
(Sonoma Toss-Ta Ranchero), 3 tsp. 3.0
(Sonoma Season-It), 2 tsp. 3.0

Tomato, dried *(cont.)*
sun-dried, in olive oil *(Christopher Ranch)*, 1 oz. 7.0
sun-dried, in olive oil *(Victoria)*, ¼ cup......................................10.0
yellow, sun-dried, chopped or halves *(Frieda's)*, ½ cup, 3 oz.....47.0
Tomato, green, raw:
1 large, 6.4 oz. 9.3
1 cup...9.2
Tomato, green, pickled, halves *(Claussen)*, 1 oz.........................1.0
Tomato, sun-dried, see "Tomato, dried"
Tomato chutney, see "Chutney"
Tomato juice, canned, 8 fl. oz., except as noted:
(Campbell's)...9.0
(Campbell's Low Sodium) 10.0
(Campbell's Healthy Request) 12.0
(Del Monte From Concentrate)...10.0
(Del Monte Not From Concentrate) 7.0
(Eden Organic) 6.0
(Muir Glen Organic), 5.5 fl. oz. 8.0
(Sacramento) 8.0
Tomato juice blend, 8 fl. oz.:
beef *(Beefmato)* 11.0
beef broth, 5.5-fl.-oz. can 14.3
and chili cocktail *(Snap-E-Tom)*, 10 fl. oz. 13.0
and chili cocktail *(Snap-E-Tom)*, 6 fl. oz. 8.0
clam:
   (Clamato Bloody Caesar)...12.0
   (Clamato Cocktail) 11.0
   5.5-fl.-oz. can 18.2
   picante *(Clamato* Cocktail)..13.0
Tomato paste, canned, 2 tbsp., except as noted:
(Contadina) 6.0
(Del Monte)..7.0
(Hunt's/Hunt's Italian/No Salt)..6.0
(Muir Glen Organic) 6.0
6-oz. can..32.8
½ cup..25.3
1 tbsp...3.2
with Italian seasoning *(Contadina)*..7.0
with roasted garlic *(Contadina)*...6.0
with tomato pesto *(Contadina)*...5.0
Tomato pesto, see "Pesto sauce"

Tomato powder *(AlpineAire)*, ½ cup...13.0
Tomato purée, canned:
(Contadina), ¼ cup 4.0
(Hunt's), 2 tbsp. 3.0
(Muir Glen Organic), ¼ cup 5.0
1 cup 23.9
Tomato relish, in jar, 1 tbsp.:
(Sonoma Spice Medley)...3.0
green *(Braswell's)* 5.0
hot *(Braswell's)* 3.0
Indian *(Patak's)* 2.0
sun-dried *(Braswell's)* 2.0
Tomato sauce, canned (see also "Pasta sauce" and
    "Tomato, canned"):
(Contadina/Contadina Extra Thick & Zesty), ¼ cup 3.0
(Del Monte/Del Monte No Salt), ¼ cup 4.0
(Goya), ¼ cup 4.0
(Hunt's/Hunt's No Salt), ¼ cup 3.0
(Muir Glen/Muir Glen No Salt Organic), ¼ cup 5.0
(Progresso), ¼ cup 4.0
1 cup 17.6
chunky *(Muir Glen* Organic), ¼ cup 4.0
with garlic and onion *(Contadina)*, ¼ cup 4.0
with herbs and cheese, ½ cup 12.5
Italian style *(Contadina)*, ¼ cup 4.0
with mushroom, 1 cup 20.7
with onion, 1 cup 24.4
with onion, green pepper, and celery, 1 cup 21.9
Spanish style, 1 cup...17.7
with tomato tidbits, 1 cup 17.3
Tomato tapenade, dried, in jar *(Sonoma)*, 1 tbsp. 4.0
Tomato toss, dried, vegetable blend *(Frieda's)*, ½ cup, 3 oz. 19.0
Tongue:
beef, raw, 1 oz...1.0
beef, simmered, 9.1 oz. (edible yield from 1 lb. raw) 9
lamb, pork, or veal (calf), braised, without added ingredients........0
Tortellini, canned or packaged:
cheese *(Chef Boyardee)*, ½ of 15-oz. can 46.0
cheese, spinach, or tri-color *(Real Torino)*, ¾ cup.....................39.0
meat *(Chef Boyardee)*, ½ of 15-oz. can 48.0
Tortellini, refrigerated, ¾ cup, except as noted:

Tortellini, refrigerated *(cont.)*

beef and roasted garlic *(Di Giorno)*, 1 cup 46.0

cheese:

    (Contadina Buitoni)...39.0

    mixed *(Contadina Buitoni)*..40.0

    three *(Contadina Buitoni)* 39.0

    three *(Di Giorno)* 37.0

herb chicken *(Contadina Buitoni)*..40.0

spinach cheese *(Contadina Buitoni)*...40.0

Tortellini dish, frozen, cheese and chicken *(Healthy Choice* Bowl), 8.7-oz. pkg. 40.0

Tortelloni, refrigerated, 1 cup, except as noted:

cheese and roasted garlic *(Contadina Buitoni)*...........................38.0

chicken and proscuitto *(Contadina Buitoni)* 45.0

lemon chicken in cracked-pepper pasta *(Di Giorno)*...................42.0

mozzarella-garlic *(Di Giorno)* 42.0

mozzarella and herb *(Contadina Buitoni)* 45.0

mozzarella and pepperoni *(Contadina Buitoni)*...........................49.0

mushroom and cheese *(Contadina Buitoni)*.................................46.0

pesto *(Di Giorno)* 46.0

portobello mushroom *(Di Giorno)*..48.0

sausage, sweet Italian *(Contadina Buitoni)* 49.0

sun-dried tomato *(Contadina Buitoni)*...46.0

Tortilla (see also "Wrap"), 1 piece:

(Cedarlane Chapati), 1.7 oz. 26.0

corn, 6" diam., .9 oz. 12.0

corn, yellow or blue *(Cedarlane* Organic Low Fat), 1.6 oz. 20.0

flour, 6" diam., 1.1 oz. 17.8

flour, whole-wheat or unbleached *(Cedarlane* Fat Free), 1.7 oz. 25.0

Tortilla chips, see "Corn chips, puffs, and similar snacks"

Tostada shell *(Ortega),* 2 shells..19.0

Trail mix:

(AlpineAire Bear Ate My Food), 4 oz...67.0

(AlpineAire Bits of Hawaii), 4 oz..84.0

(AlpineAire Can't Get Out of the Tent), 4 oz. 53.0

(AlpineAire Hawaiian Eruption), 4 oz...60.0

(AlpineAire No Fish in the Lake), 4 oz..68.0

(AlpineAire Over the Top/Stumbling Down the Trail), 4 oz.........60.0

(AlpineAire Trail Blazer), 4 oz...38.0

(Planters Flamin Cajun Crunch), ⅓ cup 19.0

1 oz.	.12.7
1 cup	.67.4
caramel nut crunch *(Planters)*, 3 tbsp.	.15.0
with chocolate chips, nuts, and seeds, 1 oz.	.12.7
with chocolate chips, nuts, and seeds, 1 cup	.65.6
nuts, seeds, and raisins *(Planters)*, 3 tbsp.	.11.0
tropical, 1 oz.	.18.6
tropical, 1 cup	.91.8

Tree fern, cooked:

1 frond, 6½" long, 1.1 oz.	.3.4
chopped, ½ cup	.7.8

Triangolo, mushroom, in bumblebee pasta *(Cafferata)*,
½ pkg., 4.5 oz.	.37.0
Triticale, whole-grain, 1 cup	.138.5
Triticale flour, whole-grain, 1 cup	.95.1

Tropical punch, see "Fruit juice blend" and "Fruit juice drink blend"

Trout, fresh or smoked, without added ingredients	0

Trout paté, smoked *(Ducktrap River/Ducktrap River Low Fat)*,
¼ cup, 2 oz.	.1.0

Tuna:

fresh or frozen, without added ingredients	0
canned, in water or oil, 2 oz.	0

"Tuna," vegetarian:

canned, drained *(Worthington Tuno)*, ⅓ cup	.4.0
frozen, drained *(Worthington Tuno)*, ½ cup	.2.0
Tuna burger, frozen *(Ocean Beauty)*, 3.2-oz. burger	.3.0

Tuna entree, dried, albacore, with noodles and cheese
(AlpineAire), 1½ cups	.40.0

Tuna entree, frozen, 1 pkg.:

casserole/noodle casserole *(Healthy Choice* Entree), 9 oz.	.33.0
noodle casserole *(Stouffer's)*, 10 oz.	.37.0
and noodles, home style *(Marie Callender's* Meals), 12 oz.	.52.0

Tuna entree mix, 1 cup*:

au gratin *(Tuna Helper)*	.37.0
cheddar, garden *(Tuna Helper)*	.36.0
cheesy broccoli *(Tuna Helper)*	.38.0
cheesy pasta *(Tuna Helper)*	.32.0
creamy broccoli *(Tuna Helper)*	.35.0
creamy pasta *(Tuna Helper)*	.31.0
fettuccine Alfredo *(Tuna Helper)*	.32.0

Tuna entree mix *(cont.)*
pasta salad *(Tuna Helper)* 25.0
pot pie *(Tuna Helper)* 40.0
Romanoff *(Tuna Helper)*...38.0
tetrazzini *(Tuna Helper)* 34.0
tuna melt *(Tuna Helper)* 34.0
Tuna salad:
with crackers:
    (Bumble Bee)...21.0
    (Bumble Bee Fat Free) 25.0
    (Bumble Bee Kit) 15.0
    (Starkist) 25.0
without crackers *(Bumble Bee)*..6.0
without crackers *(Bumble Bee* Fat Free) 10.0
Turban squash *(Frieda's)*, ¾ cup, 3 oz. 7.0
Turbot, without added ingredients 0
Turkey, fresh:
all classes:
    raw, whole, 1 turkey, 12¼ lbs. 4.4
    roasted, whole, 1 turkey, 8.9 lbs. 2.8
    without added ingredients, 4 oz. 0
hen, raw, whole, 1 turkey, 9.8 lbs. 4.9
hen, roasted, whole, 1 turkey, 7.3 lbs. 2.3
young tom, raw, whole, 1 turkey, 18.5 lbs. 6.7
young tom, roasted, whole, 1 turkey, 13.1 lbs...............6.0
Turkey, canned:
(Hormel), 2 oz..0
meat only, with broth 0
Turkey, frozen or refrigerated:
(Norbest Basted/Boneless/Family Tradition), 4 oz...........0
whole, fresh, hen or tom, cooked *(Perdue)*, 3 oz............0
all cuts *(Empire* Kosher Chill Pack), 4 oz. 0
barbecue, whole *(Empire* Kosher), 5 oz. 0
boneless *(Butterball* Young), 4 oz. 0
boneless, breast, fresh *(Butterball* Young), 4 oz. 1.0
breast, fresh *(Butterball)*, 4 oz. 1.0
breast, marinated, roasted *(Perdue* Rotisserie), 3 oz...................1.0
breast, seasoned *(Butterball)*, 4 oz. 4.0
breast or whole, stuffed, roast *(Butterball)*:
    meat, 3 oz...0
    stuffing, ¾ cup 28.0

gravy, ¼ cup..3.0
breast cutlets *(Butterball)*, 2.8-oz. cutlet.............................0
breast cutlets, cooked *(Perdue)*, 2.4 oz. 0
breast medallions *(Butterball)*, 5 pieces, 4.4 oz. 1.0
breast strips or tenderloins *(Butterball)*, 4 oz. 0
ground, see "Turkey, ground"
nuggets *(Louis Rich)*, 4 pieces, 3.25 oz..........................15.0
oven-baked *(Butterball* Young Fully Cooked), 3 oz............0
roast, light or dark meat *(Butterball* Young), 3 oz..............0
roast, light and dark meat, seasoned, boneless:
   raw, 10 oz..18.2
   roasted, 1.7 lbs...24.0
   roasted, chopped, or diced, 1 cup................................4.1
smoked:
   (Butterball Young Fully Cooked), 3 oz. 1.0
   breast, half *(Butterball* Young Fully Cooked), 3 oz. 1.0
   breast, honey-roasted *(Butterball* Young Fully Cooked), 3 oz. ..1.0
   drumsticks *(Butterball* Fully Cooked), 3 oz.................0
   honey-roasted *(Butterball* Young Fully Cooked), 3 oz. 2.0
   wing *(Butterball/Butterball* Drumettes Fully Cooked), 3 oz. 1.0
tenderloins, cracked-black-pepper seasoned, cooked
   (Perdue), 3 oz..1.0
Turkey, ground, raw:
(Butterball), 4 oz. 0
(Perdue/Perdue Fit'N Easy), 4 oz. 0
4 oz. 0
burgers:
   (Empire Kosher), 4-oz. burger.......................................0
   natural flavorings *(Butterball* Fresh), 4-oz. burger 1.0
   seasoned *(Butterball* Lean), 4-oz. burger 0
"Turkey," vegetarian:
canned, sliced *(Worthington Turkee)*, 3 slices, 3.3 oz................3.0
frozen, smoked *(Worthington* Meatless), 3 slices, 2 oz. 3.0
Turkey bacon *(Louis Rich)*, ½-oz. slice 0
Turkey bologna:
(Louis Rich 50% Less Fat), 1-oz. slice 1.0
(Louis Rich Variety-Pak), 3 slices, 2.2 oz. 3.0
2 oz. 5
Turkey dinner, frozen, 1 pkg.:
breast, with rib meat, gravy and stuffing *(Swanson Traditional
   Favorites)*, 11¾ oz...50.0

Turkey dinner *(cont.)*

breast of *(Healthy Choice* Meal) Traditional), 10.5 oz. 40.0

and gravy with dressing *(Banquet Extra Helping),* 17 oz. 54.0

with gravy and stuffing, mashed potato *(Swanson
  Hungry-Man),* 16¾ oz. 61.0

roast, country inn *(Healthy Choice* Meal), 10 oz. 28.0

Turkey entree, canned or packaged:

and dressing *(Dinty Moore American Classics),* 1 bowl 32.0

stew *(Dinty Moore),* 1 cup 19.0

stew *(Dinty Moore* Microwave), 1 cup 16.0

Turkey entree, dried:

(AlpineAire Wild Thyme), 1½ cups 47.0

mashed potatoes and gravy *(AlpineAire),* 1½ cups 56.0

Romanoff *(AlpineAire),* 1 cup 35.0

teriyaki *(AlpineAire),* 1½ cups...50.0

Turkey entree, frozen, 1 pkg., except as noted:

breast, grilled, and rice pilaf *(Marie Callender's* Meals),
  11.75 oz. 34.0

breast, roasted:

  (Lean Cuisine Cafe Classics), 9¾ oz. 49.0

  (Lean Cuisine Hearty Portions), 14 oz. 43.0

  (Lean Cuisine Skillet Sensations), ½ of 24-oz. pkg..............37.0

  (Stouffer's Hearty Portions), 16 oz. 55.0

  with sweet and sour sauce *(Empire* Kosher),
    ⅛ pkg., 5 oz. 14.0

breast medallions, oven-roasted, with gravy *(Boston
  Market),* 8 oz. 8.0

breast medallions, oven-roasted, with mashed potatoes and
  gravy *(Boston Market),* 15.5 oz..40.0

croquettes, breaded, gravy and *(Freezer Queen* Family
  Entree), ⅙ pkg. 14.0

divan *(Healthy Choice* Bowl), 9.5 oz. 31.0

and gravy:

  with dressing *(Freezer Queen* Deluxe Family Entree),
    ¼ pkg., 7 oz. 33.0

  with dressing *(Freezer Queen* Meal), 9.25 oz. 31.0

  with dressing *(Marie Callender's* Meals), 14 oz......................52.0

  with dressing and whipped potatoes *(Freezer Queen
    Homestyle),* 8.5 oz..31.0

  with mashed potatoes *(Marie Callender's* Family),
    2 pieces with gravy, ½ cup potatoes 18.0

gravy and, with dressing *(Morton)*, 9 oz. 27.0
gravy with, and dressing *(Michelina's)*, 8 oz. 23.0
home style *(Lean Cuisine Everyday Favorites)*, 9⅜ oz. 27.0
honey roast breast *(Banquet)*, 9 oz. 29.0
pie/pot pie:
    (Banquet), 7 oz. 38.0
    (Empire Kosher), 1 pie 45.0
    (Marie Callender's), 9.5 oz. 56.0
    (Marie Callender's), ½ of 16.5-oz. pkg. 45.0
    (Stouffer's), 10 oz. 39.0
    (Swanson), 7 oz. 42.0
    white meat *(Swanson Hungry-Man Deep Dish)*, 17 oz. 49.0
roast:
    (Stouffer's Homestyle), 9⅝ oz. 27.0
    breast *(Healthy Choice* Entree), 8.5 oz. 26.0
    country, with mushrooms *(Healthy Choice)*, 8.5 oz. 26.0
sliced, gravy and:
    (Banquet Family Size), 2 slices with gravy 5.0
    (Banquet Hot Sandwich Toppers), 5-oz. bag 6.0
    (Freezer Queen Cook-in-Pouch), 5 oz. 6.0
    (Freezer Queen Family Entree), ⅙ pkg., 4.5 oz. 6.0
tetrazzini *(Stouffer's)*, 10 oz. 36.0
white meat, mostly *(Banquet)*, 9.25 oz. 30.0
Turkey entree mix, frozen, with roasted potatoes
    (Birds Eye Turkey Voila!), 1 cup* 24.0
Turkey fat 0
Turkey frankfurter, see "Frankfurter"
Turkey giblets:
raw, 8.6 oz. 5.1
simmered, chopped or diced, 1 cup 3.0
Turkey gizzard:
simmered, 4 oz. 7
simmered, chopped or diced, 1 cup 9
Turkey gravy, ¼ cup, except as noted:
(Boston Market Roasted) 3.0
(Franco-American) 3.0
(Franco-American Fat Free) 4.0
(Franco-American Slow Roasted) 4.0
(Franco-American Slow Roasted Fat Free) 6.0
1 tbsp. 8
1 cup 12.2

Turkey gravy mix, roasted *(Knorr* Gravy Classics), 1 tbsp.,
   ¼ cup* 4.0
Turkey ham:
(Carl Buddig Lean), 2.5-oz. pkg. 1.0
(Hansel 'n Gretel Healthy Deli), 2 oz. 2.0
(Louis Rich Variety-Pak), 3 slices, 2.2 oz. 1.0
(Norbest), 3 oz. 2.0
honey-roasted *(Sara Lee)* 2 oz. 2.0
thigh meat, cured, 1-oz. slice.. .1
frozen, dark meat, smoked, 1 oz... .9
Turkey kielbasa, see "Kielbasa"
Turkey lunch meat (see also "Turkey bologna," etc.),
   breast, 2 oz., except as noted:
(Boar's Head Golden Skin On)......................................0
(Boar's Head Golden Skinless) ....<1.0
(Boar's Head Premium Lower Sodium)......................<1.0
(Carl Buddig Lean), 2.5-oz. pkg. 1.0
(Light & Lean 97), 1-oz. slice 0
Black Forest *(Hansel 'n Gretel Healthy Deli)*..............1.0
browned *(Healthy Choice)*...0
Cajun *(Perdue)* 1.0
cracked-pepper *(Sara Lee)*...2.0
cracked-pepper *(Sara Lee* Deli), 3 slices, 2 oz. 2.0
flame-seared *(Hansel 'n Gretel Healthy Deli)*...........2.0
glazed *(Boar's Head Maple Glazed Coat)* 2.0
golden-browned *(Norbest* Gold Label) 0
honey *(Perdue Carving)* 1.0
honey-cured, Champagne-glazed *(Black Bear)*............3.0
honey-roasted:
   (Carl Buddig Lean), 2.5-oz. pkg..............................3.0
   (Carl Buddig Premium Lean Slices), 2.5-oz. pkg...........4.0
   (Sara Lee)..1.0
   (Sara Lee Deli), 2 slices, 1.6 oz. 1.0
   cured *(Carl Buddig* Lean), 9 slices, 2 oz. 2.0
oven-roasted:
   (Black Bear Catering Style) 1.0
   (Boar's Head Ovengold Skin On) 1.0
   (Boar's Head Ovengold Skinless) 0
   (Boar's Head Salsalito) 1.0
   (Carl Buddig Premium Lean Slices), 2.5-oz. pkg...........1.0

(Hansel 'n Gretel Healthy Deli Gourmet/Less
  Sodium/Natural Shape)......................................1.0
(Healthy Choice), 1-oz. slice.................................2.0
(Healthy Choice 10 oz.), 1-oz. slice 1.0
(Healthy Choice Deli Traditions), 6 slices, 1.9 oz. 3.0
(Hebrew National 97% Fat Free), 5 slices, 2 oz.......................1.0
(Louis Rich Fat Free) 1.0
(Louis Rich Carving Board), 6 slices, 2.1 oz. 1.0
(Louis Rich Free), 1-oz. slice..............................1.0
(Louis Rich Variety-Pak Fat Free), 4 slices, 2 oz. 2.0
(Norbest Gold Label) 0
(Norbest Silver Label)...2.0
(Perdue/Perdue Carving).......................................1.0
(Perdue Healthsense) 3.0
(Russer) 2.0
(Sara Lee)...0
(Sara Lee Deli), 2 slices, 1.6 oz.............................2.0
(Spam) 1.0
cured *(Carl Buddig* Lean), 2½-oz. pkg. 1.0
cured *(Carl Buddig* Lean), 9 slices, 2 oz. 1.0
honey flavor *(Hansel 'n Gretel Healthy Deli* Gourmet) 3.0
Italian style *(Hansel 'n Gretel Healthy Deli)* 4.0
with white *(Norbest* Bronze Label) 2.0
pan-roasted:
  (Perdue Carving Classics) 0
  braised or hickory-smoked *(Perdue Carving Classics*
    Homestyle) 1.0
  cracked-pepper *(Perdue Carving Classics)*...............2.0
pepper *(Hansel 'n Gretel Healthy Deli* Tutta Bella)........................2.0
peppered *(Sara Lee)*...2.0
roasted *(Healthy Choice* Hearty Deli Flavor), 3 slices, 2 oz. 1.0
rotisserie-flavored *(Sara Lee)*.......................................1.0
rotisserie-seasoned *(Healthy Choice Deli Traditions),*
  6 slices, 1.9 oz. 4.0
salsa *(Healthy Choice)*..1.0
smoked:
  (Boar's Head Cracked Pepper Mill).............................0
  (Carl Buddig Lean), 2.5-oz. pkg................................1.0
  (Carl Buddig Lean), 9 slices, 2 oz..............................1.0
  (Carl Buddig Premium Lean Slices), 2.5-oz. pkg....................1.0
  (Healthy Choice), 1-oz. slice.................................2.0

Turkey lunch meat, smoked *(cont.)*
    (Healthy Choice 10 oz.), 1-oz. slice 1.0
    (Healthy Choice Deli Traditions), 6 slices, 1.9 oz. 3.0
    (Light & Lean 97), 1-oz. slice 0
    (Oscar Mayer Free), 4 slices, 1.8 oz. 2.0
    (Russer) 1.0
    hardwood *(Sara Lee)* 1.0
    hardwood *(Sara Lee* Deli), 2 slices, 1.6 oz. 1.0
    hickory *(Boar's Head)* ....<1.0
    hickory *(Louis Rich Variety-Pak* Fat Free), 4 slices, 2 oz.........2.0
    hickory *(Norbest* Gold Label) 0
    hickory *(Perdue)* 1.0
    honey *(Perdue)* 2.0
    honey mesquite *(Norbest* Gold Label) 3.0
    honey roast *(Healthy Choice)* 2.0
    honey roast *(Healthy Choice),* 1-oz. slice 2.0
    honey roast *(Healthy Choice Savory Selections),*
       6 slices, 1.9 oz. 4.0
    mesquite *(Boar's Head Mesquite Wood Smoked)* 1.0
    mesquite *(Healthy Choice Savory Selections),*
       6 slices, 1.9 oz. 3.0
    mesquite *(Hansel 'n Gretel Healthy Deli)* 1.0
    mesquite *(Louis Rich Carving Board),* 3 slices, 1.9 oz...........1.0
    mesquite *(Perdue)* 0
    mesquite *(Sara Lee)* 1.0
    skinless *(Healthy Choice)* 1.0
    white *(Louis Rich Variety-Pak),* 3 slices, 2.2 oz. 1.0
    white *(Norbest)* 2.0
Southwest grill *(Healthy Choice)* 1.0
TexMex *(Black Bear)* 1.0
Turkey pastrami, 2 oz.:
 (Boar's Head) 1.0
 (Hansel 'n Gretel Healthy Deli) 2.0
 (Norbest) 0
 hickory-smoked *(Perdue)* 2.0
Turkey patty, breaded, fried:
 1.5-oz. patty 6.6
 1-oz. patty 4.4
Turkey pepperoni *(Pillow Pack),* 17 slices, 1.1 oz. 0
Turkey pocket, frozen, 4.5-oz. piece:
broccoli and cheese *(Lean Pockets)* 30.0

and ham with cheddar *(Hot Pockets)*.................................43.0
and ham with cheddar *(Lean Pockets)*...............................42.0
and ham with Swiss *(Croissant Pockets)*............................39.0
Turkey roll, 2 oz.:
light meat 3
light and dark meat 1.2
Turkey salami:
cooked, sliced, 2 oz. 3
cotto *(Louis Rich Variety-Pak)*, 3 slices, 2.2 oz. 1.0
Turkey sausage, see "Sausage"
Turkey sticks, breaded, fried, 2.25-oz. stick 10.9
Turmeric, dried:
ground, 1 tbsp. 4.4
ground, 1 tsp. 1.4
Turnip, fresh or stored:
raw, 1 large, 6.5 oz. 11.4
raw, cubed, 1 cup...8.1
boiled, drained, cubed, 1 cup......................................7.6
boiled, drained, mashed, 1 cup..................................11.3
Turnip, frozen:
unprepared, mashed, 10-oz. pkg. 8.3
unprepared, mashed, ⅓ of 10-oz. pkg.........................2.8
boiled, drained, 1 cup..6.8
Turnip greens, fresh:
raw, chopped, 1 cup..3.2
boiled, drained, chopped, 1 cup..................................6.3
Turnip greens, canned
(Allens/Sunshine), ½ cup 3.0
15-oz. can 10.3
½ cup 2.8
chopped, with diced turnips *(Allens/Sunshine)*, ½ cup 5.0
Turnip greens, frozen:
unprepared:
    chopped, 10-oz. pkg..10.4
    chopped or diced, ½ cup 3.0
    with turnips, 10-oz. pkg. 9.7
boiled, drained:
    10-oz. pkg. 11.0
    1 cup 8.2
    ½ cup 4.1
    with turnips, 1 cup 4.7

Turnip greens, frozen, boiled, drained *(cont.)*

with turnips, ½ cup 2.5
chopped *(Birds Eye* Southern), 1 cup 1.0
with diced root *(Birds Eye* Southern), 1 cup 2.0

Turnover, frozen, 3.2-oz. piece:

apple *(Pepperidge Farm)* 36.0
raspberry *(Pepperidge Farm)* 35.0

Turtle beans, see "Black beans"

U-V

FOOD AND MEASURE   **CARBOHYDRATE GRAMS**

Uzbek melon *(Frieda's)*, 1 cup, 1.4 oz. 9.0
Vanilla extract, 1 tbsp. 1.6
"Vanilla" extract, imitation:
1 tbsp. 3
1 tsp. 1
nonalcoholic, 1 tbsp. 1.9
nonalcoholic, 1 tsp. 6
Veal, without added ingredients 0
Veal dinner, frozen, Parmesan, 1 pkg.:
with pasta *(Swanson Hungry-Man)*, 18¼ oz. 71.0
with spaghetti *(Swanson)*, 11¼ oz. 40.0
Veal entree, frozen, parmagiana, 1 pkg.:
(Banquet), 8.75 oz. 37.0
(Stouffer's Homestyle), 11⅝ oz. 48.0
(Stouffer's Hearty Portions), 17½ oz. 66.0
breaded *(Freezer Queen* Deluxe Family Entree), 1 patty.............15.0
with pasta in tomato sauce *(Freezer Queen* Meal), 9 oz.............37.0
with tomato sauce *(Freezer Queen* Cook-in-Pouch), 5 oz. 17.0
with tomato sauce *(Morton)*, 8.75 oz. 30.0
Vegetable chips, 1 oz., except as noted:
(Eden), 50 chips, 1.1 oz. 24.0
bell pepper *(Harry's Garden)* 19.0
beet-garlic *(Harry's Garden)* 20.0
garlic blue *(Harry's Garden)* 20.0
jalapeño bean *(Harry's Garden)* 18.0
mix, veggie *(Harry's Garden)* 19.0
mixed *(Terra Chips)* 18.0
sea *(Eden)*, 50 chips, 1.1 oz. 23.0
Vegetable dinner, frozen, 1 pkg.:
(Amy's Country Dinner), 11 oz. 60.0
(Amy's Veggie Loaf), 10 oz. 47.0
Vegetable dish, canned (see also "Vegetable entree,
    canned"), ½ cup:
sweet and sour sauce *(House of Tsang)* 40.0

Vegetable dish, canned *(cont.)*
Szechuan sauce, hot and spicy *(House of Tsang)*......................14.0
teriyaki sauce *(House of Tsang Tokyo)*.................................23.0
Vegetable dish, frozen (see also "Vegetable entree, frozen"):
Alfredo *(Green Giant)*, ¾ cup...9.0
primavera *(Green Giant)*, 9-oz. pkg...................................39.0
Vegetable entree, canned, 1½ cups:
curry *(Patak's Aloo Mattar Sabzi)*...................................25.0
curry *(Patak's Tikka Masala)* 27.0
Vegetable entree, frozen (see also specific listings),
    1 pkg., except as noted:
and beef, country *(Lean Cuisine Café Classics)*, 9 oz. 33.0
and chicken pasta bake *(Stouffer's)*, 12 oz. 46.0
pie/pot pie:
    (Amy's), 7.5 oz. 54.0
    (Amy's Country), 7.5 oz. 47.0
    (Cedarlane Mediterranean), 7.5 oz. 43.0
    (Cedarlane Santa Fe), 7.5 oz. 50.0
    with beef *(Morton)*, 7 oz. 33.0
    cheese *(Banquet)*, 7 oz..39.0
    with chicken *(Morton)*, 7 oz. 32.0
    nondairy *(Amy's)*, 7.5 oz. 50.0
    shepherd's *(Amy's)*, 8 oz. 27.0
    tamale, Mexican *(Amy's)*, 8 oz. 41.0
    with turkey *(Morton)*, 7 oz....................................29.0
    vegetable *(Cedarlane* Less Fat), 7.4 oz. 60.0
stew, country *(Yves)*, 10.6 oz. 25.0
stir-fry, with rice *(Michelina's)*, 8 oz.............................44.0
Szechuan *(Cedarlane* Veggie Chick'n), ½ of 10-oz. pkg.............40.0
teriyaki *(Cedarlane* Veggie Chick'n), ½ of 10-oz. pkg. 43.0
wrap, see "Vegetable pocket/wrap"
Vegetable entree, mix, fresh, 1 cup*:
and cheese *(Mann's Broccoli Wokly)* 8.0
lo mein stir-fry *(Mann's)* 34.0
teriyaki stir-fry *(Mann's)*.......................................26.0
Vegetable entree, mix, frozen (see also "Vegetable entree,
    frozen"):
basil herb primavera *(Birds Eye Easy Recipe Creations)*,
    2¼ cup 31.0
cashew stir-fry *(Freshlike Meal Starter)*, 2 cups 30.0
cashew stir-fry *(Freshlike Meal Starter)*, 1 cup* 20.0

cheese, cheesy *(Freshlike Meal Starter)*, 2 cups 35.0
cheese, cheesy *(Freshlike Meal Starter)*, 1 cup* 20.0
lo mein, Oriental *(Birds Eye Easy Recipe Creations)*, 2¼ cup 40.0
Parmesan, creamy *(Freshlike Meal Starter)*, 2 cups 28.0
Parmesan, creamy *(Freshlike Meal Starter)*, 1 cup* 21.0
roasted garlic Parmesan *(Birds Eye Easy Recipe Creations)*,
    2¼ cup 29.0
sesame-ginger teriyaki *(Birds Eye Easy Recipe Creations)*,
    2¼ cup 24.0
sweet and sour:
    blend *(Freshlike Meal Starter)*, 2 cups 53.0
    blend *(Freshlike Meal Starter)*, 1 cup* 35.0
    with pineapple *(Birds Eye Easy Recipe Creations)*,
        2¼ cup 45.0
Szechuan, spicy:
    (Freshlike Meal Starter), 2 cups 47.0
    (Freshlike Meal Starter), 1 cup* 32.0
    with cashews *(Birds Eye Easy Recipe Creations)*, 2¼ cup 29.0
teriyaki blend *(Freshlike Meal Starter)*, 2 cups 39.0
teriyaki blend *(Freshlike Meal Starter)*, 1 cup* 26.0
tortellini Parmigiana *(Birds Eye Easy Recipe Creations)*,
    2¼ cup 25.0
Vegetable juice, 8 fl. oz., except as noted:
(R.W. Knudsen Very Veggie Low Sodium) 11.0
(R.W. Knudsen Very Veggie Original/Organic/Spicy) 10.0
(Rocket Juice Vegi Fire), 16 fl. oz. 16.0
(V8) 10.0
(V8 Lightly Tangy/Low Sodium) 11.0
(V8 Picante/Spicy Hot) 10.0
(V8 Healthy Request) 12.0
all varieties *(Muir Glen Organic)*, 5.5 fl. oz. 10.0
green *(R.W. Knudsen Simply Nutritious Mega Green)* 30.0
Vegetable juice blend, 8 fl. oz.:
berry, strawberry-kiwi, or tropical *(V8 Splash)* 28.0
citrus *(V8 Splash)* 29.0
Vegetable juice cocktail, canned, 8 fl. oz. 11.1
Vegetable oyster, see "Salsify"
Vegetable pie, see "Vegetable entree, frozen"
Vegetable pocket/wrap (see also specific listings), frozen:
(Amy's Pie in a Pocket), 5 oz. 45.0
couscous and vegetables *(Cedarlane Veggie Wrap)*, 6 oz. 36.0

Vegetable pocket/wrap *(cont.)*
Indian style *(Ken & Robert's* Veggie Pockets), 4.5 oz. ... 40.0
Mediterranean *(Amy's* Pocket), 4.5 oz. ... 33.0
Oriental style *(Ken & Robert's* Veggie Pockets), 4.5 oz. ... 40.0
pizza *(Cedarlane* Veggie Wrap), 6 oz. ... 32.0
pot pie style *(Ken & Robert's* Veggie Pockets), 4.5 oz. ... 38.0
rice and vegetables *(Cedarlane* Veggie Wrap), 6 oz. ... 56.0
roasted *(Amy's* Pocket), 4.5 oz. ... 35.0
Santa Fe style *(Ken & Robert's* Veggie Pockets), 4.5 oz. ... 39.0
soy "cheese" *(Amy's* Pocket), 4.5 oz. ... 39.0
Vegetable wrap stuffer, frozen, 16 oz.:
mu shu *(Fantastic Foods* Veggie) ... 35.0
Santa Fe *(Fantastic Foods* Veggie) ... 45.0
Spanish *(Fantastic Foods* Veggie) ... 39.0
teriyaki *(Fantastic Foods* Veggie) ... 41.0
Vegetables, see specific vegetable listings
Vegetables, mixed, fresh, stir-fry, Asian *(Frieda's),* 3 oz. ... 3.0
Vegetables, mixed, canned, ½ cup, except as noted:
(Del Monte/Del Monte No Salt) ... 8.0
(Green Giant) ... 12.0
(Seneca) ... 9.0
1 cup ... 17.4
drained, 1 cup ... 15.1
Chinese *(La Choy)* ... 1.0
chop suey *(Chun King)* ... 3.0
chop suey *(La Choy)* ... 2.0
salad *(Hanover),* ⅓ cup ... 17.0
stir-fry *(La Choy)* ... 5.0
Vegetables, mixed, dried, ½ cup:
(AlpineAire) ... 14.0
garden mix *(AlpineAire)* ... 15.0
Vegetables, mixed, frozen:
(Birds Eye), ⅓ cup ... 12.0
(Freshlike), ⅔ cup ... 11.0
(Green Giant), ½ cup ... 12.0
(Seabrook Farms), ⅔ cup ... 13.0
(Seneca), ⅔ cup ... 11.0
unprepared, 10-oz. pkg. ... 38.2
boiled, drained, 10-oz. pkg. ... 36.0
boiled, drained, ½ cup ... 11.9
with bow tie pasta *(Birds Eye* Italian Style), 1 cup ... 12.0

gumbo blend *(Birds Eye)*, ¾ cup 10.0
Italian blend *(Seneca)*, ¾ cup 6.0
with pasta shells *(Birds Eye* New England Style), 9-oz. pkg. 29.0
Oriental blend or stir-fry *(Seneca)*, ¾ cup 5.0
Oriental style *(Birds Eye)*, ½ cup 4.0
Scandinavian blend *(Seneca)*, ¾ cup 7.0
seasoning blend *(Birds Eye* Southern), ¾ cup............................5.0
for soup *(Birds Eye/Freshlike)*, ⅔ cup 9.0
soup mix *(Seneca)*, ¾ cup 9.0
for stew *(Birds Eye)*, ¾ cup 9.0
for stew *(Freshlike)*, ⅔ cup 10.0
stir-fry style *(Birds Eye)*, ½ cup 5.0
winter blend *(Seneca)*, 1 cup 4.0
Vegetables, mixed, pickled *(Krinos* Giardinara), ¼ cup..............1.0
Vegetables, mixed, relish, drained *(Sonoma* Muffaletta),
    2 tbsp. 3.0
Vegetarian entree, see "Vegetable entree"
Vegetarian dish, canned (see also specific listings):
(Loma Linda Dinner Cuts), 2 slices, 3.2 oz. 3.0
(Loma Linda Tender Bits), 6 pieces, 3 oz. 7.0
(Loma Linda Tender Rounds), 6 pieces, 2.8 oz..............................5.0
(Loma Linda Nuteena), ⅜" slice..6.0
(Worthington Savory Slices), 3 slices, 3 oz. 6.0
(Worthington Numete/Protose), ⅜" slice 5.0
choplets *(Worthington)*, 2 slices, 3.25 oz. 3.0
cutlets *(Worthington)*, 2.2-oz. piece..3.0
cutlets, multigrain *(Worthington)*, 2 slices, 3.25 oz. 5.0
stew, country *(Worthington)*, 1 cup 20.0
Vegetarian food, frozen (see also specific listings):
croquettes *(Worthington* Golden), 4 pieces, 3 oz......................14.0
fillets *(Worthington)*, 2 pieces, 3 oz. 8.0
roast *(Worthington* Dinner), ¾" slice 5.0
Veggie burger, see "Burger, vegetarian"
Venison, meat only, without added ingredients 0
Vermicelli dish, mix, with roasted garlic and olive oil
    (Pasta Roni), about 1 cup* 48.0
Vienna sausage, see "Sausage, canned"
Vindaloo paste, see "Curry paste"
Vindaloo sauce, see "Curry sauce"
Vine spinach, raw, untrimmed, 1 lb. 15.4

Vinegar, 1 tbsp.:

all varieties *(Eden)*..0

apple cider or white distilled *(Indian Summer)*.............................0

balsamic *(Regina)* 2.0

cider.. .9

rice:

    (Nakano)...0

    seasoned *(Nakano)*...<1.0

    seasoned, balsamic blend *(Nakano)*.......................4.0

wine, all varieties *(Regina)*......................................<1.0

W

Waffle, all varieties *(Thomas')*, 1 piece.................................19.0
Waffle, frozen, 2 pieces, except as noted:
(Aunt Jemima Homestyle)..32.0
(Aunt Jemima Low Fat)..32.0
(Belgian Chef) 34.0
(Hungry Jack Homestyle)...29.0
(Kellogg's Eggo Homestyle) 29.0
(Kellogg's Eggo Homestyle Low Fat)............................31.0
(Kellogg's Eggo Minis), 3 sets of 4 pieces 38.0
(Kellogg's Eggo Nutri-Grain)...28.0
(Kellogg's Eggo Nutri-Grain Low Fat)............................28.0
(Kellogg's Eggo Special K)..26.0
apple cinnamon *(Kellogg's Eggo)*..................................30.0
banana bread *(Kellogg's Eggo)* 30.0
blueberry:
    (Aunt Jemima)..34.0
    (Hungry Jack)..33.0
    (Kellogg's Eggo) 30.0
    (Kellogg's Eggo Nutri-Grain Low Fat) 30.0
buttermilk:
    (Aunt Jemima)..33.0
    (Hungry Jack)..29.0
    (Kellogg's Eggo) 28.0
chocolate chip *(Kellogg's Eggo)*....................................32.0
cinnamon toast *(Kellogg's Eggo)*, 3 sets of 4 pieces 46.0
multibran *(Kellogg's Eggo Nutri-Grain)*...........................29.0
oat, golden *(Kellogg's Eggo)* 26.0
plain or buttermilk, 4" square, 1.2 oz. 13.5
nut and honey *(Kellogg's Eggo)*......................................30.0
sticks, 3 pieces:
    (Aunt Jemima Homestyle) 48.0
    chocolate chip *(Aunt Jemima)*...............................47.0
    cinnamon sugar *(Aunt Jemima)* 52.0
strawberry *(Kellogg's Eggo)*...30.0

Waffle mix, see "Pancake mix"
Wakame, see "Seaweed"
Walnuts, dried, shelled:
(Planters), ⅓ cup 6.0
black:
   1 oz. 3.4
   1 tbsp. 9
   chopped, 1 cup...15.1
English:
   1 oz. 3.9
   chopped, 1 cup...16.4
   ground, 1 cup..11.0
Walnuts, in syrup (Smucker's), 2 tbsp...........................20.0
Wasabi chips, hot and spicy (Eden), 50 chips, 1.1 oz..............24.0
Wasabi root, fresh, raw:
6-oz. root 39.8
sliced, 1 cup..30.6
Wasabi sauce, in jar (Sushi Chef), 1 tbsp. 0
Water chestnuts, fresh, raw:
(Frieda's), 1 tbsp., 1.1 oz. 7.0
4 chestnuts, 1.3 oz..8.6
sliced, ½ cup...14.8
Water chestnuts, canned:
whole (Chun King/La Choy), 2 pieces 2.0
whole, 4 pieces, 1 oz..3.5
sliced (La Choy), 2 tbsp..1.5
sliced, ½ cup...8.7
Watercress, fresh, raw:
(Frieda's), 1 cup, 3 oz. 1.0
chopped, 1 cup.. .4
Watermelon, fresh, raw:
1" slice, 10" diam...34.6
balls, 1 cup 11.1
diced, 1 cup 10.9
yellow, seedless (Frieda's), ½ cup, 3 oz. 6.0
Watermelon drink, 8 fl. oz.:
(Kool-Aid Splash)..30.0
(R.W. Knudsen Cooler) 29.0
Watermelon drink blend, mix, 8 fl. oz.*:
cherry (Kool-Aid) 25.0
cherry (Kool-Aid Sugar Sweetened)................................16.0

Watermelon seeds, dried:
1 oz. 4.3
1 cup 16.5
Wax beans, fresh, see "Green beans"
Wax beans, canned, ½ cup:
cut *(Del Monte* Golden) 4.0
cut *(Seneca)* 5.0
Wax gourd, fresh:
raw, cubed, 1 cup 4.0
boiled, drained, cubed, 1 cup 5.3
Welsh rarebit, frozen *(Stouffer's)*, ¼ cup 5.0
Wendy's, 1 serving:
sandwiches:
    bacon cheeseburger, Jr. 34.0
    Big Bacon Classic 46.0
    cheeseburger, Jr. 34.0
    cheeseburger, Jr., deluxe 36.0
    cheeseburger, Kids' Meal 33.0
    chicken, breaded 44.0
    chicken, grilled 35.0
    chicken, spicy 43.0
    chicken club 44.0
    hamburger, single, plain 31.0
    hamburger, single, with everything 37.0
    hamburger, Jr. 34.0
    hamburger, Kids' Meal 33.0
sandwich condiments:
    American cheese 1.0
    American cheese Jr. 0
    bacon, 1 slice 0
    honey mustard, reduced-calorie, 1 tsp. 2.0
    ketchup, 1 tsp. 2.0
    mayonnaise, ½ tsp. 1.0
    mustard, ½ tsp. 0
    onion, 4 rings 1.0
    pickles, 4 slices 0
    tomato, 1 slice 1.0
Fresh Stuffed Pitas, with dressing:
    chicken Caesar 48.0
    classic Greek 50.0
    garden ranch chicken 51.0

Wendy's, Fresh Stuffed Pitas (cont.)

garden veggie	52.0
pita dressing, Caesar vinaigrette or garden ranch, 1 tbsp.	1.0
chicken nuggets, 5 pieces	11.0
chicken nuggets, 4 pieces, Kids' Meal	9.0

chicken nuggets sauce, 1 pkt.:

barbecue	10.0
honey mustard	6.0
sweet and sour	12.0

chili:

large, 12 oz.	32.0
small, 8 oz.	21.0
cheddar cheese, shredded, 2 tbsp.	1.0
saltine crackers, 2 pieces	4.0

baked potato:

plain, 10 oz.	71.0
bacon and cheese	78.0
broccoli and cheese	80.0
cheese	78.0
chili and cheese	83.0
sour cream and chive	73.0
sour cream, 1 pkt.	1.0
whipped margarine, 1 pkt.	0

french fries:

Biggie	61.0
Great Biggie	73.0
medium	50.0
small	35.0

Garden Spot salad bar:

applesauce, 2 tbsp.	7.0
bacon bits, 2 tbsp.	0
bananas and strawberry glaze, ¼ cup	8.0
broccoli or cauliflower, ¼ cup	1.0
cantaloupe, sliced, 1 piece	4.0
carrots, ¼ cup	2.0
cheese, shredded, 2 tbsp.	1.0
chicken salad, 2 tbsp.	2.0
cottage cheese, 2 tbsp.	1.0
croutons, 2 tbsp.	4.0
cucumber, 2 slices	0
egg, hard-cooked, 2 tbsp.	0

green peas, 2 tbsp. 3.0
green pepper, 2 pieces 1.0
lettuce, iceberg and Romaine, 1 cup 2.0
mushrooms, ¼ cup 1.0
orange, sliced, 2 slices 4.0
Parmesan blend, grated, 2 tbsp. 5.0
pasta salad, 2 tbsp. 4.0
peach, sliced, 1 piece 4.0
pepperoni, sliced, 6 slices 0
potato salad, 2 tbsp. 5.0
red onion, 3 rings 1.0
sunflower seeds and raisins, 2 tbsp. 5.0
tomato, wedged, 1 piece 1.0
turkey ham, diced, 2 tbsp. 0
watermelon, wedged, 1 piece 4.0
salads-to-go, without dressing:
  Caesar side salad 8.0
  deluxe garden or grilled chicken 9.0
  grilled chicken Caesar salad 17.0
  side salad 5.0
  taco salad 28.0
  taco chips, 15 pieces 24.0
  soft bread stick, 1 piece 23.0
salad dressing, 2 tbsp., except as noted:
  blue cheese 0
  French 6.0
  French, fat-free 8.0
  Italian, reduced-fat/calorie 2.0
  Italian Caesar 1.0
  ranch, *Hidden Valley* 1.0
  ranch, *Hidden Valley,* reduced-fat/calorie 2.0
  salad oil or vinegar, 1 tbsp. 0
  Thousand Island 2.0
desserts:
  chocolate chip cookie 36.0
  Frosty, large 91.0
  Frosty, medium 73.0
  Frosty, small 56.0
  pudding, chocolate, ¼ cup 10.0
Wheat, whole-grain, 1 cup, except as noted:
durum 136.6

Wheat *(cont.)*
hard red spring 130.6
hard red winter *(Arrowhead Mills)*, ¼ cup 34.0
hard red winter..136.7
soft red winter..124.7
hard white 145.7
soft white 126.6
Wheat, parboiled, see "Bulgur"
Wheat, semolina, see "Semolina"
Wheat, sprouted, 1 cup 45.9
Wheat bran (see also "Cereal"):
(Arrowhead Mills), ¼ cup 10.0
(Hodgson Mill Miller's Bran Untoasted), ¼ cup 10.0
crude, 1 oz. 18.3
crude, 1 cup 37.4
Wheat flakes, rolled *(Arrowhead Mills)*, ⅓ cup 24.0
Wheat flour, ¼ cup, except as noted:
(Hodgson Mill 50/50), scant ¼ cup 21.0
bread:
   (Gold Medal Better for Bread Wheat Blend) 21.0
   (Hodgson Mill Best for Bread).............................22.0
   (Pillsbury Enriched)..22.0
   (Red Band) 22.0
cake, white *(Softasilk* Velvet) 23.0
cake, white *(Swans Down)*.....................................22.0
gluten *(Arrowhead Mills* Vital), 3 tbsp. 3.0
gluten *(Hodgson Mill* Vital), 1 tbsp. 2.0
pastry *(Arrowhead Mills)* 23.0
semolina, see "Semolina flour"
white:
   (Arrowhead Mills Unbleached), ⅓ cup 33.0
   (Gold Medal Organic/Unbleached/Self-rising) 22.0
   (Hodgson Mill Unbleached/Organic Unbleached), scant
     ¼ cup 23.0
   (Pillsbury Best Unbleached) 21.0
   (Red Band Self-rising).....................................22.0
   (Robin Hood Self-rising/Unbleached)..................22.0
   (Wondra) 23.0
white, all-purpose:
   (Gold Medal)..22.0
   (Pillsbury Enriched)...23.0

(Red Band) 23.0
(Robin Hood) 22.0
seasoned (Kentucky Kernel) 20.0
whole-wheat:
(Arrowhead Mills) 25.0
(Robin Hood) 21.0
graham (Hodgson Mill), scant ¼ cup 22.0
pastry (Hodgson Mill), scant ¼ cup 22.0
white (Hodgson Mill) 21.0

Wheat germ:
(Arrowhead Mills Raw), 3 tbsp. 10.0
(Hodgson Mill Untoasted), 2 tbsp. 7.0
(Kretschmer), 2 tbsp. 6.0
crude, 1 oz. 14.7
crude, 1 cup 59.6
honey crunch (Kretschmer), 1⅔ tbsp. 8.0
toasted (Kretschmer), ¼ cup 10.0

Wheat malt syrup, see "Malt syrup"
Wheat pilaf mix (Near East), 2 oz. 42.0
Wheatgrass juice, frozen (Perfect Foods), 1 oz. 2.0
Whelk, meat only:
raw, 4 oz. 8.8
boiled, poached or steamed, 4 oz. 17.6

Whey:
acid:
dry, 1 oz. 20.8
dry, 1 tablespoon 2.1
fluid, 1 cup 12.6
sweet:
dry, 1 oz. 21.1
dry, 1 tbsp. 5.6
fluid, 1 cup 12.6

Whipped topping, see "Cream topping"
Whiskey, see "Liquor"
Whiskey sour drink mixer:
(Mr & Mrs T), 4 fl. oz. 23.0
6.8-fl. oz. can 28.0
Whiskey sour mix:
bottled, 2 fl. oz. 13.8
bottled*:
3.5 fl. oz. (2 fl. oz. mix plus 1.5 oz. whiskey) 13.9

Whiskey sour mix, bottled *(cont.)*
2 fl. oz. 8.5
powder, .6-oz. packet* 16.4
White baking chips, see "Chocolate, baking"
White beans, mature:
dry, 1 cup 121.7
dry, 1 tbsp. 7.6
boiled, 1 cup 44.9
boiled, 1 tbsp. 2.8
small, dry, 1 cup 133.8
small, boiled, 1 cup 46.2
White beans, canned, mature:
(Goya Spanish Style), 7.5 oz. 29.0
1 cup 57.5
lightly seasoned *(S&W)*, ½ cup 19.0
White Castle, 1 serving:
sandwiches:
    bacon cheeseburger 12.0
    breakfast 17.0
    chicken rings 5.0
    fish 18.0
    hamburger or cheeseburger 11.0
    hamburger or cheeseburger, double 16.0
sides:
    cheese sticks, 3 pieces 19.0
    cheese sticks, 5 pieces 32.0
    fries, small 15.0
    onion rings, 8 pieces 56.0
shake, chocolate, 14 oz. 32.0
shake, vanilla, 14 oz. 35.0
White chocolate, see "Chocolate"
White sauce mix, dry, except as noted:
(Knorr Classic Sauces), 2 tsp., ¼ cup* 4.0
1¾-oz. pkt. 25.0
8 fl. oz.* 10.0
Whitefish, fresh or smoked, without added ingredients 0
Whiting, without added ingredients 0
Wiener, see "Frankfurter"
Wild rice:
raw:
    (Lundberg Organic), ¼ cup 34.0

1 oz.	21.2
1 cup	119.8
¼ cup	30.0
cooked, 1 cup	35.0
cooked, ½ cup	17.5

blends, see "Rice"
Wild rice cake, see "Rice cake"
Wild rice dish, see "Rice dish"
Wine:
dessert[1]:

3.5-fl.-oz. glass	12.2
1 fl. oz.	3.5
dry, 3.5-fl.-oz. glass	4.2
dry, 1 fl. oz.	1.2

table[2]:

red, 3.5-fl.-oz. glass	1.8
red, 1 fl. oz.	.5
rosé, 3.5-fl.-oz. glass	1.4
rosé, 1 fl. oz.	.4
white, 3.5-fl.-oz. glass	.8
white, 1 fl. oz.	.2

Wine, cooking, 2 tbsp., except as noted:

Burgundy *(Regina)*	3.0
rice *(Sun Luck* Mirin), 1 tbsp.	0
sauterne *(Regina)*	3.0
sherry *(Regina)*	5.0

Winged beans:
immature:

raw, 1 pod, .6 oz.	.7
raw, sliced, 1 cup	1.9
boiled, drained, 1 cup	2.0
boiled, drained, ½ cup	1.0
mature, raw, 1 cup	75.9
mature, boiled, 1 cup	25.7

Winged bean leaves, trimmed, 1 oz. ... 4.0
Winged bean tuber, trimmed, 1 oz. ... 8.0
Winter radish, see "Radish, black"

[1] Includes fortified wines containing more than 15% alcohol, such as port, sherry, and vermouth.
[2] Includes wines containing less than 15% alcohol, such as Burgundy, Chablis, Champagne, and Chardonnay.

Winter squash, see "Squash" and specific listings
Wolf fish, without added ingredients..0
Wonton wrappers:
(Frieda's), 4 pieces, 1 oz. 17.0
(Nasoya), 5 pieces, 1.2 oz..18.0
Worcestershire sauce, 1 tsp.:
(Crosse & Blackwell)..1.0
(D.L. Jardine's Spicy Wooster) 1.0
(French's) ....<1.0
(Heinz) 0
(Lea & Perrins) 1.0
white wine *(Lea & Perrins)* 0
Wrap stuffer, see "Vegetable wrap stuffer"
Wrap (see also "Tortilla"), unfilled, 1 piece:
all varieties *(Aladdin Bread),* 2 oz...33.0
all varieties *(Cedar's),* 2.5 oz. 36.0
6-grain *(Cedar's* Mountain Bread), 2 oz. 35.0
wheat *(Cedar's* Mountain Bread), 2 oz. 34.0
white *(Cedar's* Mountain Bread), 2 oz. 29.0
Wrap, filled, see "Vegetable pocket/wrap" and specific listings

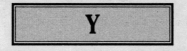

FOOD AND MEASURE **CARBOHYDRATE GRAMS**

Yam, fresh:
raw *(Frieda's* Name), ¾ cup, 3 oz. 24.0
raw, cubed, 1 cup..41.8
baked or boiled:
  1 cup 35.4
  cubed, 1 cup...37.6
  cubed, ½ cup...18.8
Yam, canned or frozen, see "Sweet potato"
Yam, mountain, Hawaiian, fresh:
raw, 14.8-lb. yam..68.5
raw, cubed, ½ cup...11.1
steamed, cubed, 1 cup..29.0
Yam bean tuber, fresh:
raw:
  (Frieda's Jicama), ¾ cup, 3 oz. 7.0
  1 cup 11.5
  sliced, ½ cup...10.6
boiled, drained, 1 oz...2.5
Yard-long beans:
fresh:
  raw *(Frieda's* Long Beans), ¾ cup, 3 oz. 7.0
  raw, 1 pod..1.0
  raw, sliced, 1 cup 7.6
  boiled, drained, 1 pod..1.3
  boiled, drained, chopped, 1 cup 9.5
mature, raw, 1 cup...103.4
mature, boiled, 1 cup 36.1
Yautier root, fresh, raw:
10¾-oz. root 72.2
1 oz. 6.7
sliced, 1 cup...32.0
Yeast:
compressed, .6-oz. cake 3.1

Yeast *(cont.)*
dry:

1 tbsp.	4.6
1 tsp.	1.5
active *(Hodgson Mill)*, 5/16 oz.	3.0
fast rise *(Hodgson Mill)*, 5/16 oz.	4.0

Yellow beans, fresh:

raw, 1 cup	7.9
boiled, drained, 1 cup	9.9

Yellow beans, canned:

½ cup	4.2
drained, 10 beans	2.8
drained, ½ cup	3.1

Yellow beans, frozen, all styles:

unprepared, 10-oz. pkg.	21.5
unprepared, 1 cup	9.4
boiled, drained, 1 cup	8.7

Yellow beans, mature:

raw, 1 cup	119.0
boiled, 1 cup	44.7

Yellow squash:
fresh or frozen, see "Crookneck squash"

canned *(Sunshine)*, ½ cup	5.0

Yellow-eyed beans, dry *(Frieda's)*, ½ cup ... 22.0

Yellowtail, without added ingredients ... 0

Yogurt:
plain:

whole-milk *(Dannon)*, 8 oz.	14.0
whole-milk *(Friendship)*, 8 oz.	18.0
whole-milk *(Stonyfield Farm* Organic 32 oz.), 1 cup	12.0
low-fat *(Colombo)*, 8 oz.	16.0
low-fat *(Dannon)*, 8 oz.	18.0
low-fat *(Stonyfield Farm* Organic 32 oz.), 1 cup	14.0
nonfat *(Colombo)*, 8 oz.	16.0
nonfat *(Dannon)*, 8 oz.	19.0
nonfat *(Stonyfield Farm)*, 8 oz.	15.0

all fruit flavors:

(Colombo Light), 8 oz.	21.0
(Dannon Light Nonfat), 4 oz.	11.0
(Jell-O Lowfat), 4.4 oz.	25.0
(Yoplait Light), 6 oz.	17.0

(Yoplait Original 99% Fat Free), 6 oz. 33.0
(Yoplait Original 99% Fat Free), 4 oz. 22.0
(Yoplait Custard Style), 6 oz. 32.0
(Yoplait Exprèsse/Yoplait Go-Gurt), 1 tube 11.0
(Yoplait Trix), 4 oz. 23.0
(Yoplait Yumsters), 4 oz. 21.0
except banana-strawberry *(Colombo* Classic), 8 oz. 42.0
apple-cinnamon *(Dannon* Fruit on the Bottom), 8 oz. 40.0
apple cobbler *(Breyers Smooth & Creamy),* 8 oz. 46.0
apple pie à la mode *(Breyers Light* Nonfat), 8 oz. 22.0
apricot-mango *(Stonyfield Farm* Nonfat), 8 oz. 31.0
apricot-mango *(Stonyfield Farm* Nonfat 32 oz.), 1 cup 34.0
banana cream pie *(Dannon Light* Nonfat), 8 oz. 21.0
banana-strawberry *(Colombo* Classic), 8 oz. 47.0
berry, mixed:
    (Breyers Low Fat), 8 oz. 43.0
    (Dannon Fruit on the Bottom), 8 oz. 40.0
    (Dannon Snap 'n Snack Fruit on the Bottom), 4 oz. 20.0
    (Stonyfield Farm Nonfat), 8 oz. 30.0
berry-banana split *(Breyers Light* Nonfat), 8 oz. 21.0
blackberry pie *(Dannon Light* Nonfat), 8 oz. 22.0
blueberries and cream flavor:
    (Breyers Light Nonfat), 8 oz. 23.0
    (Breyers Smooth & Creamy), 8 oz. 46.0
    (Breyers Smooth & Creamy), 4.4 oz. 26.0
blueberry:
    (Breyers Low Fat), 8 oz. 43.0
    (Breyers Low Fat), 4.4 oz. 25.0
    (Dannon Blended Nonfat), 4 oz. 21.0
    (Dannon Fruit on the Bottom), 8 oz. 41.0
    (Dannon Light Nonfat), 8 oz. 23.0
    (Dannon Snap 'n Snack Fruit on the Bottom), 4 oz. 20.0
    (Light n' Lively Low Fat), 4.4 oz. 25.0
    (Light n' Lively Free), 4.4 oz. 13.0
    (Stonyfield Farm Nonfat), 8 oz. 31.0
    (Stonyfield Farm Organic Low Fat), 6 oz. 23.0
    wild *(Stonyfield Farm* Organic), 6 oz. 22.0
blueberry French vanilla *(Dannon Double Delights*
    Low Fat), 6 oz. 36.0
boysenberry *(Dannon* Fruit on the Bottom), 8 oz. 40.0
cappuccino *(Dannon Light* Nonfat), 8 oz. 22.0

Yogurt *(cont.)*

cappuccino *(Stonyfield Farm* Nonfat), 8 oz. 31.0
caramel, crème *(Dannon Light* Nonfat), 8 oz. 22.0
caramel apple crunch *(Dannon Crunch* Nonfat), 8 oz. 32.0
cherry:
    (Dannon Blended Nonfat), 4 oz. 21.0
    (Dannon Fruit on the Bottom), 8 oz. 42.0
    (Dannon Danimals Low Fat), 4 oz. 21.0
    black *(Breyers* Low Fat), 8 oz. 44.0
    black *(Stonyfield Farm* Nonfat), 8 oz. 31.0
    black, jubilee *(Breyers Light* Nonfat), 8 oz. 23.0
    black, parfait *(Breyers Smooth & Creamy),* 8 oz. 46.0
    black, parfait *(Breyers Smooth & Creamy),* 4.4 oz. 26.0
cherry bonbon *(Breyers Light* Nonfat), 8 oz. 22.0
cherry cheesecake *(Dannon Double Delights* Low Fat),
    6 oz. 35.0
cherry vanilla *(Dannon Light* Nonfat), 8 oz. 23.0
cherry vanilla *(Stonyfield Farm* Nonfat), 8 oz. 43.0
chocolate *(Stonyfield Farm* Underground Nonfat), 8 oz. 46.0
chocolate, white, raspberry *(Colombo* Light), 8 oz. 21.0
chocolate, white, raspberry *(Dannon Light* Nonfat), 8 oz. 22.0
chocolate cheesecake *(Dannon Double Delights* Low Fat),
    6 oz. 46.0
coconut cream pie *(Dannon Light* Nonfat), 8 oz. 22.0
coconut cream pie *(Yoplait* Original), 6 oz. 34.0
coffee *(Dannon),* 8 oz. 37.0
cookies and cream *(Dannon Crunch* Nonfat), 8 oz. 30.0
cranberry-raspberry *(Dannon),* 8 oz. 37.0
Key lime pie *(Breyers Light* Nonfat), 8 oz. 22.0
lemon:
    (Colombo Classic), 8 oz. 32.0
    (Dannon), 8 oz. 37.0
    (Stonyfield Farm Lots Nonfat), 8 oz. 30.0
    (Stonyfield Farm Luscious Organic Low Fat), 6 oz. 23.0
    (Yoplait Original), 6 oz. 36.0
    chiffon *(Breyers Light* Nonfat), 8 oz. 22.0
    chiffon *(Dannon Light* Nonfat), 8 oz. 22.0
    meringue pie *(Dannon Double Delights* Low Fat), 6 oz. 37.0
maple, creamy *(Stonyfield Farm* Organic), 6 oz. 19.0
maple vanilla *(Stonyfield Farm* Organic Low Fat), 6 oz. 19.0
mocha *(Stonyfield Farm* Mocha-ccino Organic), 6 oz. 23.0

mocha latte *(Stonyfield Farm* Organic Low Fat), 6 oz. 20.0
peach:
    (Breyers Low Fat), 8 oz. 43.0
    (Breyers Low Fat), 4.4 oz. 26.0
    (Dannon Blended Nonfat), 4 oz. 20.0
    (Dannon Fruit on the Bottom), 8 oz.......................................40.0
    (Dannon Light Nonfat), 8 oz...23.0
    (Dannon Snap 'n Snack Fruit on the Bottom), 4 oz.............20.0
    (Light n' Lively Low Fat), 4.4 oz. 26.0
    (Light n' Lively Free), 4.4 oz...12.0
    (Stonyfield Farm Nonfat), 8 oz. 30.0
    tropical *(Dannon* Fruit on the Bottom), 8 oz.........................44.0
peaches and cream flavor:
    (Breyers Light Nonfat), 8 oz. 22.0
    (Breyers Smooth & Creamy), 8 oz. 46.0
    (Breyers Smooth & Creamy), 4.4 oz. 25.0
piña colada *(Yoplait* Original), 6 oz. 33.0
pineapple *(Breyers* Low Fat), 8 oz.......................................45.0
pineapple *(Light n' Lively* Lowfat), 4.4 oz. 26.0
orange-mango *(Dannon Light* Nonfat), 8 oz. 21.0
orange–vanilla cream flavor *(Breyers Smooth & Creamy)*,
    8 oz. 45.0
raspberries and cream flavor *(Breyers Light* Nonfat), 8 oz. 22.0
raspberries and cream flavor *(Breyers Smooth & Creamy)*,
    8 oz. 45.0
raspberry:
    (Dannon Blended Nonfat), 4 oz. 21.0
    (Dannon Fruit on the Bottom), 8 oz.......................................40.0
    (Dannon Light Nonfat), 8 oz...22.0
    (Stonyfield Farm Nonfat), 8 oz. 31.0
    (Stonyfield Farm Organic Low Fat), 6 oz. 23.0
    with granola *(Dannon Crunch* Nonfat), 8 oz..........................33.0
    red *(Breyers* Low Fat), 8 oz. 43.0
    red *(Light n' Lively* Low Fat), 4.4 oz.....................................23.0
    wild *(Dannon Danimals* Low Fat), 4 oz.................................20.0
raspberry Bavarian cream *(Dannon Double Delights*
    Low Fat), 6 oz...34.0
raspberry French vanilla *(Dannon* Fruit on the Bottom), 8 oz. 45.0
strawberries and cream *(Stonyfield Farm* Organic), 6 oz............23.0
strawberry:
    (Breyers Low Fat), 4.4 oz. 26.0

Yogurt, strawberry *(cont.)*
    (Breyers Low Fat), 8 oz. 43.0
    (Breyers Light Nonfat Classic), 8 oz. 22.0
    (Breyers Smooth & Creamy Classic), 8 oz. 45.0
    (Breyers Smooth & Creamy Classic), 4.4 oz. 25.0
    (Colombo Low Fat), 8 oz. 33.0
    (Dannon Blended Nonfat), 4 oz. 21.0
    (Dannon Fruit on the Bottom), 8 oz. 40.0
    (Dannon Danimals Low Fat), 4 oz. 22.0
    (Dannon Light Nonfat), 8 oz. 22.0
    (Dannon Snap 'n Snack Fruit on the Bottom), 4 oz. 20.0
    (Dannon Sprinkl'ins Mystery Surprise), 1 cont. 24.0
    (Light n' Lively Low Fat), 4.4 oz. 26.0
    (Light n' Lively Free), 4.4 oz. 12.0
    (Stonyfield Farm Nonfat), 8 oz. 32.0
    (Stonyfield Farm Organic Low Fat), 6 oz. 23.0
    fruit cup *(Light n' Lively* Low Fat), 4.4 oz. 25.0
    fruit cup *(Light n' Lively Free),* 4.4 oz. 13.0
strawberry, French vanilla *(Dannon* Fruit on the Bottom),
    8 oz. 44.0
strawberry-banana:
    (Breyers Low Fat), 8 oz. 44.0
    (Dannon Blended Nonfat), 4 oz. 21.0
    (Dannon Fruit on the Bottom), 8 oz. 40.0
    (Dannon Danimals Low Fat), 4 oz. 21.0
    (Dannon Light Nonfat), 8 oz. 22.0
    (Stonyfield Farm Nonfat), 8 oz. 32.0
    cream *(Light n' Lively* Low Fat), 4.4 oz. 25.0
    cream *(Light n' Lively Free),* 4.4 oz. 13.0
    split *(Breyers Smooth & Creamy),* 8 oz. 48.0
strawberry cheesecake:
    (Breyers Light Nonfat), 8 oz. 22.0
    (Breyers Smooth & Creamy), 8 oz. 46.0
    (Dannon Double Delights Low Fat), 6 oz. 33.0
strawberry-kiwi *(Dannon Light* Nonfat), 8 oz. 22.0
tangerine chiffon *(Dannon Light* Nonfat), 8 oz. 21.0
tropical punch *(Dannon Danimals* Low Fat), 4 oz. 22.0
vanilla:
    (Breyers Low Fat), 8 oz. 38.0
    (Colombo Classic/*Colombo* Fat Free), 8 oz. 32.0
    (Colombo Light), 8 oz. 21.0

(Dannon), 8 oz...36.0
(Dannon Danimals Low Fat), 4 oz. 22.0
(Dannon Light Nonfat), 8 oz.......................21.0
(Dannon Sprinkl'ins Color Creations), 1 cont. 20.0
(Stonyfield Farm Organic 32 oz.), 1 cup...............30.0
(Stonyfield Farm Organic Low Fat), 6 oz. 20.0
(Stonyfield Farm Organic Low Fat 32 oz.), 1 cup 27.0
(Yoplait Custard Style), 6 oz...........................32.0
cream flavor *(Breyers Light* Nonfat), 8 oz. 22.0
French *(Colombo* Low Fat), 8 oz. 32.0
French *(Stonyfield Farm* Nonfat), 8 oz.............30.0
French *(Stonyfield Farm* Organic), 6 oz. 23.0
truffle *(Stonyfield Farm* Organic), 6 oz. 37.0

Yogurt, frozen, ½ cup:
banana-chocolate *(Dreyer's/Edy's Bananafana)*............19.0
banana split *(Blue Bell* Nonfat)...................24.0
(Ben & Jerry's Cherry Garcia) 32.0
(Ben & Jerry's Chunky Monkey) 34.0
(Ben & Jerry's Ooey Gooey Cake)..................35.0
black raspberry *(Turkey Hill)*.......................20.0
caramel:
    crème *(Stonyfield Farm* Organic) 26.0
    crème *(Stonyfield Farm* Organic Low Fat) 23.0
    fudge *(Dreyer's/Edy's Caramel Fudge Cosmo)* 23.0
    praline crunch *(Dreyer's/Edy's* Fat Free)............23.0
cherry, black, vanilla swirl *(Dreyer's/Edy's* Fat Free) 19.0
cherry vanilla *(Stonyfield Farm* Organic).................24.0
chocolate:
    (Ben & Jerry's Chocolate Cherry Garcia)............35.0
    (Breyers All Natural)............................23.0
    (Häagen-Dazs Fat Free) 28.0
    (Stonyfield Farm Organic) 22.0
    (Stonyfield Farm Organic Nonfat).................19.0
    soft serve...17.9
    swirl, double *(Stonyfield Farm* Organic)............26.0
chocolate cherry cordial *(Turkey Hill* Nonfat) 24.0
chocolate chip cookie dough *(Ben & Jerry's)* 35.0
chocolate chip cookie dough *(Turkey Hill)* 23.0
chocolate fudge *(Edy's* Fat Free) 21.0
chocolate fudge brownie *(Ben & Jerry's)*...............36.0
chocolate-marshmallow *(Turkey Hill* Nonfat) 30.0

Yogurt, frozen *(cont.)*

chocolate mint chip *(Stonyfield Farm Organic Low Fat)* 22.0
chocolate-raspberry *(Stonyfield Farm Organic)* 25.0
chocolate toffee crunch *(Ben & Jerry's Heath Bar)*.....................35.0
coffee:
    (Häagen-Dazs Fat Free) 29.0
    cappuccino *(Turkey Hill Fat Free)* 23.0
    decaf *(Stonyfield Farm Organic)*...21.0
    decaf *(Stonyfield Farm Organic Nonfat)* 19.0
    fudge sundae *(Edy's Fat Free)* 22.0
cookies and cream *(Dreyer's/Edy's)* 19.0
(Dreyer's/Edy's Mumbo Jumbo) 21.0
dulce de leche *(Häagen-Dazs Low Fat)* 35.0
mint cookies and cream *(Turkey Hill Nonfat)* 24.0
mocha almond fudge *(Stonyfield Farm Organic Low Fat)*...........23.0
mocha biscotti fudge *(Stonyfield Farm Organic)*......................26.0
Neapolitan *(Turkey Hill Nonfat)* 22.0
peach-raspberry *(Turkey Hill)*...20.0
peanut butter caramel *(Dreyer's/Edy's Hokey Pokey)*................21.0
raspberry *(Stonyfield Farm Organic Nonfat)* 21.0
strawberry:
    (Blue Bell Nonfat) 25.0
    (Breyers All Natural) 22.0
    (Häagen-Dazs Fat Free) 31.0
    (Turkey Hill Nonfat) 21.0
    cheesecake *(Blue Bell Low Fat)* 25.0
toffee crunch *(Dreyer's/Edy's Heath)*.......................................18.0
(Turkey Hill Tin Roof Sundae) 21.0
(Turkey Hill Clark Bar) 22.0
vanilla:
    (Blue Bell Country Low Fat)..23.0
    (Breyers All Natural) 22.0
    (Dreyer's/Edy's) 17.0
    (Dreyer's/Edy's Fat Free) 19.0
    (Häagen-Dazs Fat Free) 29.0
    (Stonyfield Farm Organic) 20.0
    (Stonyfield Farm Organic Nonfat)...19.0
    bean *(Blue Bell Nonfat)*..24.0
    bean *(Turkey Hill)* 17.0
    soft serve..17.4
vanilla brownie fudge *(Stonyfield Farm Organic)* 28.0

vanilla and chocolate *(Turkey Hill)* 19.0
vanilla, chocolate, and strawberry *(Breyers* All Natural) 22.0
vanilla-chocolate swirl *(Dreyer's/Edy's* Fat Free) 19.0
vanilla fudge:
   (Turkey Hill Nonfat) 24.0
   peanut *(Dreyer's/Edy's* Ultimate Tin Roof Sundae)................20.0
   swirl *(Stonyfield Farm* Organic Nonfat) 23.0
vanilla and orange sherbet swirl *(Turkey Hill* Nonfat).................22.0
vanilla-raspberry swirl *(Häagen-Dazs* Fat Free)..........................28.0
Yogurt bar, frozen, 1 bar:
(Ben & Jerry's Cherry Garcia) 32.0
chocolate banana, cherry, chocolate, or raspberry
   (SnackWell's Low Fat) 22.0
Yogurt sandwich, frozen, vanilla, chocolate wafers
   (Turkey Hill), 1 piece...29.0
Yokan, from mature adzuki beans, .5-oz. slice 14.6
Yu choy sum, see "Greens, Chinese"
Yuca root *(Frieda's),* ⅔ cup, 3 oz. 23.0

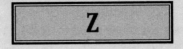

FOOD AND MEASURE   **CARBOHYDRATE GRAMS**

Ziti, see "Pasta"
Zucchini, fresh:
raw:
    with skin, sliced, 1 cup..3.3
    with skin, chopped, 1 cup 3.6
    baby *(Frieda's)*, ⅔ cup, 3 oz. 3.0
    baby, 1 large, .6 oz. 5
    baby, 1 medium, .4 oz...3
boiled, drained, with skin:
    sliced, 1 cup 7.1
    sliced, ½ cup 3.5
    mashed, ½ cup 4.7
Zucchini, breaded, frozen *(Empire* Kosher),
    7 pieces, 2.9 oz. 18.0
Zucchini, canned:
Italian style, 1 cup...15.5
Italian style tomato sauce *(Del Monte)*, ½ cup 7.0
Zucchini, frozen:
(Seneca), ⅔ cup 3.0
with skin, unprepared, 10-oz. pkg.................................10.2
with skin, boiled, drained, 1 cup 7.9
Zucchini, sun-dried, in olive oil and balsamic vinegar
    (Antica Italia), 1 oz. 2.0
Zweiback, see "Cracker"